NEUROIMAGING IN EPILEPSY

Neuroimaging in Epilepsy

Edited by

Harry T. Chugani, MD

Departments of Pediatrics and Neurology
PET Center
Children's Hospital of Michigan
Wayne State University School of Medicine
Detroit, MI

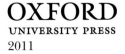
2011

OXFORD
UNIVERSITY PRESS

Oxford University Press, Inc., publishes works that further
Oxford University's objective of excellence
in research, scholarship, and education.

Oxford   New York
Auckland   Cape Town   Dar es Salaam   Hong Kong   Karachi
Kuala Lumpur   Madrid   Melbourne   Mexico City   Nairobi
New Delhi   Shanghai   Taipei   Toronto

With offices in
Argentina   Austria   Brazil   Chile   Czech Republic   France   Greece
Guatemala   Hungary   Italy   Japan   Poland   Portugal   Singapore
South Korea   Switzerland   Thailand   Turkey   Ukraine   Vietnam

Published by Oxford University Press, Inc.
198 Madison Avenue, New York, New York 10016

www.oup.com

Oxford is a registered trademark of Oxford University Press.

Library of Congress Cataloging-in-Publication Data

Neuroimaging in epilepsy/edited by Harry T. Chugani.
p. ; cm.
Includes bibliographical references and index.
ISBN 978-0-19-534276-5
1. Epilepsy—Imaging.   I. Chugani, Harry T.
[DNLM: 1. Epilepsy—diagnosis.   2. Epilepsy—therapy.
3. Magnetic Resonance Imaging—methods.   4. Tomography,
Emission–Computed—methods. WL 385 N49337 2011]
RC373.N48 2011
616.8'5307548—dc22   2010007926

The science of medicine is a rapidly changing field. As new research and clinical experience broaden
our knowledge, changes in treatment and drug therapy occur. The author and publisher of this work
have checked with sources believed to be reliable in their efforts to provide information that is
accurate and complete, and in accordance with the standards accepted at the time of publication.
However, in light of the possibility of human error or changes in the practice of medicine, neither the
author, nor the publisher, nor any other party who has been involved in the preparation or publication
of this work warrants that the information contained herein is in every respect accurate or complete.
Readers are encouraged to confirm the information contained herein with other reliable sources, and
are strongly advised to check the product information sheet provided by the pharmaceutical company
for each drug they plan to administer.

9 8 7 6 5 4 3 2 1
Printed in China
on acid-free paper

This book is dedicated to the memory of my late mother, Jamna (Janki) Chugani, and my late father, Thakurdas Chugani, in gratitude for the happiness and joy of my childhood years, as well as for the encouragement and support towards my pursuit of a medical career. I am also thankful to my wife Diane, daughter Carla Devi, and son Ryan Sunil for their support and encouragement.

Preface

One can argue with confidence that perhaps the most important achievements in the field of epileptology in the past two decades have been in the neuroimaging and genetic breakthroughs as applied to patients with epilepsy. The former has consumed much of my energy and efforts over the years because of the rapid pace with which it is moving, while the latter is moving at even a faster pace. Indeed, neuroimaging has become a vital part in the study of epilepsy, affecting broad aspects of the disorder ranging from diagnosis and classification to treatment and prognosis.

Neuroimaging in epilepsy encompasses many different approaches that have reached various levels of expertise across epilepsy centers worldwide. Depending upon the expertise of the investigators in various centers, a particular type of neuroimaging may play a more important role than others in the approach towards how they manage their patients with epilepsy. For this reason, it has been difficult to directly compare the usefulness of one imaging modality against another because, inevitably, there is an inherent bias towards the modality that has reached a higher level of sophistication than other modalities less commonly used in a particular program.

This volume does not attempt to compare the usefulness of various modalities applied to image patients with epilepsy. Rather, the purpose of this book is to present state-of-the-art accounts of all imaging modalities that are being applied and are deemed to provide useful information to improve the lives of people with epilepsy. In this undertaking, I have recruited the best international experts in the field to contribute their experience and perspectives towards this volume. Because previous books on the topic of neuroimaging in epilepsy have emphasized disproportionately the role of magnetic resonance imaging, with much less emphasis on physiologic and molecular neuroimaging (PET and SPECT) techniques, care has been taken to provide a more balanced account in this current endeavor. Indeed, this book includes seven chapters on PET and SPECT applications in epilepsy rather than the one or at most two in previous volumes. Yet the important role of MRI is not underemphasized by any means, with five chapters describing MRI applications, including an entire chapter dedicated to MRI diffusion tensor imaging not found in other volumes on neuroimaging in epilepsy.

We conclude with a chapter on multimodality neuroimaging in epilepsy, in which we describe the methods of image co-registration (including placements of intracranial EEG electrodes) and emphasize the strength of applying several imaging approaches to ask specific clinically relevant questions concerning patients with epilepsy. More and more, multimodality neuroimaging is playing an important role, and imaging devices are being manufactured that can acquire several very different imaging data sets simultaneously. For example, PET/CT scanners are already routinely used in many centers, particularly for whole-body cancer imaging, but also for evaluation of brain tumors and other intracranial lesions. Furthermore, PET/MRI scanners are on the horizon and are expected to be in the field 2 to 3 years from now. These new devices promise to greatly enhance our understanding of epilepsy mechanisms that will undoubtedly be translated to improve clinical management. It is with this enthusiasm that we now present this volume.

Harry T. Chugani, MD

Table of Contents

PREFACE   vii
CONTRIBUTORS   xi

1   Historical Perspectives of Neuroimaging in
    Epilepsy   3
    HARRY T. CHUGANI AND AJAY KUMAR

2   MRI: Overview of MR Techniques for
    Epilepsy   8
    VIVEK GUPTA AND RICHARD A. BRONEN

3   Malformations of Cortical Development   37
    RENZO GUERRINI AND FRANCESCO ZELLINI

4   Magnetic Resonance Spectroscopy   63
    HOBY HETHERINGTON

5   Functional MRI   77
    WILLIAM DAVIS GAILLARD

6   Diffusion MRI in Epilepsy   92
    RAJKUMAR MUNIAN GOVINDAN
    AND HARRY T. CHUGANI

7   Magnetoencephalography-Based Source
    Imaging for Epilepsy and Language
    Localization   106
    ROBERT C. KNOWLTON AND LAWRENCE W. VER HOEF

8   Positron Emission Tomography: Glucose
    Metabolism Studies in Temporal Lobe
    Epilepsy   122
    THOMAS R. HENRY

9   Positron Emission Tomography: Glucose
    Metabolism in Extratemporal Lobe
    Epilepsy   141
    CSABA JUHÁSZ AND HARRY T. CHUGANI

10 Positron Emission Tomography: Brain
    Glucose Metabolism in Pediatric Epilepsy
    Syndromes   156
    AIMEE F. LUAT AND HARRY T. CHUGANI

11 [^{11}C]Flumazenil Positron Emission
    Tomography   174
    MATTHIAS J. KOEPP

12 Alpha-[^{11}C]Methyl-L-Tryptophan Positron
    Emission Tomography   186
    CARLOS E. A. BATISTA, DIANE C. CHUGANI,
    AND HARRY T. CHUGANI

13 Other PET Ligands used in
    Epilepsy   199
    WILLIAM H. THEODORE

14 SPECT Scanning for Epileptic
    Seizures   210
    R. EDWARD HOGAN, ELSON L. SO, AND
    TERENCE J. O'BRIEN

15 Multimodality Neuroimaging and Future
    Directions   226
    OTTO MUZIK AND HARRY T. CHUGANI

    INDEX   247

Contributors

Carlos E. A. Batista, MD
Department of Pediatrics
PET Center
Children's Hospital of Michigan
Wayne State University School of Medicine
Detroit, MI

Richard A. Bronen, MD
Departments of Diagnostic Radiology and Neurosurgery
Yale University School of Medicine
New Haven, CT

Diane C. Chugani, PhD
Departments of Pediatrics and Radiology
PET Center
Children's Hospital of Michigan
Wayne State University School of Medicine
Detroit, MI

Harry T. Chugani, MD
Departments of Pediatrics and Neurology
PET Center
Children's Hospital of Michigan
Wayne State University School of Medicine
Detroit, MI

William Davis Gaillard, MD
Departments of Neurology and Pediatrics
George Washington University
Center for Neuroscience
Children's National Medical Center
Washington DC

Rajkumar Munian Govindan, MD
Departments of Neurology and Pediatrics
PET Center
Children's Hospital of Michigan
Wayne State University School of Medicine
Detroit, MI

Renzo Guerrini, MD
Pediatric Neurology Unit and Laboratories
Children's Hospital A. Meyer
University of Florence Medical School
Florence, Italy

Vivek Gupta, MD
Department of Diagnostic Radiology
Mayo Clinic
Jacksonville, FL

Thomas R. Henry, MD
Department of Neurology
University of Minnesota
Minneapolis, MN

Hoby Hetherington, PhD
Departments of Neurosurgery and Diagnostic Radiology
Yale University School of Medicine
New Haven, CT

R. Edward Hogan, MD
Department of Neurology
Washington University in St. Louis
St. Louis, MO

Csaba Juhász, MD, PhD
Departments of Pediatrics and Neurology
PET Center
Children's Hospital of Michigan
Wayne State University School of Medicine
Detroit, MI

Robert C. Knowlton, MD, MSPH
Department of Neurology
UAB-HSF MEG Laboratory and UAB Seizure
*   Monitoring Unit*
University of Alabama at Birmingham School of Medicine
Birmingham, AL

Matthias J. Koepp, MD, PhD
Department of Clinical and Experimental Epilepsy
UCL Institute of Neurology
National Society for Epilepsy
London, UK

Ajay Kumar, MD, PhD, DNB
Departments of Pediatrics and Neurology
Children's Hospital of Michigan
Wayne State University School of Medicine Detroit, MI

Aimee F. Luat, MD
Departments of Pediatrics and Neurology
PET Center
Children's Hospital of Michigan
Wayne State University School of Medicine Detroit, MI

Otto Muzik, PhD
Departments of Pediatrics and Neurology
PET Center
Children's Hospital of Michigan
Wayne State University School of Medicine Detroit, MI

Terence J. O'Brien, MD
Department of Medicine
The Royal Medicine Hospital
University of Melbourne
Parkville, Victoria, Australia

Elson L. So, MD
Department of Neurology
Mayo Clinic College of Medicine
Rochester, MN

William H. Theodore, MD
Clinical Epilepsy Section
National Institute of Neurological Disorders
*   and Stroke*
Bethesda, MD

Lawrence W. Ver Hoef, MD
Department of Neurology
UAB Clinical Neurophysiology and Epilepsy Fellowship
*   Program*
University of Alabama at Birmingham School of
*   Medicine*
Birmingham, AL; and
Electroencephalography Lab
Veterans Affairs Medical Center
Birmingham, AL

Francesco Zellini, MD
Pediatric Neurology Unit and
*   Laboratories*
Children's Hospital A. Meyer
University of Florence Medical School
Florence, Italy

NEUROIMAGING IN EPILEPSY

Chapter *1*

HISTORICAL PERSPECTIVES OF NEUROIMAGING IN EPILEPSY

Harry T. Chugani and Ajay Kumar

The past several decades have seen the advent and evolution of various types of high-resolution tomographic neuroimaging that has had a significant impact on the diagnosis and management of patients with epilepsy. Anatomical imaging obtained with X-ray computed tomography (CT) and magnetic resonance imaging (MRI) can readily detect gross and even subtle anatomic abnormalities. Since epilepsy is primarily a functional disturbance of the brain, functional neuroimaging modalities, such as positron emission tomography (PET), single photon emission computed tomography (SPECT), and functional MRI (fMRI), offer new methods to the study of epilepsy and can be used to complement data from anatomical neuroimaging. Magnetoencephalography (MEG), which is used to record spontaneous and evoked magnetic fields generated by brain neuronal activity, can be combined with source analysis to convert the two-dimensional scalp-recorded waveforms to three-dimensional brain location and visualized on structural or functional brain images. These multimodality neuroimaging approaches have greatly enhanced our knowledge of epilepsy in recent years and have revolutionized the treatment of epilepsy. Prior to embarking on an in-depth analysis of these various techniques, it is worthwhile to consider briefly the historical aspects and evolution of neuroimaging in epilepsy.

SKULL X-RAY

In general, skull X-rays are now of limited value in the evaluation of epilepsy. In the acute setting of head trauma, skull films may be useful in diagnosing fractures associated with brain contusion and seizures. Chronic conditions that include epilepsy as a manifestation may show calcification detectable on plain skull X-rays. For example, approximately 15% to 20% of brain tumors in children calcify; these include oligodendrogliomas, astrocytomas, ependymomas, and craniopharyngiomas. Histiocytosis may be suspected when there is bone erosion (Fig. 1.1). Various intrauterine infections, such as toxoplasmosis and cytomegalic inclusion disease, are often characterized by cerebral calcification (Fig. 1.2). Probably one of the most common causes of cerebral calcification is tuberous sclerosis, in which the skull X-ray may show calcification along the walls of the ventricles, as well as in the cortical regions. Fahr's disease probably comprises several genetic disorders associated with basal ganglia calcification, choreoathetosis, and seizures. Both Down syndrome and Cockayne disease may reveal intracranial calcification, apparent on the skull X-ray, and associated with epilepsy. Prior to the development of various CT techniques, the most common procedure used to establish the diagnosis of Sturge-Weber syndrome was the skull X-ray, which demonstrated the classical

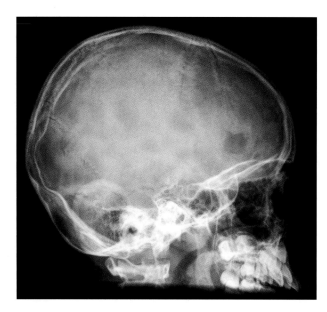

Figure 1.1 Skull X-ray of a child with seizures and histiocytosis showing bone erosion. (Courtesy of Dr. Thomas L. Slovis, Children's Hospital of Michigan)

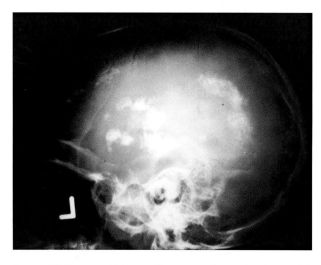

Figure 1.2 Ten-year-old boy with severe epilepsy, developmental delay, and brain calcifications shown on skull X-ray. Patient had intrauterine infection with toxoplasmosis. (Courtesy of Dr. Thomas L. Slovis, Children's Hospital of Michigan)

tramtrack-like calcifications (Fig. 1.3a,b). Cerebral angiography in patients with Sturge-Weber syndrome revealed the variable presence of arterial thromboses, absence of cortical veins, aberrant cerebral venous drainage and arteriovenous malformations, in addition to the characteristic leptomeningeal angioma commonly located in the posterior parietal distribution (Poser and Taveras 1957; Benston et al. 1971).

Conventional Nuclear Medicine Techniques

There has been minimal application of conventional nuclear medicine technology in the direct study of

epilepsy. In some conditions in which epilepsy is a manifestation, brain scanning has been used to elucidate the pathophysiology of the disorder rather than to evaluate the epilepsy. For example, Kuhl et al. (1972) performed 99m Tc-pertechnetate brain scans on 14 patients with Sturge-Weber syndrome. They found the affected hemisphere to have a smaller but more radioactive image than the unaffected side. Calcified regions showed increased uptake of the tracer. At about the time that these findings were described, CT techniques became available, and they quickly became the procedure of choice in Sturge-Weber syndrome.

CT

Cerebral imaging in patients with epilepsy became almost routine following the development and widespread availability of CT scanning, and it quickly became the standard of care in the evaluation of patients with epilepsy. For the first time, it was possible to directly visualize the brain in vivo. Various pathologic entities causing epilepsy and previously detected only postmortem could now be diagnosed in the early stages. It was discovered that about half of the large populations with epilepsy studied showed some abnormality on the CT scan. Often, these were nonspecific atrophic changes, but sometimes neoplasms (Figs. 1.4 and 1.5) and porencephalies were detected (Gastaut and Gastaut 1977). In some instances, the pattern on CT suggested intrauterine infection (Fig. 1.6). The exception, where CT scan was not required, was in patients with certain forms of primary generalized epilepsy (e.g., childhood absence epilepsy).

PARTIAL EPILEPSY   The routine application of CT scanning in intractable partial epilepsy in search of a surgically treatable lesion had a disappointingly low yield. Among 98 children with chronic epilepsy, the greatest yield of CT abnormalities was in children with partial motor epilepsy, of whom 43% showed an abnormality; however, only 2% of these could be surgically treated (Bachman, Hodges and Freeman 1976). In another large study of 143 patients with chronic seizures, in whom previous neurodiagnostic evaluations had failed to disclose abnormalities that could justify surgical intervention, CT scans revealed focal lesions that could be treated with surgery in only four. Following resection, two subjects were seizure-free and the other two showed significant improvement (Jabbari et al. 1978). Since medial temporal sclerosis is a common pathologic finding in temporal lobe epilepsy, attempts were made to detect sclerosis prior to surgery. Unfortunately, medial temporal sclerosis could not be readily detected on CT scans. The strategy developed by Wyler and Bolender (1983)

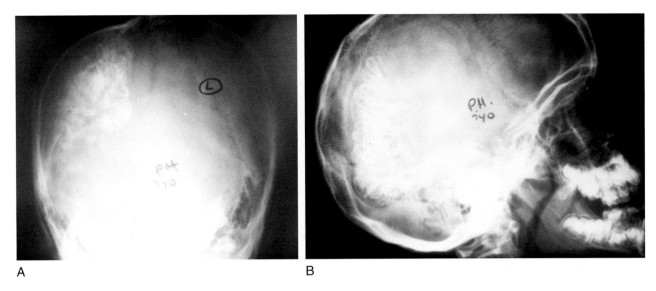

Figure 1.3 (A) AP and (B) lateral skull X-ray views of a 7-year-old boy with the Sturge-Weber syndrome showing the classic tramtrack-like calcifications. (Courtesy of Dr. Thomas L. Slovis, Children's Hospital of Michigan)

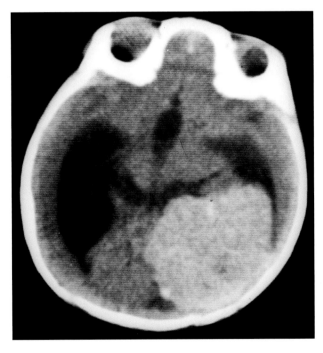

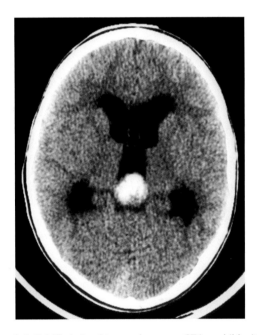

Figure 1.5 Calcified pineal tumor shown on CT in a child with epilepsy. (Courtesy of Dr. Thomas L. Slovis, Children's Hospital of Michigan)

Figure 1.4 CT scan of a child with seizures showing a large ependymoma with hydrocephalus. (Courtesy of Dr. Thomas L. Slovis, Children's Hospital of Michigan)

was to use metrizamide-enhanced CT to demonstrate abnormalities of the medial temporal structures in patients with intractable temporal lobe epilepsy. Among 25 patients examined with this technique, 17 showed close correlation between surgical findings and the high-resolution cerebrospinal fluid-enhanced CT scans. Partial epilepsy resulting from brain injury can often be predicted from CT scans obtained in the acute stage. In one study of 219 head

trauma patients, all 13 patients who later developed epilepsy had CT evidence of focal brain injury within 3 days of the traumatic event (D'Alessandro et al. 1988).

SYNDROMES ASSOCIATED WITH EPILEPSY   Early characterization of the angiomatosis distribution in Sturge-Weber syndrome was greatly aided by the advent of CT scanning. Indeed, CT has continued to play an important diagnostic role in Sturge-Weber syndrome because of its sensitivity in the detection of early calcification in

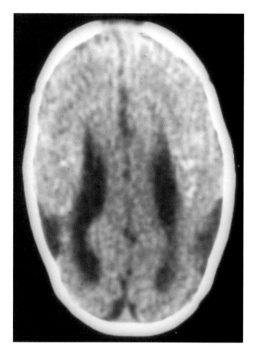

Figure 1.6 Periventricular calcifications on CT scan of a child with developmental delay and seizures suggesting TORCH infection. (Courtesy of Dr. Thomas L. Slovis, Children's Hospital of Michigan)

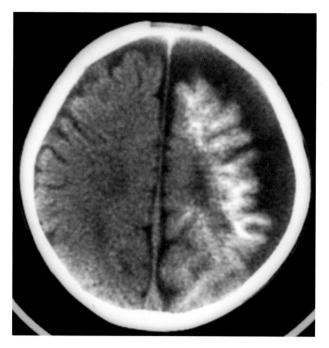

Figure 1.7 CT scan of an infant with Sturge-Weber syndrome showing advanced changes of hemispheric atrophy and calcification. (Courtesy of Dr. Thomas L. Slovis, Children's Hospital of Michigan)

the brain (Maki and Semba, 1979). In infants younger than about 1 or 2 years of age, CT scanning may show the affected hemisphere to be enlarged, with small arachnoid spaces and lateral ventricles. Following the administration of contrast medium, CT may reveal opacification of the angioma and adjacent regions of the hemisphere. The choroid plexus on the involved side is typically enlarged. In some cases, contrast infusion may reveal enhancement of the affected cerebral convolutions. Calcifications may also be seen within the angioma. As the disease progresses and the angioma is progressively excluded from the circulation, large areas of calcification may be seen on the CT (Fig. 1.7). This is accompanied by focal or generalized cerebral atrophy, presumably secondary to chronic ischemia (see also Chapter 10). When bilateral occipital cortico-subcortical calcifications are present in the absence of cutaneous stigmata of Sturge-Weber syndrome in patients with epilepsy (Gobbi et al. 1988), the diagnosis may be folate deficiency and celiac disease (Bye et al. 1993). The calcifications are best shown with CT scanning.

Thirty-eight children with Lennox-Gastaut syndrome underwent CT scanning, and two were shown to have focal lesions that were amenable to surgical treatment; these consisted of tuberous sclerosis and temporal lobe astrocytoma (Zimmerman, Niedermeyer and Hodges 1977). In several other epilepsy syndromes of childhood, such as hemimegalencephaly and other gross malformations of the brain, CT continues to be

useful in establishing the diagnosis early in the course of epilepsy.

CURRENT APPLICATIONS OF CT IN EPILEPSY   Although MRI has replaced CT as the neuroimaging procedure of choice in the evaluation of patients with epilepsy, there are a number of instances where brain CT scans continue to be performed. These are reviewed in Chapter 2.

REFERENCES

Bachman, D. S., F. J. Hodges, and J. M. Freeman. 1976. Computerized axial tomography in chronic seizure disorders of childhood. *Pediatrics* 58: 828–31.

Benston, J. R., G. H. Wilson, and T. H. Newton. 1971. Cerebral venous drainage pattern of the Sturge-Weber syndrome. *Radiology* 101: 111–8.

Bye, A. M. E., F. Andermann, T. Robitaille, et al. 1993. Cortical vascular abnormalities in the syndrome of celiac disease, epilepsy, bilateral occipital calcifications, and folate deficiency. *Annals of Neurology* 34: 399–403.

D'Alessandro, R., R. Ferrara, G. Benassi, et al. 1988. Computed tomographic scans in post-traumatic epilepsy. *Archives of Neurology* 45: 42–3.

Gastaut, H., and J. L. Gastaut. 1977. Computerized axial tomography in epilepsy. In *Epilepsy, the Eighth International Symposium*, ed. J. K. Penry. New York: Raven Press, 5–15.

Gobbi, G., G. Sorrenti, M. Santucci, et al. 1988. Epilepsy with bilateral occipital calcifications: a benign onset with progressive severity. *Neurology* 38: 913–20.

Jabbari, B., A. D. Huott, G. DiChiro, et al. 1978. Surgically correctable lesions detected by CT in 143 patients with chronic epilepsy. *Surgical Neurology* 10: 319–22.

Kuhl, D. E., J. E. Bevilacqua, M. M. Mishkin, and T. P. Sanders. 1972. The brain scan in Sturge-Weber syndrome. *Radiology* 103: 621–6.

Maki, Y., and A. Semba. 1979. Computed tomography of Sturge-Weber disease. *Childs Nervous System* 5: 51–61.

Poser, C. M., and J. M. Taveras. 1957. Cerebral angiography in encephalotrigeminal angiomatosis. *Radiology* 68: 327–36.

Wyler, A. R., and N. F. Bolender. 1983. Preoperative CT diagnosis of mesial temporal sclerosis for surgical treatment of epilepsy. *Annals of Neurology* 13: 59–64.

Zimmerman, A. W., E. Niedermeyer, and F. J. Hodges. 1977. Lennox-Gastaut syndrome and computerized axial tomography findings. *Epilepsia* 18: 463–4.

Chapter *2*

MRI: OVERVIEW OF MR TECHNIQUES FOR EPILEPSY

Vivek Gupta and Richard A. Bronen

Modern neuroimaging, particularly magnetic resonance (MR), has revolutionized the science and clinical practice of epilepsy and seizure disorders. This is most evident in the surgical management of chronic refractory epilepsy. Prior to the advent of cross-sectional imaging, evaluation and classification of seizure disorders were based solely on electroencephalographic (EEG) data and clinical features. This is reflected in the most recent International League Against Epilepsy (ILAE) classification (1981), in which etiology, anatomical localization, and pathways of spread are not considered even though they are critical in the neurosurgical management of epilepsy. Since then, new insights into mechanisms of neuronal hyperexcitability and developments in molecular genetics have radically changed our view of seizures and epilepsy. In addition to having a tremendous impact on the diagnosis and management of epilepsy, MR has led to a greater understanding of epilepsy syndromes. In essence, it has shifted the emphasis from purely clinical and electrophysiologic diagnosis to include structural brain abnormalities underlying the electrophysiologic and clinical features (Jackson et al. 1996b). In this chapter, we will discuss the more general aspects of MR imaging in epilepsy. The following four chapters are dedicated to malformations of cortical development (Chapter 3), MR spectroscopy (Chapter 4),

functional MRI (Chapter 5), and diffusion tensor imaging (Chapter 6) as applied to epilepsy.

IMAGING OF EPILEPSY

Computed tomography (CT) and MR have become standard in the evaluation of unexplained seizure(s) in children and adults. Neuroimaging is not indicated in patients with primary idiopathic generalized epilepsy and infants with new-onset typical febrile seizures and benign rolandic epilepsy (1998). For typical childhood febrile seizures, the American Academy of Pediatrics also does not recommend neuroimaging (1996b). Although MRI is more informative, CT may be appropriate in the acute emergency setting for evaluation of new-onset seizure patients with symptomatic causes (i.e., focal deficits, persistent altered mental status, fever, trauma, persistent headaches, history of cancer, anticoagulation, ventriculoperitoneal shunts, or acquired immunodeficiency syndrome) and for the elderly, in whom acute stroke and tumors are the most likely causes (Greenberg et al. 1996, 1996a; Hirstz et al. 2000; Maytal et al. 2000). CT, however, has very little role in preoperative evaluation of intractable epilepsy and pediatric new-onset seizures without apparent symptomatic cause. In these groups, MR is the neuroimaging study of choice (Bronen et al. 1996,

Table 2.1 Indications for Imaging in Seizure Disorders

Imaging typically not indicated

Primary (idiopathic) generalized epilepsy (grand mal or absence)

Simple febrile seizures

Juvenile myoclonic epilepsy

Benign rolandic epilepsy of childhood

Imaging typically indicated

Localization related seizures

Focal history, neurologic (or neuropsychological) deficits, focal EEG abnormalities

Developmental regression

Symptomatic generalized epilepsy syndromes

Increased intracranial pressure

History of status epilepticus

Onset of seizures in the first 2 years of life or adulthood

Medically refractory epilepsy

Change in pattern of seizures

1997c,d; Laster et al. 1985; Latack et al. 1986) because of its excellent soft tissue contrast allowing detailed depiction of anatomy, and multiplanar capability (Bronen et al. 1997c, Brooks et al. 1990; Kuzniecky et al. 1987; Laster et al. 1985; Lesser et al. 1986; Ormson et al. 1986; Schörner et al. 1987; Sperling et al. 1986; Theodore et al. 1990). Other modalities for preoperative evaluation of surgical candidates with intractable epilepsy include single photon emission computed tomography (SPECT), positron emission tomography (PET) and magnetoencephalography, all of which are discussed in detail elsewhere in this volume. Indications for imaging in the evaluation of seizure disorders is summarized in Table 2.1.

ROLE OF MRI IN EPILEPSY AND EPILEPSY SURGERY

The goal of epilepsy surgery is to remove or functionally disconnect the epileptogenic cortex responsible for the generation of seizures. For surgical remediation, seizures must typically have focal origin with reliable preoperative localization of the epileptogenic cortex. Localization of the epileptogenic cortex by anatomical or functional means, therefore, is the primary task in preoperative evaluation of surgical candidates. Attempts are directed towards building consensus among data from a variety of localizing modalities, beginning with the least invasive. These modalities include electrographic studies (scalp and intracranial EEG), magnetic source imaging (MSI or MEG), and neuroimaging with MRI, CT, PET, and SPECT. Scalp EEG is the standard initial localization and characterization step;

however, alone it is neither sufficiently sensitive nor reliably localizing for surgical decision making. Intracranial EEG (subdural and parenchymal depth recording), although considered the gold standard in seizure localization, is an expensive and invasive procedure not without risks and, therefore, not practical for universal application in epilepsy patients. Moreover, by its nature, intracranial EEG can sample a limited part of the brain, invariably requiring some preliminary localization data to guide the electrode placement, often not obtainable from scalp EEG alone. Intracranial EEG is therefore usually reserved for confirming the epileptogenicity of indeterminate structural lesion(s) seen on MRI, and validating the results of alternative methods of functional localization such as SPECT, PET, and MEG in MR-negative epilepsy.

Detection of structural abnormalities has provided a practical, highly valuable approach to localization since, in the overwhelming majority of localization-related epilepsy, structural abnormalities constitute the niche for epileptogenesis. Strategies for surgical treatment typically depend upon and begin with the identification of a structural abnormality detected on MRI. The goals of neuroimaging in presurgical evaluation of epilepsy patients include delineation of a structural or alternatively functional abnormality in the putative epileptogenic region; subsequently, mapping of sensorimotor, language, and memory functions in the epileptogenic and adjacent regions of the brain is attempted. Establishing the epileptogenicity of the abnormality detected on imaging by electrophysiologic studies is crucial to a successful surgical outcome. The algorithm for localization of the seizure focus and assessment of resectability varies according to institutional practice and resources. Based on extensive multicenter experience, patients with circumscribed lesions on MRI with convergent semiology, scalp EEG, and neuropsychological findings are considered for surgery without invasive electrographic recording. The widely accepted initial approach is to correlate clinical features, scalp EEG, and MRI; if concordant, no further seizure localization studies are usually necessary (Spencer et al. 1996). Nonconcordance of EEG and MRI, or indeterminate epileptogenicity of the MR-identified lesion, usually warrants intracranial EEG recordings using subdural or parenchymal depth electrodes (Spencer et al. 1996). Invasive electrophysiologic studies are also indicated in cases with normal MRI, more than one potentially epileptogenic MR abnormality, a large atrophic region or developmental abnormality, and when functional mapping of cortex is warranted based on MR findings or other reasons (Spencer et al. 1996).

The sensitivity of MRI for detecting epileptogenic lesions varies with the clinical profile of the patients. The positivity of MR is significantly lower in new-onset seizures than in chronic intractable epilepsy. In patients presenting with first seizure, King et al. (1998) found epileptogenic abnormality in 38 of 265 (14%) patients who underwent MRI. No epileptogenic lesions were found in patients with generalized seizures in their study. Similarly, in another study of 50 patients with late-onset epilepsy, Kilpatrick et al. (1991) reported MR to be positive in 32% of cases of partial/focal seizures compared to none in generalized epilepsy. In a study of newly diagnosed epilepsy, Berg et al. (2000) reported an etiologically relevant abnormality on MR imaging in 12.9% of the 389 children. Almost all subjects with positive relevant neuroimaging findings had partial or focal epilepsy. Neuroimaging is therefore recommended in all children with newly diagnosed epilepsy except those with idiopathic generalized epilepsy. Occasionally in symptomatic generalized epilepsy, such as infantile spasms and Lennox-Gastaut syndrome, surgically remediable abnormalities may be found on MRI (Berg et al. 2000). In adult patients with newly diagnosed partial seizures, MR abnormalities have been found in 24% (10% hippocampal sclerosis [HS] and 14% other abnormalities), a higher percentage than groups comprising unspecified new-onset seizure patients (Van Paesschen et al. 1997a). The sensitivity of MR for detecting epileptogenic abnormalities in children undergoing epilepsy surgery has been found to be 75% or higher (Cascino et al. 1992; Grattan et al. 1993; Kuzniecky et al. 1993; Wyllie et al. 1993, 1996). Therefore, the data overwhelmingly support obtaining MRI in partial and symptomatic epilepsies.

An overall sensitivity of 82% to 86% has been reported for MRI of intractable epilepsy (Bronen et al. 1996, 1997c,d; Brooks et al. 1990; Kuzniesky et al. 1987, 1993; Laster et al. 1985; Latack et al. 1986; Lesser et al. 1986; Ormson et al. 1986; Scott et al. 1999; Schörner et al. 1987; Sperling et al. 1986; Theodore et al. 1990). Approximately 90% of patients with clinically typical mesial temporal lobe epilepsy (MTLE) have a relevant structural lesion defined on high-resolution MRI studies. In MTLE, sensitivity of 75% to 100% for MRI detection of HS and over 90% for other focal lesions has been reported (Ashtari et al. 1991; Bronen et al. 1995a, 1997b; Brooks et al. 1990; Cascino et al. 1992; Cendes et al. 1993b; Cook et al. 1992; Grattan et al. 1993; Jack et al. 1990; Jack C et al. 1996; Jackson et al. 1990, 1993b; Kuzniesky et al. 1987, 1993; Lee et al. 1998; Schörner et al. 1987; Spencer et al. 1993, 1994; Theodore et al. 1990; Wyllie et al. 1993). By contrast, in patients with extratemporal or neocortical TLE, the detection rate is somewhat lower, as the abnormalities are often cortical dysplasia. Dysplasias may be unresectable or incompletely resectable. Incomplete resection is associated with a high rate of seizure recurrence. Detection of a dysplastic lesion

therefore adversely alters the surgical options and prognosis, particularly when surgery is aimed at cure of seizures (Edwards et al. 2000; Francione et al. 2003; Hader et al. 2004; Terra-Bustamante 2005; Wyllie et al. 1996). Low-grade neoplasms and dysembryoplastic neuroepithelial tumors (DNETs), on the other hand, are associated with excellent prognosis for seizure control when completely resected (Daumas-Duport et al. 1988; Morris et al. 1998).

The convergence of anatomic MR abnormality and epileptogenic pathology in partial epilepsies has led to development of a "lesion" or "substrate" concept in partial epilepsies (Spencer D et al. 1994, Spencer et al. 1998). An epileptogenic lesion signifies a structural pathology believed to be responsible for epileptogenesis. Identification of a structural brain lesion in an epileptic patient implies a relatively poor chance of achieving seizure freedom with antiepileptic medications alone (Spooner et al. 2006). On the other hand, the likelihood of postoperative seizure freedom is higher if a lesion is found on preoperative MRI and successfully resected. Even with reliable localization of focal seizure origin in imaging-negative or "nonlesional" epilepsy, the surgical results are less favorable compared with those from lesionectomies and temporal lobectomies with a definable lesion (Alarcón et al. 2006; Chapman et al. 2005; Holmes et al. 2000; Scott et al. 1999). Postsurgical seizure freedom is reported in only 47% of nonlesional cases (Alarcón et al. 2006). Many other investigators have found MR to be useful in prognosticating postoperative seizure control. A successful outcome in TLE is achieved in 70% to 95% patients with MR findings of HS compared with 40% to 55% of patients in whom the MR is normal (Alarcón et al. 2006; Berkovic et al. 1995; Bronen et al. 1997b,c; Chapman et al. 2005; Garcia et al. 1994; Holmes et al. 2000; Jack et al. 1992; Lee et al. 1998). Berkovic et al. (1995) found the postoperative outcome to depend both on identification of a lesion by MRI and the nature of MRI abnormality—a seizure-free state in 80% with focal lesions other than HS, 62% in patients with HS, and only 36% with normal MRI. In a recent study of 210 patients rendered seizure-free after epilepsy surgery, those with normal preoperative MRI had a higher rate of postoperative seizure recurrence after discontinuation of antiepileptic medication (Schiller et al. 2000). As mentioned above, lesion characteristics also affect the surgical prognosis. HS, cavernous angioma, and certain cortical neoplasms (such as DNET) are epileptogenic lesions with a high degree of convergence of the anatomic pathology with the epileptogenic zone. Consequently, removal of the MRI abnormality or lesionectomy leads to seizure freedom in a high proportion of cases. Other epileptogenic lesions often may not have intrinsic epileptogenicity. Gliomas, for example, may induce seizures by mass effect and metabolic changes in the adjacent cerebral cortex. Nonetheless, removal of the lesion renders most of these patients seizure-free. In focal cortical dysplasia, however, removal of the visible anatomic lesion alone frequently does not lead to seizure freedom, indicating that the epileptogenic zone extends beyond the lesion defined by structural imaging. Consequently, the distinction between "lesional" and "nonlesional" epilepsy, and hence characterization of the lesion, has become quite relevant in management and prognosis of individual patients (Spencer et al. 1998), thereby promoting MRI as an essential evaluation in modern epilepsy practice. A major challenge for the current epilepsy classification scheme is a framework to incorporate MRI, and efforts are under way to overcome this limitation.

The role of MRI in epilepsy surgery (Table 2.2), in addition to its principal value of identifying the epileptogenic lesion, also lies in its ability to depict topographic relationships between the epileptogenic lesion and the eloquent regions of brain. Co-registration of PET and SPECT abnormalities with MR facilitates their precise anatomical localization in relation to functional cortex in nonlesional epilepsy (O'Brien et al. 1999). Functional MRI (discussed in Chapter 5) can greatly facilitate assessments of the eloquent brain regions. This information, among other factors, is key in assessing the appropriateness and type of surgery, and minimizing postoperative neurologic deficits. MRI influences the need for invasive EEG and is also useful in planning the placement of subdural and parenchymal depth electrodes.

MRI and surgical navigation

MRI is increasing being used for surgical navigation using frameless image guidance for real-time localization during resections in relation to the preoperative imaging (Braun et al. 2001; Kratimenos et al. 1993; Mahvash et al. 2006; Mehta et al. 2005; Murphy et al. 2001; Oertel et al. 2004; Rezai et al. 1997; Scellig et al. 2008; Shenai et al. 2007; Stapelton et al. 1997; Wurm et al. 2003). MR-based multimodality image-guided navigation incorporates data from fMRI, PET, SPECT, and diffusion tensor imaging (DTI) and is particularly valuable for small or deep-seated lesions to facilitate the most direct and least damaging trajectory to the target, thus avoiding injury to eloquent cortex (Braun et al. 2001; Rezai et al. 1997; Scellig et al. 2008; Stapelton et al. 1997). Depth electrodes placement with image-guided techniques has been demonstrated to be accurate, and absence of the head frame permits placement of subdural electrodes during the same session. MRI guidance also reduces complications of depth electrode placement. In selective amygdalo-hippocampectomy, these methods are useful to precisely define the craniotomy and guide the route to the anterior portion of the temporal horn, minimizing the risk of postoperative visual field deficit by avoiding Meyer's loop. Due to the variability of the anterior limit of Meyer's loop, there is a risk of contralateral superior visual field deficit following anterior temporal lobe resection (Yogarajah et al. 2009). Fiber-tracking by DTI (see also Chapter 6) superimposed on the preoperative imaging could, therefore, further contribute in minimizing the risk of damage to optic radiations. Image guidance can also serve to predefine or standardize amygdalo-hippocampectomy and the posterior extent of resection in temporal lobectomy (Schwartz et al. 2002). Intraoperative MRI is increasingly being used in epilepsy surgery, allowing direct intraoperative localization of the lesion, extent of lesion resection, and direct overall visualization of the brain, eliminating the issues related to brain shifts inherent in navigation based on preoperative imaging.

Postoperative MRI

Accurate information regarding the position of the subdural grid relative to the cortex is very important in planning resective surgery. MRI is one method to verify the precise anatomical localization of the contacts, and it can help with precise determination of the seizure focus and the extent of surgical resection

Table 2.2 Role of MRI in Surgical Management of Refractory Epilepsy

Localize epilepsy

1. Identify epileptogenic pathology
2. Define topographic relationship of epileptogenic lesion to functional cortex (fMRI), and critical white matter tracts (MR tractography)
3. Co-register PET & SPECT for precise anatomic localization

Intracranial EEG

1. Determine strategy of subdural grids/strips and depth electrodes placement
2. Guide electrode placement: MR-guided frame or frameless stereotaxy
3. Verify precise location of contacts after placement

Intraoperative

1. MRI-based navigation in resections and corticography
2. Intraoperative imaging for real-time assessment of surgical changes

Postoperative

1. Assess adequacy of resection, postoperative complications
2. Follow-up for tumor recurrence

(Davis et al. 1999; Brooks et al. 1992). However, obtaining MRI soon after grid implantation is not very practical, especially in pediatric cases; instead, post-implantation multiplanar radiographs or CT scans can be fused with the pre-implantation MR images. Following resective epilepsy surgery, MRI may help detect reasons for failure such as inadequate resection and monitor tumor recurrence on follow-up imaging.

MRI: STRATEGIES AND TECHNICAL ISSUES

The age at onset of the seizure disorder affects the probability of a particular epilepsy substrate (Table 2.3). The superiority of a dedicated MRI protocol in detecting epileptogenic lesions has been demonstrated (Von Oertzen et al. 2002). Therefore, the clinical MR acquisition protocols must be optimized to maximize the diagnostic yield (Table 2.3). In older children and adults, the optimized imaging protocol,

Table 2.3 Recommended MRI Protocol for Seizure Evaluation

Age (yr)	Probable etiologies	Dedicated sequences
≤2	Hypoxia Metabolic abnormalities Developmental malformations Neurocutaneous syndromes Congenital or acquired infections	Ax SE PD and T2W Ax, cor SE T1W Cor long-TR FSE T2[a] High-res 3D T1 GRE, or FSE T2 Ax DWI Optional: MRS
2-50	Hippocampal sclerosis Tumor and vascular lesions Developmental malformations Infection Posttraumatic	Oblique cor high-res FSE T2 through temporal lobes Cor FSE FLAIR 3D hi-res (IR) T1 GRE T2* W GRE, SWI Ax DWI Optional: volumetry, T2 relaxometry, DTI, MRS, fMRI
≥50	Stroke Tumor	Ax DWI Ax FSE T2 Cor FSE FLAIR Optional: fMRI MRS DTI

Ax, axial; Cor, coronal; SE, spin echo; PD, proton density; FSE, fast spin echo; FLAIR, fluid attenuated inversion recovery; GRE, gradient recalled echo; SWI, susceptibility weighted imaging DWI, diffusion weighted imaging; T1W, T1 weighted; T2W, T2 weighted; MRS, magnetic resonance spectroscopy; DTI, diffusion tensor imaging; fMRI, functional MRI

[a]Useful under 2 years of age for incomplete myelination of white matter

in addition to the standard imaging sequences, includes coronal T2-weighted and fluid-attenuated inversion recovery (FLAIR) and a high-resolution, T1-weighted, gradient echo isotropic three-dimensional (3D) volume acquisition (MPRAGE, SPGR). The first sequence allows detail of the hippocampus. The latter provides multiplanar views for better anatomical localization and helps avoid partial volume effects in the detection of malformations of cortical development; it also can be used to correct for head rotation in the coronal plane. In a majority of adult surgical cases, the region of interest is temporal lobe, primarily hippocampus. Hippocampal pathology is characterized often by subtle volume and signal changes. Whereas FSE T2-weighted imaging provides the best combination of structural detail and signal changes from gliosis-related T2-prolongation, ultra-high-resolution 3D spoiled gradient-recalled echo (GRE) adds to the structural detail, and FLAIR enhances the perception of signal changes. Thus, the MR imaging of hippocampus (and amygdala) is best performed using 2- to 3-mm FSE T2, FSE FLAIR sequences in a slightly oblique coronal plane, perpendicular to the long axis of the hippocampus (Fig. 2.1). Rigorous attention must be paid to correct for head rotation to allow accurate comparison with the contralateral hippocampus (Fig. 2.2).

The PROPELLER (**P**eriodically **R**otated **O**verlapping **P**arall**EL** **L**ines with **E**nhanced **R**econstruction) technique of k-space filling (referred to as BLADE in the MR system of Siemens Medical Systems) is quite valuable in improving T2 image detail by minimizing the artifact from gross and microscopic head motion,

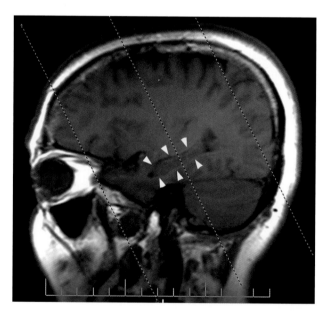

Figure 2.1 Oblique coronal plane for optimal imaging of the medial temporal lobe structures: dotted lines orthogonal to the long axis of hippocampus (*arrowheads*) on sagittal T1 scout.

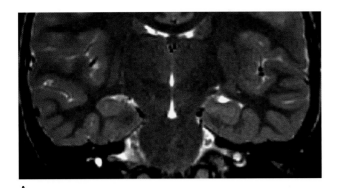

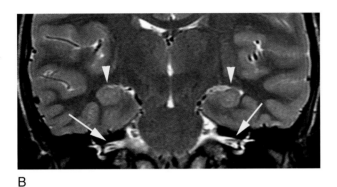

Figure 2.2 Effect of head rotation on hippocampal symmetry. (A) Head rotation (evident from internal acoustic canal and vestibular structures) causing slightly anterior sectioning of the left hippocampus and making it appear larger. (B) Upon correction of the head position, the internal acoustic canals (*arrows*), and hippocampi (*arrowheads*) appear symmetric.

even in cooperative subjects (Eriksson et al. 2008, Fig. 2.3). The motion correction in PROPELLER emerges from rotation of concentric rectangular strips (or blades) about the k-space origin. The consequent

oversampling of the central region of k-space allows correction of misregistration of position, rotation, and phase between acquisitions by rejecting uncorrelated data (Forbes et al. 2001). Priming the volumetric 3D spoiled GRE with an appropriately timed inversion pulse (TI~300-450 ms for IR-SPGR, and TI~600-900 for MPGR) enhances gray–white matter contrast and may be routinely employed. Optimal gray–white differentiation can also be obtained from high-resolution T2-weighted images, which can be gray scale inverted to resemble T1 weighting if desired. In neonates and infants up to 6 months, longer TR (≥6000 ms) on the T2-weighted sequence helps to improve the contrast between gray and nonmyelinated white matter. Susceptibility-weighted or T2*GRE sequence is also recommended in the routine epilepsy protocol as it enhances detection of occult hemorrhage, calcified lesions, and vascular malformations that may be responsible for seizures.

High-field MRI in epilepsy

High-field MRI (3 Tesla or greater) is increasingly being explored in the evaluation of epilepsy (Knake et al. 2005; Phal et al. 2008; Strandberg et al. 2008). MRI at 3T with its intrinsically greater signal-to-noise ratio combined with advances in parallel acquisition (sensitivity encoding) has the potential to add diagnostic utility. The increased signal-to-noise ratio allows faster imaging for a given resolution, higher resolution for a given imaging time, or a combination of both. Shorter acquisitions help to reduce motion artifacts, which is important in imaging ill or less cooperative subjects. In structural MRI, the application of

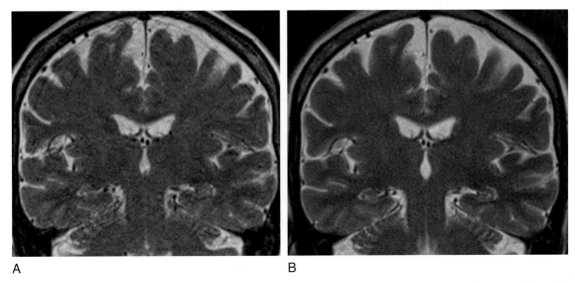

Figure 2.3 Improvement of image degradation cause by head motion on PROPELLER. Marked improvement of image quality on PROPELLER T2-weighted (B) as compared FSE T2-weighted (A) in an uncooperative subject. PROPELLER obtained immediately after the FSE sequence.

higher field is primarily aimed at increasing detection rates of focal structural lesions. As noted above, the surgical outcomes are superior when lesionectomy is possible. Enhanced lesion detection by MRI at higher fields could therefore more often permit lesionectomy, thereby improving the prognosis. Equally important, it may reduce the need for invasive electrographic monitoring, or facilitate better brain targeting and coverage during invasive monitoring. MRI applications with inherently low signals, such as fMRI, MRS, diffusion and perfusion imaging, derive greater benefit from higher field strengths (Barker et al. 2001; Bartha et al. 2000; Kruger et al. 2001; Li et al. 2001).

At higher field strengths, a few important technical considerations that affect image quality and contrast need to be addressed. Standing wave (dielectric resonance) effects result in signal and contrast non-uniformity. At 3T, radiofrequency (RF) wavelength is of the order of the head size. The constructive and destructive interference patterns from standing RF waves manifest as relative hyperintensity of the deep structures and hypointensity of the cortex and superficial structures. The effect is largely negated by phased-array head coils and signal intensity uniformity correction routinely employed in general clinical imaging. The issues related to high RF energy deposition and specific absorption ratio also arise at high-field. The RF energy deposition and consequent tissue heating can be reduced by decreasing the flip angles of the excitation and/or refocusing pulses in spin-echo techniques. These modifications may be limited to peripheral k-space sampling, thereby unaffecting the

tissue-contrast characteristics. In addition to maintaining specific absorption ratio, they tend to improve gray–white contrast on T1-weighted imaging, but at the cost of slightly reduced signal-to-noise ratio. Conventional spin-echo is generally preferred over FSE in T1-weighted imaging due to higher contrast and less image blurring. Enhanced magnetic susceptibility at 3T increases the sensitivity of T2*-weighted sequences for detection of calcification and hemorrhage (Fig. 2.4). The image distortion in echo-planar and gradient-echo sequences resulting from increased susceptibility adjacent to the skull base and sinuses can usually be effectively addressed by routine use of parallel imaging (spatial sensitivity encoding). Due to inherent prolongation of tissue T1 at higher field strength, the TR and TI (inversion time) need appropriate upward adjustment for optimal gray–white matter contrast.

Thus far, the data pertaining to added value of high-field MRI in epilepsy are somewhat limited. There appears to be a trend towards slightly increased lesion detection on 3T compared to 1.5T, particularly of subtle cortical dysplasia (Knake et al. 2005; Phal et al. 2008; Strandberg et al. 2008). Improved detection of HS on 3T is anecdotal so far (Iwasaki et al. 2009; Sawaishi et al. 2005). It is unclear whether this improvement results from higher field strength or application of phased-array coils, which are standard on 3T. Improved lesion detection has been reported with the use of dedicated phased-array surface coils at 1.5T (Goyal et al. 2004; Grant et al. 1997). The clinical utility of higher field strength in functional MR localization

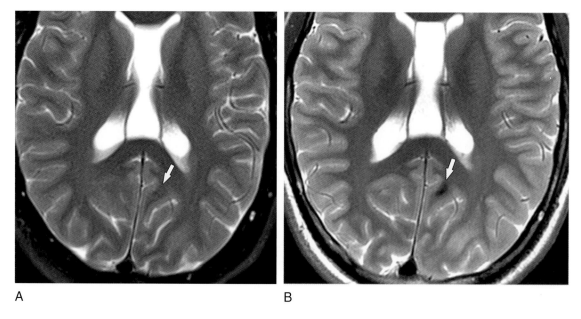

A   B

Figure 2.4 Enhanced magnetic susceptibility at 3T helps detection of focal siderosis (B, arrow), which is not appreciated at 1.5T (A, arrow).

techniques such as DTI and MRS is yet to be evaluated in epilepsy (Chen et al. 2008). These techniques could be of significant value in targeting of intracranial EEG in nonlesional (negative structural MRI) epilepsy.

MRI OF COMMON EPILEPTOGENIC ABNORMALITIES

Hippocampal sclerosis

Medial temporal or hippocampal sclerosis is the most important single cause of intractable MTLE found in surgical series. A large body of data confirms the validity of structural abnormalities detected on MRI in pathologically proven HS. HS is histologically characterized by gliosis and neuronal loss (pyramidal and granule cells) in the Ammon's horn and dentate regions of the hippocampus. Hoever, extrahippocampal pathology is often also found elsewhere in the temporal lobe, including white matter (Wieser et al. 2004). Such pathology frequently affects the amygdala, with neuronal cell loss and gliosis (sclerosis) in the amygdala (Van Paesschen et al. 1997b). In addition, ectopic neurons and perivascular oligodendrocytic infiltrates have been found in the temporal lobe white matter (Wieser et al. 2004). Retrospective data from surgical series often implicate "initial precipitating incidents," including febrile seizures, trauma, hypoxia, and intracranial infection in the first 5 years of life (Wieser et al. 2004). A "silent" period between the first habitual seizure and the onset of intractability exists in a majority of patients (Berg et al. 2003). The typical onset of intractable complex partial seizures is during the first two decades of life (Wieser et al. 2004). Even in patients with medically controlled complex partial epilepsy, HS has been reported on MRI (Kim et al. 1999). A detailed description of the epidemiology and clinico-pathological aspects of HS can be found in the ILAE Commission report on MTLE with HS (Wieser et al. 2004).

Overview of medial temporal lobe anatomy

The hippocampus (Figs. 2.5 and 2.6) is a curved structure in the medial temporal lobe consisting of U-shaped layers of the *dentate gyrus* and *cornu ammonis*, which are interlocked. The cornu ammonis (also known as the endfolium) comprises four regions, namely CA1 through CA4, enveloped by the dentate gyrus. The cornu ammonis continues into the *subiculum*, which represents the transition to the neocortex of *parahippocampal gyrus*. The hippocampus lies above the *subiculum* and medial part of parahippocampal gyrus, forming a 4- to 4.5-cm-long convexity in the floor of the temporal horn. Three regions of the

hippocampus can be defined based on morphology and relationship to the midbrain. The most anterior expanded part, the *hippocampal head* or *pes hippocampus* (Fig. 2.5A), is recognized by three or four digitations on its superior surface. The cylindrical body extends posteriorly about the midbrain. The posterior portion—the tail of hippocampus—tapers behind the brain stem. Along the convex ventricular surface, tangential white matter tracts, known as *alveus*, pass medially and converge into the *fimbria*, which runs in the temporal horn and continues posteriorly as *fornix*. The *amygdala* (Figs. 2.5A and 2.7) is a gray matter structure

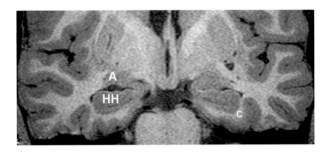

A

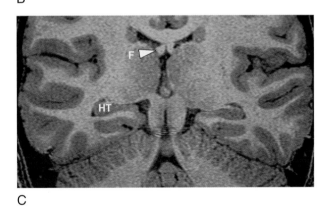

B

C

Figure 2.5 Normal anatomy of medial temporal structures at 3T: Coronal T1-weighted (spoiled) GRE, anterior to posterior. (A) Hippocampal head, HH, separated by temporal horn from amygdala, labeled A. Note the undulations on the superior surface of the hippocampal head, which are known as digitations. Collateral white matter, C, is inferolateral to the hippocampus. (B) Hippocampal body containing cornu ammonis (*arrow*) and dentate gyrus (*arrowhead*). The transition from parahippocampal gyrus to hippocampus, called subiculum, is indicated on the left by the long arrow. (C) Hippocampal tail, HT; fornix, F.

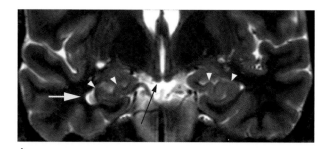

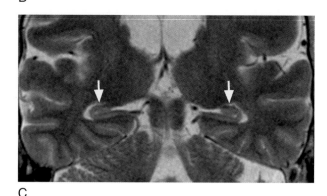

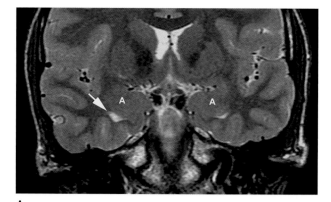

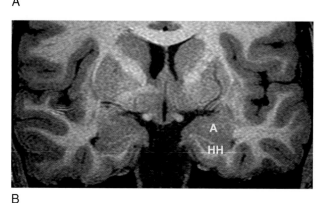

Figure 2.7 (A) Coronal T2-weighted FSE: amygdala (labeled A) in its relationship to uncal recess (*arrow*). (B) Coronal T1-weighted GRE image showing amygdala immediately superior to hippocampal head (HH) on a slightly posterior plane.

Figure 2.6 Normal anatomy of medial temporal structures, anterior to posterior. Coronal T2-weighted FSE at 1.5T. (A) Digitations of the hippocampal head (*arrowheads*), normal asymmetry of the temporal horn (*arrow*), symmetric mammillary bodies (*long black arrow*). (B) Body of hippocampus. Cornu ammonis (CA1 region, *arrowhead*), alveus (*short arrow*), temporal horn (*long arrow*). (C) Hippocampal tail (*arrows*).

located superomedial to the anterior end of the temporal horn of the lateral ventricle (*uncal recess*), separating it from the hippocampal head (Fig. 2.5A). For volumetric assessment, the criteria for anatomical boundaries of hippocampus and amygdala described by Watson et al. (1992) are usually employed.

A number of imaging modalities have been shown to provide reliable localizing information in MTLE-HS. Structural MRI is highly sensitive and specific in patients with electroclinical features of MTLE and is currently the gold standard for in vivo detection of HS (N4). Other modalities helpful in localization of MTLE, however, without a specific diagnosis of HS,

include (1) interictal proton magnetic resonance spectroscopy (proton-MRS), primarily using reduced N-acetyl-aspartate (NAA) as a marker of neuronal loss and dysfunction, (2) ictal/interictal SPECT using perfusion-based tracers such as [Tc-99m]technetium-hexamethylpropyleneamine oxime (HMPAO) or [99mTc] technetium-ethylene cysteine dimer (ECD), to study ictal and interictal regional perfusion changes, (3) interictal PET with [18F]fluoro-2-deoxyglucose (FDG), to detect glucose hypometabolism associated with epileptogenesis, and (4) interictal PET with [11C]flumazenil, to assess altered density of benzodiazepine receptors. Nonlesional MTLE typically is not distinguishable from MTLE-HS preoperatively when MRI is negative for HS.

MRI of normal and sclerotic hippocampus

The amygdala and hippocampus are isointense to gray matter on all MR pulse sequences, except FLAIR, on which the hippocampus is usually slightly hyperintense to gray matter, presumably due to incomplete suppression of cerebrospinal fluid (CSF) (Fig. 2.8) (Hirai et al. 2000). High-resolution, thin-section FSE and

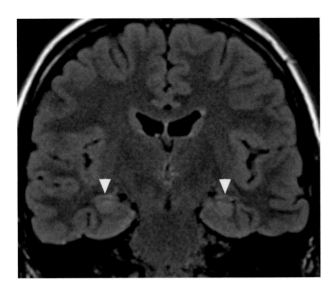

Figure 2.8 Normal appearance of hippocampus (*arrowheads*) on FLAIR. Note slight hyperintensity relative to cortex elsewhere.

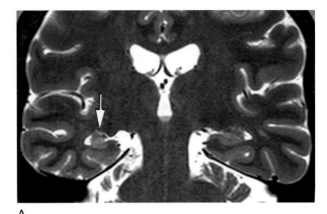

A

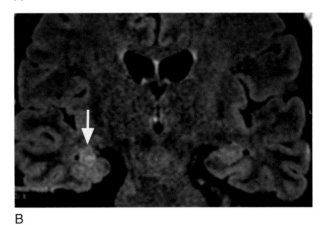

B

Figure 2.9 Hippocampal sclerosis at 1.5T, atrophy and increased signal in the body of right hippocampus (*arrow*). (A) Coronal high-resolution T2 FSE. (B) Coronal FLAIR.

inversion recovery (IR) sequences are most important in the depiction of hippocampal architecture (Jack et al. 1994b; Jackson et al. 1993a, 1995; Tien et al. 1993). Conventional or fast spin echo T2-weighted acquisitions are sensitive for assessing hippocampal signal changes (Fig 2.9A) and for detecting signal abnormalities in the rest of the brain. FLAIR may provide better T2-weighted signal detection (Spencer D et al. 1994, Fig. 2.9B). Coronal high-resolution 3D T1-weighted spoiled gradient echo is optimally suited for quantitative volumetry. The 3D data can be reformatted to obtain true coronal images of the hippocampus orthogonal to its long axis for optimal delineation in volumetric analysis.

The key MR abnormalities in HS are hippocampal atrophy and hyperintense signal on T2-weighted images (Figs. 2.9 and 2.10) (Ashtari et al. 1991; Berg et al. 2003; Bronen et al. 1991b, 1997b; Cendes et al. 1993a,b; Cook et al. 1992, 1994; Jack et al. 1990; Jackson et al. 1990; Kuzniecky et al. 1987; Lee et al. 1998; Lencz et al. 1992; Spencer et al. 1993, 1994). These findings occur in a large majority of surgically proven cases of HS. Loss of the internal architecture is a frequent corroborative finding. MRI also often shows atrophy and signal alteration outside of the hippocampus, usually ipsilateral to the sclerotic hippocampus. Other MR findings associated with HS (Table 2.4) include loss of ipsilateral hippocampal head digitations, widening of the temporal horn (Fig. 2.10C), and loss of the white matter adjacent to the collateral sulcus (Fig. 2.11). The commonly identified extrahippocampal abnormalities in surgically treated MTLE-HS are atrophy and signal changes in the ipsilateral amygdala, temporal neocortex and white matter, fornix, mammillary body, insula, thalamus, and basifrontal cortex.

Diffuse hemispheric atrophy may rarely occur ipsilaterally. Sclerosis of the contralateral hippocampus is often seen but is typically less severe than that affecting the hippocampus ipsilateral to epileptogenesis. Increased T2 signal in the ipsilateral anterior temporal white matter and atrophy of the ipsilateral fornix (Fig. 2.10B) and mammillary body (Fig. 2.10B) result from degeneration of hippocampal tracts and can be well seen on coronal images (Baldwin et al. 1994; Bronen et al. 1995b, 1997a, 1998; Duncan et al. 1997; Jackson et al. 1996a; Meiners et al. 1994, 1999; Oppenheim et al. 1998). Quantitative measurements of T2 decay (T2 relaxometry) obtained on a single-slice multiecho or FSE sequence through the hippocampal body can reliably reveal abnormal T2 prolongation in sclerotic hippocampi (Bartlett et al. 2007; Jackson et al. 1993b; Okujava et al. 2002). One of the challenges with T2 relaxometry in young children and infants is the variable degree of hypomyelination of the brain, resulting in higher T2 relaxation times, thus making assessment difficult. Normative data on the immature brain are limited, and each center performing T2 mapping needs to determine its

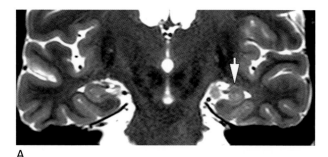

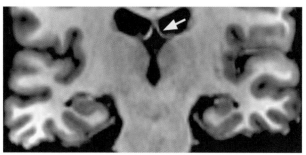

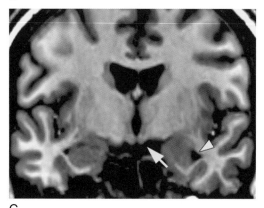

Figure 2.10 Left HS at 3T. (A) Hippocampal atrophy and increased signal(*arrow*) on coronal high-resolution T2 FSE. Coronal T1 GRE. (B) Atrophy of left hippocampus and fornix (*arrow*). (C) Atrophy of the left mammillary body (*arrow*) and enlargement of left temporal horn (*arrowhead*). Note the detail of normal hippocampal anatomy at 3T in A, compared to that at 1.5 T in Figure 2.9A.

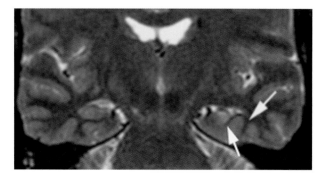

Figure 2.11 Collateral white matter atrophy in HS (*arrows*; compare with the normal right side).

Table 2.4 MRI Findings in Hippocampal Sclerosis

Primary (hippocampal) findings

Atrophy

Signal alterations

Loss of internal architecture

Secondary (extrahippocampal) findings

Temporal lobe

    Loss of hippocampal head digitations

    Dilation of temporal horn

    Temporal lobe atrophy

    Collateral white matter atrophy

    Anterior temporal white matter signal changes

Extratemporal lobe

    Fornix atrophy

    Mammillary body atrophy

    Thalamic atrophy

    Caudate atrophy

own normal controls to evaluate the results. The typical FDG-PET finding in HS is ipsilateral, or less commonly bilateral, temporal lobe hypometabolism (see Chapter 8). PET confirmation can be valuable in cases of subtle or equivocal HS findings and negative MRI in MTLE, and potentially avoid invasive EEG (Fig. 2.12).

Quantitative hippocampal volumetry slightly adds to the sensitivity over visual scrutiny (90%–95% vs. 80%–90%) in detection of hippocampal atrophy (Bronen et al. 1994; Jack et al. 1990, 1994a; Jack C et al. 1993). The MRI abnormalities in HS are typically unilateral, or unambiguously asymmetrical when bilateral; however, rarely they can be symmetrical. Hippocampal volumetry and T2 relaxometry are quite useful in cases of symmetric bilateral hippocampal atrophy without visually appreciable signal changes. Quantitative methods are also an important tool in epilepsy research, when measurable anatomical data are required for statistical correlation with clinical and pathologic indices. Routine clinical quantitative MR volumetry, however, is usually not practical due to demands of operator time; dedicated personnel, workstations, and software; and reliable normative data from matched control subjects.

A less common hippocampal lesion associated with MTLE is endfolium sclerosis, which is characterized by sclerotic changes limited to or predominantly in the CA4 region (endfolium) of the Ammon's horn. Endfolium sclerosis has been variably reported in MTLE and shows less specific correlation as the etiology of temporal lobe seizures. Endfolium sclerosis is typically undetectable on standard MR imaging (including T2-relaxometry and MR volumetry) and is identified in many of the resected hippocampi in MR-negative MTLE (also sometimes referred to as

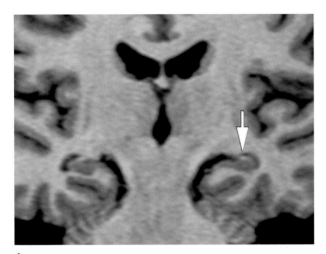

A

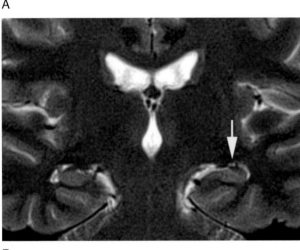

B

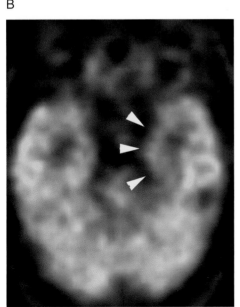

C

paradoxical TLE). Paradoxical TLE is characterized by less frequent history of febrile seizures, onset of epilepsy later in life, and poorer postoperative seizure outcome compared with typical HS (Cohen-Gadol et al. 2005). With increasing application of high-field (3T or higher) MRI in clinical epilepsy, there is the potential for increased presurgical detection of this entity (Eriksson et al. 2008; Fatterpekar et al. 2002; Iwasaki et al. 2009).

The combination of HS with another potentially epileptogenic macroscopic extrahippocampal abnormality, referred to as dual pathology (Fig. 2.13), has been observed in 15% of surgical epilepsy cases with

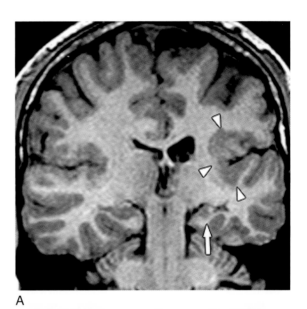

A

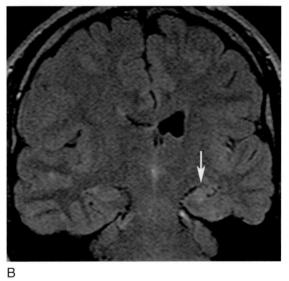

B

Figure 2.12 Medial temporal lobe epilepsy: value of PET. (A) Coronal T1-weighted SPGR showing subtle hippocampal volume loss (*arrow*). (B) Equivocal hyperintensity of left hippocampus on FSE T2 (*arrow*). (C) Left medial temporal lobe hypometabolism on axial PET (*arrowheads*) supports hippocampal sclerosis.

Figure 2.13 Dual pathology: left temporoparietal focal cortical dysplasia indicated by cortical thickening on coronal SPGR (A, *arrowheads*), and left HS (*arrow*) evident from atrophy (A and B) and increased signal on coronal FLAIR (B).

MR imaging (Cendes et al. 1995; Wieser et al. 2004). Dual pathology is associated with a less favorable surgical outcome and requires intracranial EEG to determine whether seizures originate in the hippocampus, outside the hippocampus, or at both sites. For successful control of seizures, both abnormalities usually need to be resected (Li et al. 1997, 1999; Sisodiya et al. 1997; Wieser et al. 2004). Therefore, a search for additional abnormalities must be continued after detection of a possible epileptogenic lesion on MR. The most often encountered abnormality associated with HS is cortical dysplasia. In complex partial epilepsy, dual pathology consisting of HS and an extrahippocampal lesion of the same temporal lobe is more common than dual pathology consisting of HS and an extratemporal lesion (Wieser et al. 2004).

MR imaging findings, along with EEG data, strongly guide the workup of TLE patients. Anterior temporal lobectomy or selective amygdalo-hippocampectomy can be performed if there is concordance of MR with EEG and if there are no conflicting results from other seizure or memory lateralization tests, such as PET, SPECT, magnetoencephalography, neuropsychological testing, functional MR, or intracarotid amytal procedure.

Neoplasms and vascular malformations

Most tumors associated with chronic recurrent seizures tend to be relatively small, superficial, and well localized, making them suitable for resection, unless located in critical regions of cerebral cortex (Bronen et al. 1995a). Routine MRI has nearly 100% sensitivity for detecting epileptogenic neoplastic and vascular lesions (Bronen et al. 1995a). Most epileptogenic neoplasms occur in the temporal lobe, in or adjacent to the cerebral cortex. Mass effect is not observed in greater than one third of neoplasms associated with epilepsy. Resection of the tumor with or without amygdalo-hippocampectomy provides a high rate of seizure-free outcome (Adachi et al. 2008; Aronica et al. 2001; Burneo et al. 2008; Cataltepe et al. 2005; Giulioni et al. 2005,2006; Jooma et al. 1995; Khajavi et al. 1995; Minkin et al. 2008; Nolan et al. 2004; Radhakrishnan et al. 2006; Urbach et al. 2008). In intractable tumor-related epilepsy in children and young adults, low-grade indolent neoplasms such as DNET (Fig.2.14), ganglioglioma (Fig. 2.15), and low-grade gliomas are most commonly encountered (Adachi et al. 2008; Aronica et al. 2001; Burneo et al. 2008; Cataltepe et al. 2005; Giulioni et al. 2005,2006; Jooma et al. 1995; Khajavi et al. 1995; Minkin et al. 2008; Nolan et al. 2004; Radhakrishnan et al. 2006; Urbach et al. 2008). In the elderly population, cerebral metastasis is the most frequent neoplastic lesion associated with new-onset seizures (Bronen et al. 1995a).

Seizures are the chief clinical presentation of intracranial vascular malformations, occurring in 24% to 69% of arteriovenous malformations (Forster et al. 1972; Ondra et al. 1990) and 34% to 51% of cavernous

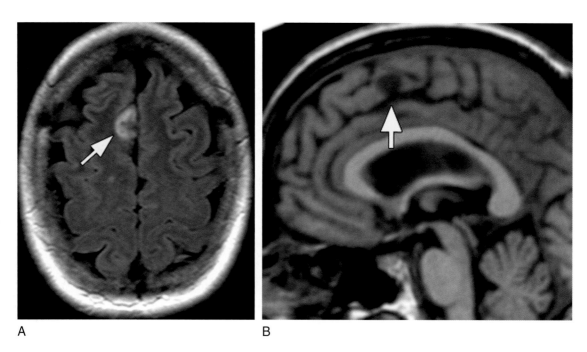

A   B

Figure 2.14 DNET. (A[1]) Axial FLAIR and (B) sagittal reformatted volumetric SPGR, showing well-demarcated intracortical lesion (*arrow*) in the right superior medial frontal region.

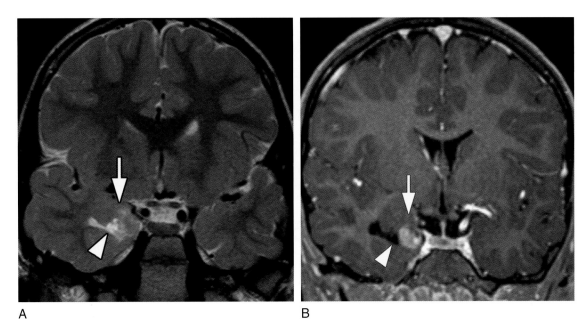

A   B

Figure 2.15 Ganglioglioma: medial temporal lesion with cystic (*arrowhead*) and solidly enhancing (*arrow*) components. (A) Coronal T2-weighted FSE. (B) Coronal gadolinium-enhanced T1-weighted image. (Images courtesy of Dr. Carlos Bazan, University of Texas Health Science Center, San Antonio, TX)

hemangiomas (Fig. 2.16) (also referred to as cavernous angiomas or cavernous malformations) (Kapacki et al. 1990; Requena et al. 1991; Topper et al. 1999). However, the vast majority of capillary telangiectasias and venous angiomas are clinically silent and incidental in epilepsy subjects, although the association of venous malformations with cavernous angioma is well known (Jackson et al. 1994).

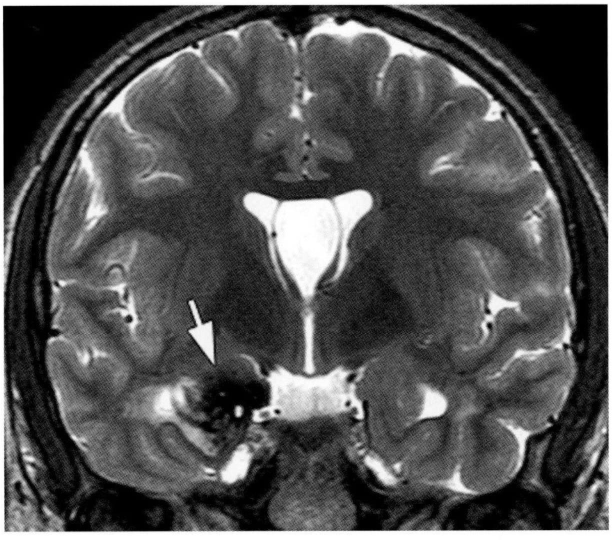

For tumors and vascular lesions located in or near eloquent cortex, fMRI and DTI techniques provide useful information regarding functionally eloquent cortical regions and important white matter tracts for surgical planning and navigation as described earlier. For critically located lesions, this information may be crucial for resectability.

Developmental abnormalities

Developmental disorders of cortex constitute 4% to 25% of all epileptogenic lesions in adults and 10% to 50% in pediatric epilepsy series (Brodtkorb et al. 1992; Jackson et al. 1994; Kuzniecky et al. 1996; Raymond et al. 1995; Wyllie et al. 1998). These abnormalities are highly epileptogenic, and the resulting partial epilepsy is usually refractory. These lesions are described in detail in the following chapter and will not be considered further here with the exception of hypothalamic hamartoma.

Hypothalamic hamartomas are categorized into two types, intrahypothalamic and parahypothalamic (Arita et al. 1999). The intrahypothalamic variety lies within the hypothalamus, deforming the third ventricle, and carries intrinsic epileptogenicity (Kuzniecky et al. 1997a). These lesions may present with both intractable seizures and precocious puberty (Arita et al. 1999). The parahypothalamic hamartoma, found either in the floor of third ventricle or tuber cinereum, may present with precocious puberty but not seizures.

Figure 2.16 [2]Medial temporal cavernoma. Coronal FSE T2 showing marked hypointensity of right amygdala, hippocampal head, and parahippocampal gyrus (arrow) due to siderosis.

Gliosis and miscellaneous abnormalities

Cortical gliosis can result from a variety of inflammatory, posttraumatic, and cerebrovascular brain insults. Irrespective of the etiology, gliosis usually appears as a region of increased signal change on T2-weighted images and decreased signal on T1-weighted images, often associated with focal volume loss. Resective surgery is usually not as successful for neocortical gliosis as it is for HS.

Traumatic brain injury accounts for 20% of symptomatic epilepsy cases in the general population and 5% of all epilepsy cases (Angeleri et al. 1999; Asikainen et al. 1999; Englander et al. 2003; Kobayashi et al. 1997; Temkin et al. 2003; Wang et al. 2008). Late-onset or delayed *posttraumatic seizures* are defined as seizures occurring 1 week after the initial trauma. Although early posttraumatic seizures have a favorable prognosis, as many as 25% of patients with late-onset seizures develop intractable drug-resistant epilepsy. Antiepileptic drugs are usually only effective in preventing early posttraumatic seizures. No beneficial effect of antiepileptic drugs has been demonstrated for patients with late posttraumatic seizures, and phenytoin may have negative cognitive effects in this population. The pathologic mechanisms for late-onset posttraumatic epilepsy include deposition of tissue hemosiderin, which is a potent epileptogenic agent, and cortical gliosis (Willmore et al. 1990, 1993). Risk factors for posttraumatic seizures include posttraumatic amnesia lasting more than 24 hours, intracranial hemorrhage, penetrating brain trauma, depressed skull fractures, and residual intracerebral foreign bodies (Asikainen et al. 1999; Jennett et al. 1960). The surgical evaluation of posttraumatic epilepsy is made challenging by the frequent multifocality of traumatic abnormalities, making determination of the epileptogenic lesion difficult, multifocality of epileptogenesis, and lack of concordance between imaging abnormalities and epileptogenic zone. FLAIR is highly sensitive for detection of subtle particularly superficial gliosis and should be routine in MR imaging of posttraumatic epilepsy. Susceptibility-weighted imaging is very sensitive in detecting focal parenchymal siderosis and should also be included in the MR protocol.

Beyond age 50 years, stroke is the most common cause of seizures (Luhdorf et al. 1986). Similar to posttraumatic epilepsy, delayed-onset seizures after an acute stroke carry a higher risk of developing into chronic epilepsy (Fish et al. 1989; Hauser et al. 1981; Kilpatrick et al. 1990; Kotila et al. 1992). The pathologic mechanism is possibly similar to that of posttraumatic epileptogenesis (Kilpatrick et al. 1990; Kotila et al. 1992).

Central nervous system infections, including viral, bacterial, mycobacterial, and fungal, and helminthic lesions may present with seizures, most of which occur in the acute phase of illness. Chronic epilepsy, however, may result from post-inflammatory glial scarring. In certain developing regions of the world, neurocysticercosis is one of the most common causes of new-onset partial seizures. Inflammation surrounding the cerebral lesions of cysticercosis manifests as acute seizure disorder. In the inflammatory stage provoked by the dying parasite, the cerebral lesions of cysticercosis appear as small enhancing rings on CT and MR with a variable degree of edema in the surrounding brain (Zee et al. 2000). The lesions usually spontaneously resolve and often calcify upon healing.

Widespread cortical gliosis and atrophy, typified by entities such as infantile hemiplegia, Sturge-Weber syndrome, or end-stage Rasmussen encephalitis, is easily appreciated both on MR and CT. Rasmussen encephalitis syndrome is clinically characterized by intractable partial seizures, progressive hemiplegia, and cognitive decline (Rasmussen et al. 1958, 1978). This rare syndrome results from chronic, unilateral, immune-mediated cortical inflammation with progressive cortical atrophy and gliosis. It typically presents in children under the age of 15 with epilepsia partialis continua. MR findings in early stages include high-intensity cortical foci extending into subcortical white matter on FLAIR and T2-weighted sequences (Fig 2.17). Lobar or hemispheric atrophy is seen in end-stage disease (Geller et al. 1998; Tien et al. 1992). Antiepileptic drugs are usually not effective in seizure control or in halting progression of cerebral atrophy. Resective epilepsy surgery in the form of lobectomy or

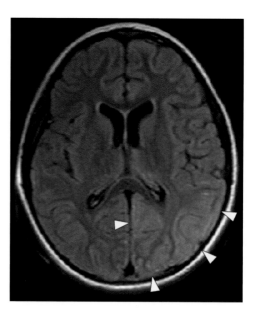

Figure 2.17 Rasmussen encephalitis, axial FLAIR: cortical swelling and increased signal (*arrowheads*), typical in early stages of the disease.

hemispherectomy is typically considered (Terra-Bustamante et al. 2009; Topçu et al. 1999; Tubbs et al. 2005). This condition is also discussed in Chapter 10.

Recurrent seizures are the most common and clinically important symptom of *Sturge-Weber syndrome,* also known as encephalotrigeminal angiomatosis (Kotagal et al. 1993). This syndrome consists of a facial port-wine nevus in the trigeminal nerve distribution, leptomeningeal angiomatosis, epilepsy, mental retardation, and other neurologic deficits. The brain involvement is typically unilateral, although a bilateral form is also known (Yeakley et al. 1992). Characteristic tramtrack gyriform calcification is seen on CT (Fig. 2.18), appearing as linear low signal on MR. The involved hemisphere is atrophic, often with overlying calvarial thickening. Early onset of epilepsy (less than 1 year of age) is associated with worse seizure control and neurologic outcome. Hemispherectomy is very effective for the control of seizures (Bourgeois et al. 2007; Kossoff et al. 2002) (see also Chapter 10).

Postoperative findings

Postoperative imaging is typically performed to assess the extent of resection and postoperative complications. Complete resection of lesions, and somewhat equivocally adequate resection of mesial temporal lobe, are predictors of successful seizure outcome (Abosch et al. 2002; Hader et al. 2004; Krsek et al.

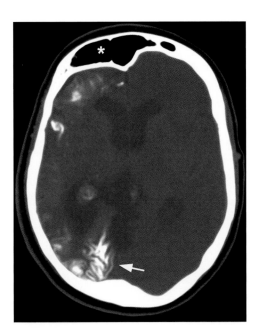

Figure 2.18 Sturge-Weber syndrome. Axial noncontrast CT. Characteristic unilateral tramtrack cortical calcification (*arrow*), right hemispheric atrophy and compensatory enlargement of right frontal sinus (*).

2009; Schramm et al. 2008; Van Rijckevorsel et al. 2005; Wyler et al. 1995). Awareness of the typical normal postoperative signal changes and contrast enhancement after lesionectomy and anterior temporal lobectomy is important to avoid misinterpretation of benign changes (Dietrich et al. 1991; Harris et al. 1989; Laohaprasit et al. 1990; Saluja et al. 2000; Sato et al. 1997). In the first postoperative week, thin linear enhancement is observed at the resection margin, which may subsequently become thick or nodular, and should not be interpreted as pathologic. An extra-axial fluid collection may be seen after temporal lobectomy, lasting 1 to 2 months. During the first postoperative week, enlargement and intense enhancement of the ipsilateral choroid plexus occurs normally and may also mimic tumor (Saluja et al. 2000). Punctate hyperintense foci on T2-weighted images have been reported in the tracts of the intraparenchymal depth electrodes (Merriam et al. 1993).

SUCCESSFUL INTERPRETATION: NORMAL VARIATIONS, INCIDENTAL FINDINGS, AND PITFALLS

MR imaging of epilepsy is usually more challenging than routine brain imaging, as the epileptogenic abnormalities are often subtle and incidental abnormalities are more often detected due to high-resolution imaging and greater variety of sequences in the MR protocols. Lesions often manifest as subtle asymmetry of brain structure, and normal anatomical variations and asymmetries can mimic pathology.

An important normal variant that occurs in 10% to 15% of normal hippocampi, known as the hippocampal sulcus remnant, should be distinguished from tumor and HS (Sasaki et al. 1993). It results from failure of normal involution of the embryonic hippocampal sulcus and appears as a tiny round or ovoid CSF intensity cyst between the dentate gyrus and cornu ammonis (Fig. 2.19) (Bronen et al. 1991a; Sasaki et al. 1993). The uncal recess, the anterior end of the temporal horn, is asymmetric in about half of routine MR scans and can be misinterpreted as local atrophy (Fig. 2.6A). Venous angioma, arachnoid cysts, and choroid fissure cysts (Fig. 2.20) are often incidentally found in patients with seizure disorders and bear no relationship to seizures. Rarely, venous anomalies are associated with other potentially epileptogenic abnormalities, such as cavernous angioma and malformations of cortical development such as polymicrogyria. Arachnoid and choroidal fissure cysts remain isointense to CSF on all MR sequences and demonstrate no contrast enhancement. Perivascular (Virchow-Robin) spaces are more frequently observed in epilepsy imaging because the thin-slice, higher-resolution imaging

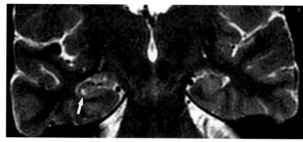

A

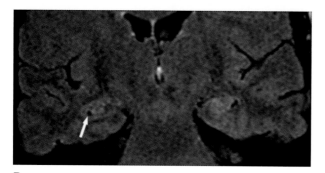

B

Figure 2.19 (A) Coronal T2-weighted FSE and (B) coronal FLAIR showing postictal swelling of left hippocampus resulting from prolonged seizure. Incidental right hippocampal sulcus remnant appears as CSF signal structure between cornu ammonis and dentate gyrus (*arrows*).

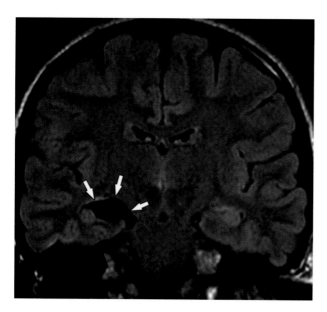

Figure 2.20 Choroid fissure cyst. Coronal FLAIR image: CSF signal cyst expands the right choroid fissure (*arrows*) and compresses the hippocampus. Note lack of signal change in right hippocampus, which remains isointense to its left counterpart, thus allowing distinction from HS.

sequences provide better anatomical detail and reduce volume averaging (Song et al. 2000). Dilated feather-like subcortical Virchow-Robin spaces between the extreme and external capsules can mimic lesion on

T2-weighted FSE sequences (Song et al. 2000). FLAIR usually confirms their CSF composition by suppressing the signal.

Artifactual hippocampal size asymmetry can easily be caused by head rotation as the hippocampus is largest anteriorly, tapering progressively on posterior sections (Fig. 2.2A). Correct interpretation requires accurate head positioning (Fig. 2.2B) and accounting for any rotation. Normally somewhat brighter signal of the hippocampus on FLAIR (Fig. 2.8) can mislead the less experienced observer to a diagnosis of bilateral HS. Identification of intact internal hippocampal architecture on high-resolution coronal T1- and T2-weighted images (Figs. 2.2B, 2.6B) helps avoid this pitfall. The variable configuration of the hippocampus may also cause difficulties in interpretation. The hippocampus infrequently has a more vertical orientation (Fig. 2.21), erroneously suggesting hippocampal dysplasia.

Normal variations of gyral and sulcal morphology must be taken into account when assessing cortical malformations. The cortex bordering the superior temporal sulcus on the right is usually slightly thicker than that of the left hemisphere and can be easily misinterpreted as dysplasia. The normal folding of the cortex may cause apparent thickening if the gyrus is parallel and the cortex is oblique or tangential to the MR slice. Dysplasia should be entertained only when cortical thickening persists in the orthogonal planes. In the rolandic region, the gray–white matter junction is often indistinct. This appearance results from parallel, coronal orientation of the rolandic (central) sulcus and normally thinner cortex lining it. Therefore, careful examination of the axial or axial reformatted images should be routine when evaluating this region for dysplasia.

In addition to the normal variations, misinterpretation in epilepsy imaging could arise from transient abnormalities resulting from, and not causing, seizures

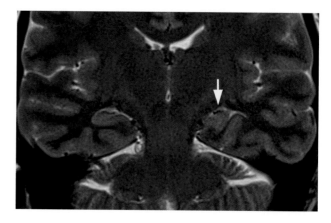

Figure 2.21 Normal variant of vertically oriented hippocampus on coronal T2-weighted FSE (*arrow*). Note otherwise normal morphology, volume, and signal of the hippocampus.

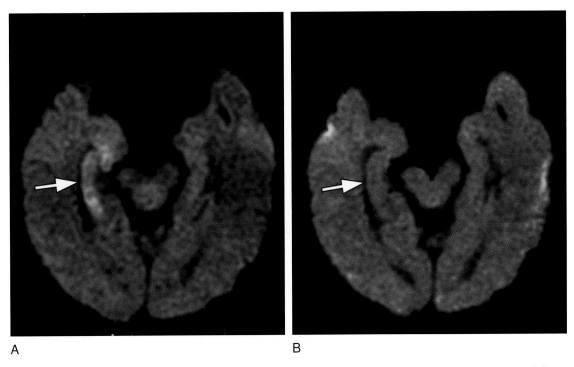

A   B

Figure 2.22 Transient postictal changes, axial diffusion-weighted image. (A) Right hippocampal hyperintensity (*arrow*) following status epilepticus. (B) Complete resolution one week later (*arrow*).

(Figs. 2.19, 2.22, 2.23). Acute, particularly prolonged and repetitive seizures can result in focal or regional signal changes in the cortex and hippocampus. The characteristic findings include hyperintensity on FLAIR (Figs. 2.19B and 2.23), T2-weighted (Fig. 2.19A), and diffusion-weighted images (Fig. 2.22), sometimes with abnormal focal contrast enhancement involving the cortex and hippocampus (Chan et al. 1996; Horowitz et al. 1992; Jayakumar et al. 1985; Kramer et al. 1987; Meierkord et al. 1997; Riela et al. 1991). Hippocampal enlargement and increased signal during the acute phase may be followed by atrophy on subsequent scans (Tien et al. 1995; VanLandingham et al. 1998). Therefore, a history check for recent seizure activity should be performed in cases of cortical or hippocampal swelling and signal alteration. Due caution must be exercised in MR interpretation, as hippocampal swelling more frequently results from immediate postictal changes than neoplasms, and may occasionally be encountered in truly sclerotic hippocampus following status epilepticus. Rarely, when the abnormal hippocampal signal is not accompanied by atrophy, findings favoring neoplasm over sclerosis include heterogeneity and extension of signal changes beyond the hippocampus into the parahippocampal white matter. In Rasmussen encephalitis, signal changes may not only be transient, but also shift from one location to another. Differentiating neoplasms from focal cortical dysplasia is occasionally difficult.

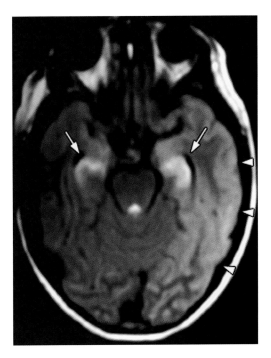

Figure 2.23 Bilateral hippocampal (*arrows*) and left temporal cortical (*arrowheads*) postictal signal changes on axial FLAIR image.

Findings suggestive of cortical dysplasia (particularly the Taylor type) include cortical thickening, presence of a radial band extending to the ventricle, and homogeneous appearance of the subcortical hyperintensity

(Fig. 2.24). The presence of multiple subcortical lesions should raise the possibility of tuberous sclerosis, and a search for subependymal nodules should be carried out (Fig. 2.25). Finally, HS is not infrequent in cases of developmental cortical anomalies (Fig. 2.13) and periventricular heterotopia.

MAGNETIC RESONANCE SPECTROSCOPY (MRS)

The topic of MRS as applied in epilepsy is discussed in detail in Chapter 4. At the risk of some redundancy, a brief technical account will be presented here. Most studies have evaluated proton MRS in epilepsy because of the widespread availability of this technique, although phosphorus MRS has also been found useful in providing insight into the metabolic alterations (Kuzniecky et al. 1999). Two MRS techniques are generally used. Single-voxel spectroscopy acquiring a single spectrum has been predominantly targeted at the hippocampal regions and the comparison of metabolite concentrations in ipsi- and contralateral hippocampus by using the coefficient of asymmetry (Connelly et al. 1998; Garcia et al. 1995; Kuzniecky et al. 1998; Woermann et al. 1999). In extratemporal epilepsies, the epileptogenic zone is frequently larger and more difficult to delineate in comparison with TLE. This makes voxel positioning difficult, and studies on the use of single-voxel proton MRS in extratemporal epilepsy have, therefore, been limited. Multivoxel MRS, also called chemical shift imaging or MR spectroscopic imaging, collects spectroscopic data from a large volume of interest in a single measurement and enables the creation of two- or three-dimensional maps of metabolites. The advent of chemical shift imaging has enabled use of MR spectroscopic imaging in localization of the epileptogenic zone outside of the temporal lobes. In both techniques, NAA has been the most commonly studied metabolite. NAA appears to be a dynamic marker of epileptic activity and not simply a reflector of neuronal number. Reduction in NAA:creatine or decreased NAA:(creatine + choline) ratios, signifying neuronal loss and/or metabolic dysfunction, has been shown to lateralize TLE in 65% to 96% of patients with bilateral temporal lobe structural abnormalities on MRI (Garcia et al. 1995; Kuzniecky et al. 1999).

In nonlesional epilepsy, MRS can potentially detect metabolic changes corresponding to the epileptogenic zone. In cases of TLE with normal MRI, NAA ratios can lateralize the seizure focus in 20% of patients (Connelly et al. 1998; Woermann et al. 1999). Few reports have described MRS abnormalities in patients with frontal or parietal lobe epilepsy, with or without MRI-detected lesions (Kuzniecky et al. 1997b; Simone

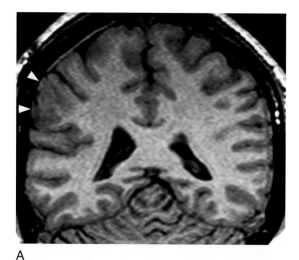

A

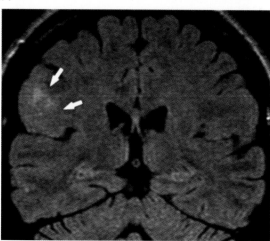

B

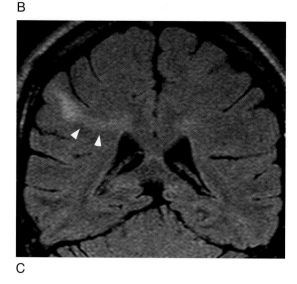

C

Figure 2.24 Balloon-cell focal cortical dysplasia, Taylor type II. (A) Gyral enlargement with thickened cortex (*arrowheads*) on coronal T1-weighted GRE. On coronal FLAIR (B and C), homogeneous increased cortical and subcortical signal (B, *arrows*) and radiating band of hyperintensity towards the ventricle (C, *arrowheads*). The radiating band helps differentiate type II focal cortical dysplasia from low-grade glioma.

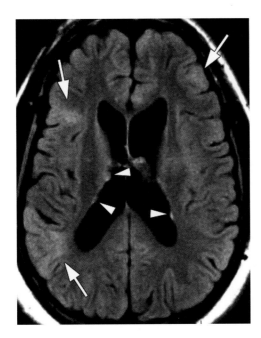

Figure 2.25 Tuberous sclerosis, axial FLAIR. Multiple tubers are indicated by regions of increased cortical and subcortical increased signal (*arrows*), which individually appear identical to Taylor-type focal cortical dysplasia. Note subependymal nodules (*arrowheads*) characteristic of tuberous sclerosis.

et al. 1999; Stanley et al. 1998; Widjaja et al. 2003; Woermann et al. 2001). Widespread hemispheric alterations in metabolite concentrations have usually been seen in these studies. Proton MRS, thus, may help in the hemispheric lateralization of extratemporal epilepsy. However, it is unclear whether it is truly useful in the localization of the epileptogenic zone. There are few data evaluating the relationship of proton MRS abnormalities with the epileptogenic zone as identified by intracranial monitoring and histopathologic changes in resected brain tissue in nonlesional epilepsy.

Proton MRS has also been used to estimate concentrations of neurotransmitters, including gamma amino-butyric acid, glutamate, and glutamine, using spectral editing techniques (Novotny et al. 1999; Petroff et al. 1996a,b; Rothman et al. 1992a,b, 1993). This approach holds promise for characterizing neurochemical derangements associated with epilepsy and monitoring pharmacokinetics of antiepileptic drugs. This application is discussed in greater depth in Chapter 4.

DIFFUSION MR IN EPILEPSY

Chapter 6 is fully dedicated to diffusion-weighted MR and DTI as applied to the evaluation of epilepsy.

Diffusion anisotropy in tissues has been investigated with DTI (Arfanakis et al. 2002; Assaf et al. 2003; Chen et al. 2008; Eriksson et al. 2001; Gross et al. 2005; Kimiwada et al. 2006; Lee et al. 2006; Rugg-Gunn et al. 2001; Thivard et al. 2005) and is beginning to play an increasingly important role in both clinical and research investigations of epilepsy. For example, DTI in malformations of cortical development has demonstrated reduced fractional anisotropy and increased mean diffusivity in the white matter adjacent to the malformation visible on MRI. Hence, regional alteration of these parameters in white matter may help draw attention to otherwise unappreciated malformations of cortical development. DTI has been useful in assessing the integrity of the white matter adjacent to cortical dysplasias. The disorganization of the underlying white matter tracts can be detected with DTI fiber tractography (Fig. 2.26) (Lee et al. 2005; Widjaja et al. 2007). In addition, areas of increased diffusivity and reduced FA have also been detected beyond the margins of malformations of cortical development visible on MR imaging (Eriksson et al. 2001). This finding may explain, at least partly, the poorer surgical outcome in this group of disorders.

DTI fiber-tracking has been used to map the major motor and sensory tracts in surgical planning of both lesional and nonlesional epilepsy. In temporal lobe resections, preoperative mapping of Meyer's loop can help minimize postoperative visual field defects (Taoka et al. 2008; Yogarajah et al. 2009). Similarly, asymmetry of the arcuate fasciculus on DTI could be of value in lateralizing language dominance (Matsumoto et al. 2008). DTI has revealed reduced fractional anisotropy values in uncinate fasciculus ipsilateral to HS, suggesting a role of this pathway in spread of TLE (Rodrigo et al. 2007; Takahashi et al. 2007) (see Chapter 6 for a more comprehensive discussion of DTI).

MRI POST-PROCESSING TECHNIQUES FOR ENHANCED DETECTION OF EPILEPTOGENIC PATHOLOGY

Attempts to improve detection of epileptogenic abnormalities by MRI are not limited to scanner hardware and image acquisition techniques. Several MR image post-processing methods have been developed to facilitate lesion detection. These include curvilinear reformatting quantification of regional distribution of gray and white matter, statistical parametric mapping, quantification of thickness of cerebral cortex, and texture or morphometric analysis (Antel et al. 2003; Bastos et al. 1995; Bernasconi et al. 2001, 2003; Besson et al. 2008; Colliot et al. 2006a,b; Huppertz et al. 2005, 2008; Kassubek et al. 2002; Montenegro et al. 2003). Detailed description of these techniques is beyond the

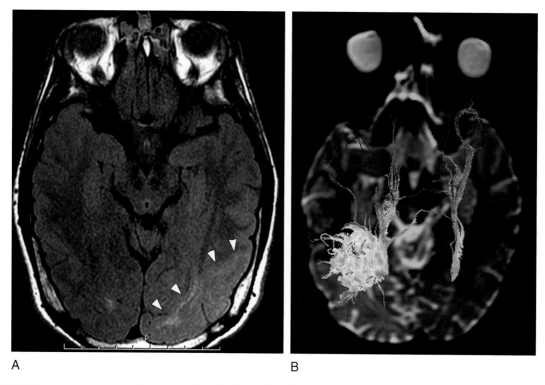

A   B

Figure 2.26 Diffusion tensor changes in focal cortical dysplasia. (A) Left temporo-occipital balloon-cell cortical dysplasia (*arrowheads*). (B) Absent normal arborization of tracts on diffusion tensor tractography in left temporo-occipital white matter due to markedly reduced fractional anisotropy. Compare with normal appearance of white matter tracts on the right side.

scope of this chapter, and only a general outline is presented here.

Focal cortical dysplasia is frequently undetected by visual inspection of conventional MRI due to its subtlety and the complexity of the cortical convolutions. Standard rectilinear slices are limited in addressing the complex convolutional pattern of the brain. Due to convexity of the brain surface, rectilinear slices allow only localized orthogonal sectioning of the gyri and create an apparent impression of cortical thickening when the plane of section is not perpendicular to the gyral orientation. Apparent blurring of the gray–white matter interface can result from volume averaging effects on rectilinear multiplanar reformatting. Curvilinear reformatting of three-dimensional MRI data parallel to the cerebral convexities addresses these limitations and improves the anatomical display of the gyri. It minimizes the asymmetric sampling of gray and white matter and reduces artifactual cortical thickening, which is inherent in rectilinear slicing of curved surfaces.

Voxel-based post-processing methods, such as texture analysis and morphological processing, are modeled on known MRI features of focal cortical dysplasia such as thickening of gray matter, hyperintense signal, and blurring of the gray–white interface (Bernasconi et al. 2003; Bernasconi N et al. 2004; Besson et al. 2008; Bonilha et al. 2006; Bruggemann

et al. 2007; Huppertz et al. 2005; Kassubek et al. 2003; Keller et al. 2004, 2008; Labate et al. 2008; Mueller et al. 2006; Pell et al. 2008). These methods allow automated generation of reproducible color- or brightness-coded 3D maps of cortical thickness, hyperintensity, and gray–white interface gradient. Voxel-based morphometry (VBM) is an automated technique to identify regional differences in the proportion of grey and white matter. VBM analysis involves spatial normalization, tissue segmentation, and spatial smoothing of 3D MR images. After the above spatial processing stages have been applied to MR images, voxel-wise statistical analyses can be undertaken to make inferences about differences in brain morphology between cohorts of subjects. This technique has been applied in the detection of not only cortical dysplasia but also HS, with variable success (Bernasconi et al. 2004; Keller et al. 2004, 2008; Labate et al. 2008; Mueller et al. 2006; Pell et al. 2008). The basic parameter of interest for detecting HS in patients with TLE include reduction in gray matter concentration or gray matter volume, whereas an increase or excess of these measures is used to detect focal cortical dysplasia. The VBM analysis in TLE associated with HS has shown reduced gray matter volume not only in the hippocampus but also in extrahippocampal regions (Bernasconi et al. 2004; Labate et al. 2008; Mueller et al. 2006; Pell et al. 2008).

REFERENCES

Abosch, A., N. Bernasconi, W. Boling, et al. 2002. Factors predictive of suboptimal seizure control following selective amygdalo hippocampectomy. *Journal of Neurosurgery* 97: 1142–51.

Adachi, Y., and A. Yagishita. 2008. Gangliogliomas: Characteristic imaging findings and role in the temporal lobe epilepsy. *Neuroradiology* 50(10): 829–34.

Alarcón, G. A. Valentín, C. Watt C, et al. 2006. Is it worth pursuing surgery for epilepsy in patients with normal neuroimaging? *Journal of Neurology Neurosurgery & Psychiatry* 77: 474–80.

Angeleri, F., J. Majkowski, G. Cacchiò, et al. 1999. Posttraumatic epilepsy risk factors: one-year prospective study after head injury. *Epilepsia* 40(9): 1222–30.

Antel, S. B., D. L. Collins, N. Bernasconi, et al. 2003. Automated detection of focal cortical dysplasia lesions using computational models of their MRI characteristics and texture analysis. *Neuroimage* 19(4): 1748–59.

Arfanakis, K., B. P. Hermann, B. P. Rogers, et al. 2002. Diffusion tensor MRI in temporal lobe epilepsy. *Magnetic Resonance Imaging* 20(7): 511–9.

Arita, K., F. Ikawa, K. Kurisu, et al. 1999. The relationship between magnetic resonance imaging findings and clinical manifestations of hypothalamic hamartoma. *Journal of Neurosurgery* 91: 212–20.

Aronica, E., S. Leenstra, C. W. van Veelen, et al. 2001. Glioneuronal tumors and medically intractable epilepsy: a clinical study with long-term follow-up of seizure outcome after surgery. *Epilepsy Research* 43(3): 179–91.

Ashtari, M., W. B. Barr, N. Schaul N, et al. 1991. Three-dimensional fast low-angle shot imaging and computerized volume measurement of the hippocampus in patients with chronic epilepsy of the temporal lobe. *AJNR American Journal of Neuroradiology* 12: 941–7.

Asikainen, I., M. Kaste, S. Sarna. 1999. Early and late post-traumatic seizures in traumatic brain injury rehabilitation patients: brain injury factors causing late seizures and influence of seizures on long-term outcome. *Epilepsia* 40: 584–9.

Assaf, B. A., F. B. Mohamed, K. J. Abou-Khaled, et al. 2003. Diffusion tensor imaging of the hippocampal formation in temporal lobe epilepsy. *AJNR American Journal of Neuroradiology* 24(9): 1857–62.

Baldwin, G. N., J. S. Tsuruda, K. R. Maravilla, et al. 1994. The fornix in patients with seizures caused by unilateral hippocampal sclerosis: detection of unilateral volume loss on MR images. *AJR American Journal of Roentgenology* 162: 1185–9.

Barker, P. B., D. O. Hearshen, and M. D. Boska. 2001. Single-voxel proton MRS of the human brain at 1.5 T and 3.0 T. *Magnetic Resonance in Medicine* 45: 765–9.

Bartha, R., D. J. Drost, R. S. Menon, et al. 2000. Comparison of the quantification precision of human short echo time (1)H spectroscopy at 1.5 and 4.0 tesla. *Magnetic Resonance in Medicine* 44: 185–92.

Bartlett, P. A., M. R. Symms, S. L. Free, et al. 2007. T2 relaxometry of the hippocampus at 3T. *AJNR American Journal of Neuroradiology* 28(6): 1095–8.

Bastos, A. C., I. P. Korah, F. Cendes, et al. 1995. Curvilinear reconstruction of 3D magnetic resonance imaging in patients with partial epilepsy: a pilot study. *Magnetic Resonance Imaging* 13(8): 1107–12.

Berg, A., F. M. Testa, S. R. Levy, et al. 2000. Neuroimaging in children with newly diagnosed epilepsy: a community-based study. *Pediatrics* 106: 527–32.

Berg, A. T., J. Langfitt, S. Shinnar, et al. 2003. How long does it take for partial epilepsy to become intractable? *Neurology* 60: 186–90.

Berkovic, S. F., A. M. McIntosh, R. M. Kalnins, et al. 1995. Preoperative MRI predicts outcome of temporal lobectomy: an actuarial analysis. *Neurology* 45: 1358–63.

Bernasconi, A., S. B. Antel, D. L. Collins, et al. 2001. Texture analysis and morphological processing of magnetic resonance imaging assist detection of focal cortical dysplasia in extra-temporal partial epilepsy. *Annals of Neurology* 49(6): 770–5.

Bernasconi, A. 2003. Advanced MRI analysis methods for detection of focal cortical dysplasia. *Epileptic Disorders* 5 (Suppl 2): S81–4.

Bernasconi, N., S. Duchesne, A. Janke, et al. 2004. Whole-brain voxel-based statistical analysis of gray matter and white matter in temporal lobe epilepsy. *Neuroimage* 23(2): 717–23.

Besson, P, N. Bernasconi, O. Colliot, et al. 2008. Surface-based texture and morphological analysis detects subtle cortical dysplasia. *Med Image Comput Comput Assist Interv Int Conf Med Image Comput Comput Assist Interv* 11(Pt 1): 645–52.

Bonilha, L., M. A. Montenegro, C. Rorden, et al. 2006. Voxel-based morphometry reveals excess gray matter concentration in patients with focal cortical dysplasia. *Epilepsia* 47(5): 908–15.

Bourgeois, M., D. W. Crimmins, R. S. de Oliveira, et al. 2007. Surgical treatment of epilepsy in Sturge–Weber syndrome in children. *Journal of Neurosurgery* 106: 20–8.

Braun, V., S. Dempf, R. Tomczak, et al. 2001. Multimodal cranial neuronavigation: direct integration of functional magnetic resonance imaging and positron emission tomography data: technical note. *Neurosurgery* 48: 1178–82.

Brodtkorb, E., G. Nilsen, O. Smevik, et al. 1992. Epilepsy and anomalies of neuronal migration: MRI and clinical aspects. *Acta Neurologica Scandinavica* 86: 24–32.

Bronen, R., A. Anderson, and D. Spencer. 1994. Quantitative MR for epilepsy: a clinical and research tool? *AJNR American Journal of Neuroradiology* 15: 1157–60.

Bronen, R. A., and G. Cheung. 1991a. MRI of the temporal lobe: normal variations with special reference toward epilepsy. *Magnetic Resonance Imaging* 9: 501–7.

Bronen, R. A., G. Cheung, J. T. Charles, et al. 1991b. Imaging findings in hippocampal sclerosis: correlation with pathology. *AJNR American Journal of Neuroradiology* 12: 933–940.

Bronen, R. A., R. K. Fulbright, D. D. Spencer, et al. 1995a. MR characteristics of neoplasms and vascular malformations associated with epilepsy. *Magnetic Resonance Imaging* 13: 1153–62.

Bronen, R. A., R. K. Fulbright, J. H. Kim, et al. 1995b. Regional distribution of MR findings in hippocampal sclerosis. *AJNR American Journal of Neuroradiology* 16: 1193–1200.

Bronen, R. A., R. K. Fulbright, D. D. Spencer, et al. 1996. Refractory epilepsy: comparison of MR imaging, CT, and histopathologic findings in 117 patients. *Radiology* 201: 97–105.

Bronen, R. A., R. K. Fulbright, J. H. Kim, et al. 1997a. A systematic approach for interpreting MR images of the seizure patient. *AJR American Journal of Roentgenology* 169: 241–7.

Bronen, R. A., R. F. Fulbright, D. King, et al. 1997b. Qualitative MR imaging of refractory temporal lobe epilepsy requiring surgery: correlation with pathology and seizure outcome after surgery. *AJR American Journal of Roentgenology* 169: 875–82.

Bronen, R. A., R. F. Fulbright, S. S. Spencer, et al. 1997c. Comparison of MR and CT imaging of refractory epilepsy: correlation with postoperative seizure outcome in 109 patients. *International Journal of Neuroradiology* 3: 140–6.

Bronen, R. A., R. F. Fulbright, S. S. Spencer, et al. 1997d. Economic impact of replacing CT with MR imaging for refractory epilepsy. *Magnetic Resonance Imaging* 15: 857–62.

Bronen, R. A. 1998. MR imaging of mesial temporal sclerosis: how much is enough? AJNR *American Journal of Neuroradiology* 19: 15–7.

Brooks, B. S., D. W. King, T. El Gammal, et al. 1990. MR imaging in patients with intractable complex partial epileptic seizures. *AJNR American Journal of Neuroradiology* 11: 93–9.

Brooks, M. L., M. J. O'Connor, M. R. Sperling, et al. 1992. Magnetic resonance imaging in localization of EEG depth electrodes for seizure monitoring. *Epilepsia* 33: 888–91.

Bruggemann, J. M., M. Wilke, S. S. Som, et al. 2007. Voxel-based morphometry in the detection of dysplasia and neoplasia in childhood epilepsy: combined grey/white matter analysis augments detection. *Epilepsy Research* 77(2-3): 93–101.

Burneo, J. G., J. Tellez-Zenteno, D. A. Steven, et al. 2008. Adult-onset epilepsy associated with dysembryoplastic neuroepithelial tumors. *Seizure* 17(6): 498–504.

Cascino, G. D., C. J. Jack, J. E. Parisi, et al. 1992. MRI in the presurgical evaluation of patients with frontal lobe epilepsy and children with temporal lobe epilepsy: pathologic correlation and prognostic importance. *Epilepsy Research* 11: 51–9.

Cataltepe, O., G. Turanli, D. Yalnizoglu, et al. 2005. Surgical management of temporal lobe tumor-related epilepsy in children. *Journal of Neurosurgery* 102(3 Suppl): 280–7.

Cendes, F., F. Andermann, P. Gloor, et al. 1993a. Atrophy of mesial structures in patients with temporal lobe epilepsy: cause or consequence of repeated seizures? *Annals of Neurology* 34: 795–801.

Cendes, F., F. Leproux, D. Melanson, et al. 1993b. MRI of amygdala and hippocampus in temporal lobe epilepsy. *Journal of Computer Assisted Tomography* 17: 206–10.

Cendes, F., M. J. Cook, C. Watson, et al. 1995. Frequency and characteristics of dual pathology in patients with lesional epilepsy. *Neurology* 45: 2058–64.

Chan, S., S. S. Chin, K. Kartha, et al. 1996. Reversible signal abnormalities in the hippocampus and neocortex after prolonged seizures. *AJNR American Journal of Neuroradiology* 17: 1725–31.

Chapman, K., E. Wyllie, I. Najm, et al. 2005. Seizure outcome after epilepsy surgery in patients with normal preoperative MRI. *Journal of Neurology, Neurosurgery, and Psychiatry* 76: 710–713.

Chen, Q., S. Lui, C. X. Li, et al. 2008. MRI-negative refractory partial epilepsy: role for diffusion tensor imaging in high field MRI. *Epilepsy Research* 80(1): 83–9.

Cohen-Gadol, A. A., C. C. Bradley, A. Williamson, et al. 2005. Normal magnetic resonance imaging and medial temporal lobe epilepsy: the clinical syndrome of paradoxical temporal lobe epilepsy. *Journal of Neurosurgery* 102: 902–9.

Colliot, O., S. B. Antel, V. B. Naessens, et al. 2006a. In vivo profiling of focal cortical dysplasia on high-resolution MRI with computational models. *Epilepsia* 47(1): 134–42.

Colliot, O., N. Bernasconi, N. Khalili, et al. 2006b. Individual voxel-based analysis of gray matter in focal cortical dysplasia. *Neuroimage* 29(1): 162–71.

Commission on Classification and Terminology of the International League Against Epilepsy. 1981. Proposal for revised clinical and electroencephalographic classification of epileptic seizures. *Epilepsia* 22: 489–501.

Commission on Neuroimaging of the International League Against Epilepsy. 1989. Guidelines for neuroimaging evaluation of patients with uncontrolled epilepsy considered for surgery. *Epilepsia* 39: 1375–6.

Connelly, A., W. Vanpaesschen, D. A. Porter, et al. 1998. Proton magnetic resonance spectroscopy in MRI-negative temporal lobe epilepsy. *Neurology* 51: 61–6.

Cook, M. J., D. R. Fish, S. D. Shorvon, et al. 1992. Hippocampal volumetric and morphometric studies in frontal and temporal lobe epilepsy. *Brain* 115: 1001–15.

Cook, M. J. 1994. Mesial temporal sclerosis and volumetric investigations. *Acta Neurologica Scandinavica Supplementum* 152: 109–14.

Daumas-Duport, C., B. W. Scheithauer, J. P. Chodkiewicz, et al. 1988. Dysembryoplastic neuroepithelial tumour: a surgically curable tumour of young patients with intractable partial seizures. *Neurosurgery* 23: 545–56.

Davis, L. M., D. D. Spencer, S. S. Spencer, et al. 1999. MR imaging of implanted depth and subdural electrodes: is it safe? *Epilepsy Research* 35: 95–8.

Dietrich, R. B., S. el Saden, H. T. Chugani, et al. 1991. Resective surgery for intractable epilepsy in children: radiologic evaluation. *AJNR American Journal of Neuroradiology* 12: 1149–58.

Duncan, J. S. 1997. Imaging and epilepsy. *Brain* 120: 339–77.

Edwards, J. C., E. Wyllie, P. M. Ruggoieri, et al. 2000. Seizure outcome after surgery due to malformation of cortical development. *Neurology* 55: 1110–4.

Englander, J., T. Bushnik, T. T. Duong, et al. 2003. Analyzing risk factors for late posttraumatic seizures: a prospective, multicenter investigation. *Archives of Physical Medicine & Rehabilitation* 84(3): 365–73.

Eriksson, S. H., F. J. Rugg-Gunn, et al. 2001. Diffusion tensor imaging in patients with epilepsy and malformations of cortical development. *Brain* 124(Pt 3): 617–26.

Eriksson, S. H., M. Thom, P. A. Bartlett, et al. 2008. PROPELLER MRI visualizes detailed pathology of hippocampal sclerosis. *Epilepsia* 49: 33–9.

Fatterpekar, G. M., T. P. Naidich, B. N. Delman, et al. 2002. Cytoarchitecture of the human cerebral cortex: MR microscopy of excised specimens at 9.4 Tesla. *AJNR American Journal of Neuroradiology* 23: 1313–21.

Fish, D. R., D. H. Miller, R. C. Roberts, et al. 1989. The natural history of late-onset epilepsy secondary to vascular disease. *Acta Neurologica Scandinavica* 80: 524–6.

Forbes, K. P., J. G. Pipe, C. R. Bird, et al. 2001. PROPELLER MRI: clinical testing of a novel technique for quantification and compensation of head motion. *Journal of Magnetic Resonance Imaging* 14(3): 215–22.

Forster, D., L. Steiner, S. Hakanson. 1972. Arteriovenous malformations of the brain. A long-term clinical study. *Journal of Neurosurgery* 37: 562–70.

Francione, S., P. Vigliano, L. Tassi, et al. 2003. Surgery for drug-resistant partial epilepsy in children with focal cortical dysplasia: anatomical–clinical correlations and neurophysiological data in 10 patients. *Journal of Neurology, Neurosurgery and Psychiatry* 74: 1493–1501.

Garcia, P. A., K. D. Laxer, N. M. Barbaro, et al. 1994. Prognostic value of qualitative magnetic resonance imaging hippocampal abnormalities in patients undergoing temporal lobectomy for medically refractory seizures. *Epilepsia* 35: 520–4.

Garcia, P. A., K. D. Laxer, and T. Ng. 1995. Application of spectroscopic imaging in epilepsy. *Magnetic Resonance Imaging* 13: 1181–5.

Geller, E., E. Faerber, A. Legido, et al. 1998. Rasmussen encephalitis: complementary role of multitechnique neuroimaging. *AJNR American Journal of Neuroradiology* 9: 445–9.

Giulioni, M., E. Galassi, M. Zucchelli, et al. 2005. Seizure outcome of lesionectomy in glioneuronal tumors associated with epilepsy in children. *Journal of Neurosurgery* 102(3 Suppl): 288–93.

Giulioni, M., E. Gardella, G. Rubboli, et al. 2006. Lesionectomy in epileptogenic gangliogliomas: seizure outcome and surgical results. *Journal of Clinical Neuroscience* 13(5): 529–35.

Goyal, M., B. A. Bangert, J. S. Lewin, et al. 2004. High-resolution MRI enhances identification of lesions amenable to surgical therapy in children with intractable epilepsy. *Epilepsia* 45(8): 954–9.

Grant, P. E., A. J. Barkovich, L. L. Wald, et al. 1997. High-resolution surface-coil MR of cortical lesions in medically refractory epilepsy: a prospective study. *AJNR American Journal of Neuroradiology* 18(2): 291–301.

Grattan, S. J., A. S. Harvey, P. M. Desmond, et al. 1993. Hippocampal sclerosis in children with intractable temporal lobe epilepsy: detection with MR imaging. *AJR American Journal of Roentgenology* 161: 1045–8.

Greenberg, M. K., Barsan, W. G., and S. Starkman. 1996. Neuroimaging in the emergency patient presenting with seizure. *Neurology* 47: 26–32.

Gross, D. W., A. Bastos, and C. Beaulieu. 2005. Diffusion tensor imaging abnormalities in focal cortical dysplasia. *Canadian Journal of Neurologic Science* 32(4): 477–82.

Hader, W. J., M. Mackay, H. Otsubo, et al. 2004. Cortical dysplastic lesions in children with intractable epilepsy: role of complete resection. *Journal of Neurosurgery (Pediatrics 2)* 100: 110–7.

Harris, R. D., D. W. Roberts, and L. D. Cromwell. 1989. MR imaging of corpus callosotomy. *AJNR American Journal of Neuroradiology* 10: 677–80.

Hauser, W. A., and J. F. AnnegersF. 1991. Risk factors for epilepsy [Review]. *Epilepsy Research Supplement* 4: 45–52.

Hirai, T., Y. Korogi, K. Yoshizumi, et al. 2000. Limbic lobe of the human brain: evaluation with turbo fluid-attenuated inversion-recovery MR imaging. *Radiology* 215: 470–5.

Hirtz, D., S. Ashwal, A. Berg, et al. 2000. Practice parameter: evaluating a first nonfebrile seizure in children. Report of the quality standards subcommittee of the American Academy of Neurology, the Child Neurology Society, and the American Epilepsy Society. *Neurology* 55: 616–23.

Holmes, M. D., D. E. Born, R. L. Kutsy, et al. 2000. Outcome after surgery in patients with refractory temporal lobe epilepsy and normal MRI. *Seizure* 9: 407–11.

Horowitz, S. W., M. Merchut, M. Fine, et al. 1992. Complex partial seizure-induced transient MR enhancement. *Journal of Computer Assisted Tomography* 16: 814–6.

Huppertz, H. J., C. Grimm, S. Fauser, et al. 2005. Enhanced visualization of blurred gray-white matter junctions in focal cortical dysplasia by voxel-based 3D MRI analysis. *Epilepsy Research* 67(1-2): 35–50.

Huppertz, H. J., J. Kassubek, D. M. Altenmüller, et al. 2008. Automatic curvilinear reformatting of three-dimensional MRI data of the cerebral cortex. *Neuroimage* 39(1): 80–6.

Iwasaki, M., N. Nakasato, H. Suzuki, et al. 2009. Endfolium sclerosis in temporal lobe epilepsy diagnosed preoperatively by 3-tesla magnetic resonance imaging. *Journal of Neurosurgery* 110: 1124–6.

Jack, C. J., F. W. Sharbrough, C. K. Twomey, et al. 1990. Temporal lobe seizures: lateralization with MR volume measurements of the hippocampal formation. *Radiology* 175: 423–9.

Jack, C. J., F. W. Sharbrough, G. D. Cascino, et al. 1992. Magnetic resonance image-based hippocampal volumetry: correlation with outcome after temporal lobectomy. *Annals of Neurology* 31: 138–46.

Jack, C. J. 1994a. MRI-based hippocampal volume measurements in epilepsy. *Epilepsia* 35(Suppl 6): S21–9.

Jack, C. J., K. N. Krecke, P. H. Luetmer, et al. 1994b. Diagnosis of mesial temporal sclerosis with conventional versus fast spin-echo MR imaging. *Radiology* 192: 123–7.

Jack, C. R. 1993. Epilepsy: surgery and imaging. *Radiology* 189: 635–46.

Jack, C. R. Jr, C. H. Rydberg, K. N. Krecke, et al. 1996. Mesial temporal sclerosis: diagnosis with fluid-attenuated inversion-recovery versus spin-echo MR imaging. *Radiology* 199: 367–73.

Jackson, G. D., S. F. Berkovic, B. M. Tress, et al. 1990. Hippocampal sclerosis can be reliably detected by magnetic resonance imaging. *Neurology* 40: 1869–75.

Jackson, G. D., S. F. Berkovic, J. S. Duncan, et al. 1993a. Optimizing the diagnosis of hippocampal sclerosis using MR imaging. *AJNR American Journal of Neuroradiology* 14: 753–62.

Jackson, G. D., A. Connelly, J. S. Duncan, et al. 1993b. Detection of hippocampal pathology in intractable partial epilepsy: increased sensitivity with quantitative magnetic resonance T2 relaxometry. *Neurology* 43: 1793–9.

Jackson, G. D. 1994. New techniques in magnetic resonance and epilepsy. *Epilepsia* 35 (Suppl 6): S2–13.

Jackson, G. D. 1995. The diagnosis of hippocampal sclerosis: other techniques. *Magnetic Resonance Imaging* 13: 1081–93.

Jackson, G. D. 1996a. Visual analysis in mesial temporal sclerosis. In: G. D. Cascino, C. R. Jack Jr, eds. *Neuroimaging in epilepsy: Principles & practice*. Newton, MA: Butterworth-Heinemann, 73–110.

Jackson, G. D., and A. Connelly. 1996b. Magnetic resonance imaging and spectroscopy. *Current Opinion in Neurology* 9: 82–8.

Jayakumar, P. N., A. B. Taly, and P. K. Mohan. 1985. Transient computerised tomographic (CT) abnormalities following partial seizures. *Acta Neurologica Scandinavica* 72: 26–9.

Jennett, W., and W. Lewin. 1960. Traumatic epilepsy after closed head injuries. *Journal of Neurosurgery* 23: 295–256.

Jooma, R., H. S. Yeh, M. D. Privitera, et al. 1995. Lesionectomy versus electrophysiologically guided resection for temporal lobe tumors manifesting with complex partial seizures. *Journal of Neurosurgery* 83(2): 231–6.

Kassubek, J., H. J. Huppertz, J. Spreer, et al. 2002. Detection and localization of focal cortical dysplasia by voxel-based 3-D MRI analysis. *Epilepsia* 43(6): 596–602.

Keller, S. S., M. Wilke, U. C. Wieshmann, et al. 2004. Comparison of standard and optimized voxel-based morphometry for analysis of brain changes associated with temporal lobe epilepsy. *Neuroimage* 23(3): 860–8.

Keller, S. S., and N. Roberts. 2008. Voxel-based morphometry of temporal lobe epilepsy: an introduction and review of the literature. *Epilepsia* 49(5): 741–57.

Khajavi, K., Y. G. Comair, R. A. Prayson, et al. 1995. Childhood ganglioglioma and medically intractable epilepsy. A clinicopathological study of 15 patients and a review of the literature. *Pediatric Neurosurgery* 22(4): 181–8.

Kilpatrick, C. J., S. M. Davis, B. M. Tress, et al. 1990. Epileptic seizures in acute stroke. *Archives of Neurology* 47: 157–60.

Kilpatrick, C. J., B. M. Tress, C. O'Donnell, et al. 1991. Magnetic resonance imaging and late-onset epilepsy. *Epilepsia* 32: 358–64.

Kim, W. J., Park, S. C., Lee, S. J., et al. 1999. The prognosis for control of seizures with medications in patients with MRI evidence for mesial temporal sclerosis. *Epilepsia* 40: 290–3.

Kimiwada, T., C. Juhasz, M. Makki, et al. 2006. Hippocampal and thalamic diffusion abnormalities in children with temporal lobe epilepsy. *Epilepsia* 47(1): 167–75.

King, M. A., M. R. Newton, G. D. Jackson, et al. 1998. Epileptology of the first-seizure presentation: a clinical, electroencephalographic, and magnetic resonance imaging study of 300 consecutive patients. *Lancet* 352: 1007–11.

Knake, S., C. Triantafyllou, L. L. Wald, et al. 2005. 3T phased array MRI improves the presurgical evaluation in focal epilepsies: a prospective study. *Neurology* 11;65(7): 1026–31.

Kobayashi, M., T. Ohira, M. Ishihara, et al. 1997. Cooperative multicentre study on posttraumatic epilepsy. *No To Shinkei* 49(8): 723–7.

Kossoff, E. H., Buck, C., and J. M. Freeman. 2002. Outcomes of 32 hemispherectomies for Sturge–Weber syndrome worldwide. *Neurology* 59: 1735–8.

Kotagal, P., and A. D. Rothner. 1993. Epilepsy in the setting of neurocutaneous syndromes. *Epilepsia* 4 (Suppl 3): S71–8.

Kotila, M., and O. Waltimo. 1992. Epilepsy after stroke. *Epilepsia* 33: 495–8.

Kramer, R. E., H. Luders, R. P. Lesser, et al. 1987. Transient focal abnormalities of neuroimaging studies during focal status epilepticus. *Epilepsia* 28: 528–32.

Kratimenos, G. P., D. G. Thomas, and S. D. Shorvon. 1993. Stereotactic insertion of intracerebral electrodes in the investigation of epilepsy. *British Journal of Neurosurgery* 7(1): 45–52.

Krsek, P., B. Maton, P. Jayakar, et al. 2009. Incomplete resection of focal cortical dysplasia is the main predictor of poor postsurgical outcome. *Neurology* 20;72(3): 217–23.

Kruger, G., A. Kastrup, and G. H. Glover. 2001. Neuroimaging at 1.5 T and 3.0 T: comparison of oxygenation-sensitive magnetic resonance imaging. *Magnetic Resonance in Medicine* 45: 595–604.

Kuzniecky, R., V. de la Sayette, R. Ethier, et al. 1987. Magnetic resonance imaging in temporal lobe epilepsy: pathological correlations. *Annals of Neurology* 22: 341–7.

Kuzniecky, R., S. Burgard, E. Faught, et al. 1993. Predictive value of magnetic resonance imaging in temporal lobe epilepsy surgery. *Archives of Neurology* 50: 65–9.

Kuzniecky, R., B. Guthrie, J. Mountz, et al. 1997a. Intrinsic epileptogenesis of hypothalamic hamartomas in gelastic epilepsy. *Annals of Neurology* 42: 60–7.

Kuzniecky, R., H. Hetherington, J. Pan, et al. 1997b. Proton spectroscopic imaging at 4.1 tesla in patients with malformations of cortical development and epilepsy. *Neurology* 48: 1018–24.

Kuzniecky, R., J. W. Hugg, H. Hetherington, et al. 1998. Relative utility of H-1 spectroscopic imaging and hippocampal volumetry in the lateralization of mesial temporal lobe epilepsy. *Neurology* 51: 66–71.

Kuzniecky, R. 1999. Magnetic resonance spectroscopy in focal epilepsy: P-31 and H-1 spectroscopy. *Rev Neurol* 155: 495–8.

Kuzniecky, R. I. 1996. Magnetic resonance imaging in cerebral developmental malformations and epilepsy. In G. D. Cascino and C. R. Jack Jr, eds. *Neuroimaging in epilepsy: principles & practice*. Newton, MA: Butterworth-Heinemann, 51–63.

Labate, A., A. Cerasa, A. Gambardella, et al. 2008. Hippocampal and thalamic atrophy in mild temporal lobe epilepsy: a VBM study. *Neurology* 71(14): 1094–101.

Laohaprasit, V., D. L. Silbergeld, G. A. Ojemann, et al. 1990. Postoperative CT contrast enhancement following lobectomy for epilepsy. *Journal of Neurosurgery* 73: 392–5.

Laster, D. W., J. K. Penry, D. R. Ball, et al. 1985. Chronic seizure disorders: contribution of MR imaging when CT is normal. *AJNR American Journal of Neuroradiology* 6: 177–80.

Latack, J. T., B. W. Abou-Khalil, G. J. Siegel, et al. 1986. Patients with partial seizures: evaluation by MR, CT, and PET imaging. *Radiology* 159: 159–63.

Lee, D. H., F. Q. Gao, J. M. Rogers, et al. 1998. MR in temporal lobe epilepsy: analysis with pathologic confirmation. *AJNR American Journal of Neuroradiology* 19: 19–27.

Lee, S. K., D. I. Kim, J. Kim, et al. 2005. Diffusion-tensor MR imaging and fiber tractography: a new method of describing aberrant fiber connections in developmental CNS anomalies. *Radiographics* 25(1): 53–68.

Lencz, T., G. McCarthy, R. A. Bronen, et al. 1992. Quantitative magnetic resonance imaging in temporal lobe epilepsy: relationship to neuropathology and neuropsychological function. *Annals of Neurology* 31: 629–37.

Lesser, R. P., M. T. Modic, M. A. Weinstein, et al. 1986. Magnetic resonance imaging (1.5 Tesla) in patients with intractable focal seizures. *Archives of Neurology* 43: 367–71.

Li, B. S., J. Regal, and O. Gonen. 2001. SNR versus resolution in 3D 1H MRS of the human brain at high magnetic fields. *Magnetic Resonance in Medicine* 46: 1049–53.

Li, L. M., F. Cendes, C. Watson, et al. 1997. Surgical treatment of patients with single and dual pathology: relevance of lesion and of hippocampal atrophy to seizure outcome. *Neurology* 48: 437–44.

Li, L. M., F. Cendes, F. Andermann, et al. 1999. Surgical outcome in patients with epilepsy and dual pathology. *Brain* 122: 799–805.

Luhdorf, K., L. K. Jensen, and A. M. Plesner. 1986. Etiology of seizures in the elderly. *Epilepsia* 27: 458–63.

Mahvash, M., R. Konig, H. Urbach, et al. 2006. FLAIR-/T1-/T2-co-registration for image-guided diagnostic and resective epilepsy surgery. *Neurosurgery* 58: 69–75.

Matsumoto, R., T. Okada, N. Mikuni, et al. 2008. Hemispheric asymmetry of the arcuate fasciculus: a preliminary diffusion tensor tractography study in patients with unilateral language dominance defined by Wada test. *Journal of Neurology* 255(11): 1703–11.

Maytal, J., J. M. Krauss, G. P. Novak, et al. 2000. The role of brain computed tomography in evaluating children with new onset of seizures in the emergency department. *Epilepsia* 41: 950–4.

Mehta, A. D., D. Labar, A. Dean, et al. 2005. Frameless stereotactic placement of depth electrodes in epilepsy surgery. *Journal of Neurosurgery* 102(6): 1040–5.

Meierkord, H., U. Wieshmann, L. Niehaus, et al. 1997. Structural consequences of status epilepticus demonstrated with serial magnetic resonance imaging. *Acta Neurologica Scandinavica* 96: 127–32.

Meiners, L., A. van Gils, G. Jansen, et al. 1994. Temporal lobe epilepsy: the various MR appearances of histologically proven mesial temporal sclerosis. *AJNR American Journal of Neuroradiology* 15: 1547–55.

Meiners, L. C., T. D. Witkamp, G. A. P. De Kort, et al. 1999. Relevance of temporal lobe white matter changes in hippocampal sclerosis—magnetic resonance imaging and histology. *Investigative Radiology* 34: 38–45.

Merriam, M. A., R. A. Bronen, D. D. Spencer, et al. 1993. MR findings after depth electrode implantation for medically refractory epilepsy. *AJNR American Journal of Neuroradiology* 14: 1343–6.

Minkin, K., O. Klein, J. Mancini, et al. 2008. Surgical strategies and seizure control in pediatric patients with dysembryoplastic neuroepithelial tumors: a single-institution experience. *J Neurosurg Pediatr* 1(3): 206–10.

Montenegro, M. A., L. M. Li, M. Guerreiro, et al. 2002. Focal cortical dysplasia: improving diagnosis and localization with magnetic resonance imaging multiplanar and curvilinear reconstruction. *Journal of Neuroimaging* 12(3): 224–30.

Morris, H. H., Z. Matkovic, M. L. Estes, et al. 1998. Ganglioglioma and intractable epilepsy: clinical and neurophysiologic features and predictors of outcome after surgery. *Epilepsia* 39: 307–13.

Mueller, S. G., K. D. Laxer, N. Cashdollar, et al. 2006. Voxel-based optimized morphometry (VBM) of gray and white matter in temporal lobe epilepsy (TLE) with and without mesial temporal sclerosis. *Epilepsia* 47(5): 900–7.

Murphy, M., T. J. O'Brien, K. Morris, et al. 2001. Multimodality image-guided epilepsy surgery. *Journal of Clinical Neuroscience* 8: 534–8.

Nolan, M. A., R. Sakuta, N. Chuang, et al. 2004. Dysembryoplastic neuroepithelial tumors in childhood: long-term outcome and prognostic features. *Neurology* 62(12): 2270–6.

Novotny, E. J., F. Hyder, M. Shevell, et al. 1999. GABA changes with vigabatrin in the developing human brain. *Epilepsia* 40: 462–6.

O'Brien, T. J., E. L. So, B. P. Mullan, et al. 1999. Subtraction SPECT co-registered to MRI improves postictal SPECT localization of seizure foci. *Neurology* 52(1): 137–46.

Oertel, J., M. R. Gaab, U. Runge, et al. 2004. Neuronavigation and complication rate in epilepsy surgery. *Neurosurgery Review* 27: 214–7.

Okujava, M., R. Schulz, A. Ebner, et al. 2002. Measurement of temporal lobe T2 relaxation times using a routine diagnostic MR imaging protocol in epilepsy. *Epilepsy Research* 48(1-2): 131–42.

Ondra, S., H. Troupp, E. George, et al. 1990. The natural history of symptomatic arteriovenous malformations of the brain: a 24-year follow-up assessment. *Journal of Neurosurgery* 73: 387–91.

Oppenheim, C., D. Dormont, A. Biondi, et al. 1998. Loss of digitations of the hippocampal head on high-resolution fast spin-echo MR: a sign of mesial temporal sclerosis. *AJNR American Journal of Neuroradiology* 19: 457–63.

Ormson, M. J., D. B. Kispert, F. W. Sharbrough, et al. 1986. Cryptic structural lesions in refractory partial epilepsy: MR imaging and CT studies. *Radiology* 160: 215–9.

Pell, G. S., R. S. Briellmann, H. Pardoe, et al. 2008. Composite voxel-based analysis of volume and T2 relaxometry in temporal lobe epilepsy. *Neuroimage* 39(3): 1151–61.

Petroff, O. A., D. L. Rothman, K. L. Behar, et al. 1996a. Human brain GABA levels rise rapidly after initiation of vigabatrin therapy. *Neurology* 47: 1567–71.

Petroff, O. A., D. L. Rothman, K. L. Behar, et al. 1996b. Low brain GABA level is associated with poor seizure control. *Annals of Neurology* 40: 908–11.

Petroff, O. A., and D. L. Rothman. 1998. Measuring human brain GABA in vivo: effects of GABA-transaminase inhibition with vigabatrin. *Molecular Neurobiology* 16: 97–121.

Petroff, O. A., Hyder, F., Mattson, R. H., et al. 1999. Topiramate increases brain GABA, homocarnosine, and pyrrolidone in patients with epilepsy. *Neurology* 52: 473–8.

Petroff, O. A. C., F. Hyder, T. Collins, et al. 1999a. Acute effects of vigabatrin on brain GABA and homocarnosine in patients with complex partial seizures. *Epilepsia* 40: 958–64.

Petroff, O. A. C., D. L. Rothman, K. L. Behar, et al. 1999b. Effects of valproate and other antiepileptic drugs on brain glutamate, glutamine, and GABA in patients with refractory complex partial seizures. *Seizure* 8: 120–7.

Phal, P. M., A. Usmanov, G. M. Nesbit, et al. 2008. Qualitative comparison of 3-T and 1.5-T MRI in the evaluation of epilepsy. *AJR American Journal of Roentgenology* 191(3): 890–5.

Practice parameter. 1996a. Neuroimaging in the emergency patient presenting with seizure. Summary statement. *Neurology* 47: 288–91.

Practice parameter. 1996b. The neurodiagnostic evaluation of the child with a first simple febrile seizure. *Pediatrics* 97: 769–75.

Radhakrishnan, A., M. Abraham, V. V. Radhakrishnan. et al. 2006. Medically refractory epilepsy associated with temporal lobe ganglioglioma: characteristics and postoperative outcome. *Clinical Neurology & Neurosurgery* 108(7): 648–54.

Rapacki, T. F., M. J. Brantley, T. J. Furlow, et al. 1990. Heterogeneity of cerebral cavernous hemangiomas diagnosed by MR imaging. *Journal of Computer Assisted Tomography* 14: 18–25.

Rasmussen, T., J. Olszweski, and D. Lloyd-Smith. 1958. Focal seizures due to chronic localized encephalitis. *Neurology* 8: 435–55.

Rasmussen, T. 1978. Further observations on the syndrome of chronic encephalitis and epilepsy. *Applied Neurophysiology* 41: 1–12.

Raymond, A. A., D. R. Fish, S. M. Sisodiya, et al. 1995. Abnormalities of gyration, heterotopias, tuberous sclerosis, focal cortical dysplasia, microdysgenesis, dysembryoplastic neuroepithelial tumour and dysgenesis of the archicortex in epilepsy. Clinical, EEG and neuroimaging features in 100 adult patients*Brain* 118: 629–60.

Requena, I., M. Arias, I. L. Lopez, et al. 1991. Cavernomas of the central nervous system: clinical and neuroimaging manifestations in 47 patients. *Journal of Neurology Neurosurgery & Psychiatry* 54: 590–4.

Rezai, A. R., A. Y. Mogilner, J. Cappell, et al. 1997. Integration of functional brain mapping in image-guided neurosurgery. *Acta Neurochirgica Supplementum* (Wien) 68: 85–9.

Riela, A. R., B. P. Sires, and J. K. Penry. 1991. Transient magnetic resonance imaging abnormalities during partial status epilepticus. *J Child Neurology* 6: 143–5.

Robinson, J. R., I. A. Awad, and J. R. Little. 1991. Natural history of the cavernous angioma. *Journal of Neurosurgery* 75: 709–14.

Rodrigo, S., C. Oppenheim, F. Chassoux, et al. 2007. Uncinate fasciculus fiber tracking in mesial temporal lobe epilepsy. Initial findings. *European Radiology* 17: 1663–8.

Rothman, D. L., C. C. Hanstock, O. A. Petroff, et al. 1992a. Localized 1H NMR spectra of glutamate in the human brain. *Magnetic Resonance Medicine* 25: 94–106.

Rothman, D. L., E. J. Novotny, G. I. Shulman, et al. 1992b. 1H-(13C) NMR measurements of (4-13C) glutamate turnover in human brain. *Proceedings of the National Academy of Sciences of the USA* 89: 9603–6.

Rothman, D. L., O. A. Petroff, K. L. Behar, et al. 1993. Localized 1H NMR measurements of gamma-aminobutyric acid in human brain in vivo. *Proceedings of the National Academy of Sciences of the USA* 90: 5662–6.

Rugg-Gunn, F. J., S. H. Eriksson, M. R. Symms, et al. 2001. Diffusion tensor imaging of cryptogenic and acquired partial epilepsies. *Brain* 124(Pt 3): 627–36.

Saluja, S., N. Sato, Y. Kawamura, et al. 2000. Choroid plexus changes after temporal lobectomy. *AJNR American Journal of Neuroradiology* 21: 1650–3.

Sasaki, M., M. Sone, S. Ehara, et al. 1993. Hippocampal sulcus remnant: potential cause of change in signal intensity in the hippocampus. *Radiology* 188(3): 743–6.

Sato, N., R. A. Bronen, G. Sze, et al. 1997. Postoperative changes in the brain: MR imaging findings in patients without neoplasms. *Radiology* 204: 839–46.

Sawaishi, Y., M. Sasaki, T. Yano, et al. 2005. A hippocampal lesion detected by high-field 3 tesla magnetic resonance imaging in a patient with temporal lobe epilepsy. *Tohoku Journal of Experimental Medicine* 205(3): 287–91.

Scellig, S. D., M. Stone, and James T. Rutka. 2008. Utility of neuronavigation and neuromonitoring in epilepsy surgery: a review. *Neurosurgery Focus* 25(3):

Schiller, Y., G. Cascino, E. So, et al. 2000. Discontinuation of antiepileptic drugs after successful epilepsy surgery. *Neurology* 54: 346–9.

Schörner, W., H. J. Meencke, and R. Felix. 1987. Temporal-lobe epilepsy: comparison of CT and MR imaging. *AJR American Journal of Roentgenology* 149: 1231–9.

Schramm, J. 2008. Temporal lobe epilepsy surgery and the quest for optimal extent of resection: a review. *Epilepsia* 49(8): 1296–307.

Schwartz, T. H., D. Marks, J. Pak, et al. 2002. Standardization of amygdalohippocampectomy with intraoperative magnetic resonance imaging: preliminary experience. *Epilepsia* 43: 430–6.

Scott, C. A., D. R. Fish, S. J. Smith, et al. 1999. Presurgical evaluation of patients with epilepsy and normal MRI: role of scalp video-EEG telemetry. *Journal of Neurology Neurosurgery & Psychiatry* 66: 69–71.

Shenai, M. B., D. A. Ross, and O. Sagher. 2007. The use of multiplanar trajectory planning in the stereotactic placement of depth electrodes. *Neurosurgery* 60(4 Suppl 2): 272–6.

Simone, I. L., F. Federico, C. Tortorella, et al. 1999. Metabolic changes in neuronal migration disorders: evaluation by combined MRI and proton MR spectroscopy. *Epilepsia* 40: 872–9.

Sisodiya, S. M., N. Moran, S. L. Free, et al. 1997. Correlation of widespread preoperative magnetic resonance imaging changes with unsuccessful surgery for hippocampal sclerosis. *Annals of Neurology* 41: 490–6.

Song, C. J., J. H. Kim, E. L. Kier, et al. 2000. MR and histology of subinsular T2-weighted bright spots: Virchow-Robin spaces of the extreme capsule and insula cortex. *Radiology* 214: 671–7.

Spencer, D. D. 1994. Classifying the epilepsies by substrate. *Clin Neurosci* 2: 104–9.

Spencer, S. S., G. McCarthy, and D. D. Spencer. 1993. Diagnosis of medial temporal lobe seizure onset: relative specificity and sensitivity of quantitative MRI. *Neurology* 43: 2117–24.

Spencer, S. S. 1994. The relative contributions of MRI, SPECT, and PET imaging in epilepsy. *Epilepsia* 35[Suppl 6]: S72–89.

Spencer, S. S. 1996. Selection of candidate for invasive monitoring. In G. D. Cascino and C. R. Jack Jr, eds. *Neuroimaging in epilepsy: Principles & practice.* Newton, MA: Butterworth-Heinemann, 219–34.

Spencer, S. S. 1998. Substrates of localization-related epilepsies: biologic implications of localizing findings in humans. *Epilepsia* 39: 114–23.

Sperling, M. R., G. Wilson, J. J. Engel, et al. 1986. Magnetic resonance imaging in intractable partial epilepsy: correlative studies. *Annals of Neurology* 20: 57–62.

Spooner, C. G., S. F. Berkovic, L. A. Mitchell, et al. 2006. New-onset temporal lobe epilepsy in children. Lesion on MRI predicts poor seizure outcome. *Neurology* 67: 2147–53.

Stanley, J. A., F. Cendes, F. Dubeau, et al. 1998. Proton magnetic resonance spectroscopic imaging in patients with extratemporal epilepsy. *Epilepsia* 39(3): 267–73.

Stapleton, S. R., E. Kiriakopoulos, D. Mikulis, et al. 1997. Combined utility of functional MRI, cortical mapping, and frameless stereotaxy in the resection of lesions in eloquent areas of brain in children. *Pediatric Neurosurgery* 26: 68–82.

Strandberg, M., E. M. Larsson, S. Backman, et al. 2008. Presurgical epilepsy evaluation using 3T MRI. Do surface coils provide additional information? *Epileptic Disorders* 10(2): 83–92.

Takahashi, E., K. Ohki, and D. S. Kim. 2007. Diffusion tensor studies dissociated two frontotemporal pathways in the human memory system. *Neuroimage* 34(2): 827–38.

Taoka, T., M. Sakamoto, H. Nakagawa, et al. 2008. Diffusion tensor tractography of the Meyer loop in cases of temporal lobe resection for temporal lobe epilepsy: correlation between postsurgical visual field defect and anterior limit of Meyer loop on tractography. *AJNR American Journal of Neuroradiology* 29(7): 1329–34.

Temkin, N. R. 2003. Risk factors for posttraumatic seizures in adults. *Epilepsia* 44 Suppl 10: 18–20.

Terra-Bustamante, V. C., R. M. Fernandes, L. M. Inuzuka, et al. 2005. Surgically amenable epilepsies in children and adolescents: clinical, imaging, electrophysiological, and post-surgical outcome data. *Child's Nervous System* 21: 546–50.

Terra-Bustamante, V. C., H. R. Machado, R. dos Santos Oliveira, et al. 2009. Rasmussen encephalitis: long-term outcome after surgery. *Childs Nerv Syst* 25(5): 583–9.

Theodore, W. H., D. Katz, C. Kufta, et al. 1990. Pathology of temporal lobe foci: correlation with CT, MRI, and PET. *Neurology* 40: 797–803.

Thivard, L., S. Lehericy, A. Krainik, et al. 2005. Diffusion tensor imaging in medial temporal lobe epilepsy with hippocampal sclerosis. *Neuroimage* 28(3): 682–90.

Tien, R. D., B. C. Ashdown, D. J. Lewis, et al. 1992. Rasmussen's encephalitis: neuroimaging findings in four patients. *AJR American Journal of Roentgenology* 158: 1329–32.

Tien, R. D., G. J. Felsberg, C. Castro, et al. 1993. Complex partial seizures and mesial temporal sclerosis: evaluation with fast spin-echo MR imaging. *Radiology* 189: 835–42.

Tien, R. D., and G. J. Felsberg. 1995. The hippocampus in status epilepticus: demonstration of signal intensity and morphologic changes with sequential fast spin-echo MR imaging. *Radiology* 194: 249–56.

Topçu, M., G. Turanli, F. M. Aynaci, et al. 1999. Rasmussen encephalitis in childhood. *Child's Nervous System* 15(8): 395–402.

Topper, R., E. Jurgens, J. Reul, et al. 1999. Clinical significance of intracranial developmental venous anomalies. *Journal of Neurology Neurosurgery & Psychiatry* 67: 234–8.

Tubbs, R. S., S. M. Nimjee, and W. J. Oakes. 2005. Long-term follow-up in children with functional hemispherectomy for Rasmussen's encephalitis. *Child's Nervous System* 21(6): 461–5.

Urbach, H. 2008. MRI of long-term epilepsy-associated tumors. *Seminars in Ultrasound CT MR* 29(1): 40–6.

Van Paesschen, W., J. S. Duncan, J. M. Stevens, et al. 1997a. Etiology and early prognosis of newly diagnosed partial seizures in adults: a quantitative hippocampal MRI study. *Neurology* 49: 753–7.

Van Paesschen, W., T. Revesz, J. S. Duncan, et al. 1997b. Quantitative neuropathology and quantitative magnetic resonance imaging of the hippocampus in temporal lobe epilepsy. *Annals of Neurology* 42: 756–66.

Van Rijckevorsel, K., C. Grandin C, M. de Tourtchaninoff, et al. 2005. Selective amygdalo-hippocampectomy: seizure outcome in 26 consecutive cases compared to the amount of resection. *Epilepsia* 46: 253–60.

VanLandingham, K. E., E. R. Heinz, J. E. Cavazos, et al. 1998. Magnetic resonance imaging evidence of hippocampal injury after prolonged focal febrile convulsions. *Annals of Neurology* 43: 413–26.

Von Oertzen, J., H. Urbach, S. Jungbluth, et al. 2002. Standard magnetic resonance imaging is inadequate for patients with refractory focal epilepsy. *Journal of Neurology Neurosurgery & Psychiatry* 73: 643–7.

Wang, H. C., W. N. Chang, H. W. Chang, et al. 2008. Factors predictive of outcome in posttraumatic seizures. *J Trauma* 64(4): 883–8.

Watson, C., F. Andermann, P. Gloor, et al. 1992. Anatomic basis of amygdaloid and hippocampal volume measurement by magnetic resonance imaging. *Neurology* 42: 1743–50.

Widjaja, E., P. D. Griffiths, and I. D. Wilkinson. 2003. Proton MR spectroscopy of polymicrogyria and heterotopia. *AJNR American Journal of Neuroradiology* 24(10): 2077–81.

Widjaja, E., S. Blaser, E. Miller, et al. 2007. Evaluation of subcortical white matter and deep white matter tracts in malformations of cortical development. *Epilepsia* 48(8): 1460–9.

Wieser, H. G.; ILAE Commission on Neurosurgery of Epilepsy. 2004. ILAE Commission Report: Mesial temporal lobe epilepsy with hippocampal sclerosis. *Epilepsia* 45(6): 695–714.

Willmore, L. 1990. Post-traumatic epilepsy: cellular mechanisms and implications for treatment. *Epilepsia* 31: 67–73.

Willmore, L. 1993. Post-traumatic seizures. *Neurol Clin* 11: 823–34.

Woermann, F. G., M. A. McLean, P. A. Bartlett, et al. 1999. Short echo time single-voxel H-1 magnetic resonance spectroscopy in magnetic resonance imaging negative temporal lobe epilepsy: different biochemical profile compared with hippocampal sclerosis. *Annals of Neurology* 45: 369–76.

Woermann, F. G., M. A. McLean, P. A. Bartlett, et al. 2001. Quantitative short echo time proton magnetic resonance spectroscopic imaging study of malformations of cortical development causing epilepsy. *Brain* 124(Pt 2): 427–36.

Wurm, G., H. Ringler, F. Knogler, et al. 2003. Evaluation of neuronavigation in lesional and non-lesional epilepsy surgery. *Comput Aided Surg* 8: 204–14.

Wyler, A. R., B. P. Hermann, and G. Somes. 1995. Extent of medial temporal resection on outcome from anterior temporal lobectomy: a randomized prospective study. *Neurosurgery* 37: 982–91.

Wyllie, E., M. Chee, M. L. Granstrom, et al. 1993. Temporal lobe epilepsy in early childhood. *Epilepsia* 34: 859–68.

Wyllie, E., Y. G. Comair, P. Kotagal, et al. 1996. Epilepsy surgery in infants. *Epilepsia* 37: 625–37.

Wyllie, E., Y. G. Comair, P. Kotagal, et al. 1998. Seizure outcome after epilepsy surgery in children and adolescents. *Annals of Neurology* 44: 740–8.

Yeakley, J. W., M. Woodside, and M. J. Fenstermacher. 1992. Bilateral neonatal Sturge–Weber–Dimitri disease: CT and MR findings. *AJNR American Journal of Neuroradiology* 13: 1179–82.

Yogarajah, M., N. K. Focke, S. Bonelli S, et al. 2009. Defining Meyer's loop-temporal lobe resections, visual field deficits and diffusion tensor tractography. *Brain* 132(6): 1656–68.

Zee, C., J. Go, P. Kim, et al. 2000. Imaging of neurocysticercosis. *Neuroimag Clinics of North America* 10: 391–407.

Chapter 3

MALFORMATIONS OF CORTICAL DEVELOPMENT

Renzo Guerrini and Francesco Zellini

INTRODUCTION

Abnormal cortical development represents a major cause of epilepsy. Most such abnormalities may now be detected using magnetic resonance imaging (MRI), although some remain undetectable even with the best imaging techniques.

Although the formation of the cerebral cortex is extremely complex, it can be grossly schematized in three main, partially overlapping steps: cell proliferation, cell migration, and cortical organization (Barkovich 2005). Cells proliferate in the germinal zones, within and adjacent to the walls of the lateral ventricles, then migrate along various pathways to the developing cortex, where they disengage from the guide cell. Either during migration or after migrating into the proper cortical layer, cells extend neurites and establish synaptic connections (ten Donkelaar 2006). Disruption of any or all of these processes produces characteristic morphologic disturbances, typically abnormal sulcation and gyral patterns, with irregular cortical thickness, that allow them to be classified into distinct entities, which have been designated malformations of cortical development (MCD) (Table 3.1) (Barkovich 2005).

As a rule, thin-section T1- and T2-weighted MR images should be acquired when evaluating for MCD. For T1-weighted images, a volumetric spoiled gradient echo sequence (such as SPGR or MP-RAGE) should be acquired with partition size of 1 to 1.5 mm to allow the data to be reformatted in any plane. At a minimum, sagittal, coronal, and axial images are necessary. For T2-weighted images, contrast between gray and white matter is best appreciated when using conventional spin echo images. However, in the interest of reducing scanning time, fast spin echo (FSE; also called turbo spin echo) images might be better, especially if acquired as a 3D data set that can be reformatted (Guerrini et al. 2008). To study disturbances of white matter connectivity associated with MCD, it will become progressively more important to apply sophisticated diffusion imaging techniques (diffusion tensor imaging, high-angular-resolution diffusion imaging, q-ball imaging) (Hosey et al. 2005; Perrin et al. 2005) that allow mapping of the major white matter tracts. In neonates and infants less than 10 months old (before significant myelination), thin-section (1.5–3 mm) heavily T2-weighted spin echo images are optimal, whereas between the ages of 10 and 24 months, thin partitions of T1-weighted volumetric spoiled gradient echo images with heavy T1 weighting are best. Beyond age 2 years, standard adult protocols should be used.

The following section reviews the most common disorders of cortical development and their associated clinical characteristics, with special reference to epilepsy.

Table 3.1 Classification Scheme

I. Malformations due to abnormal neuronal and glial proliferation or apoptosis

  A. Decreased proliferation/increased apoptosis or increased proliferation/decreased apoptosis—abnormalities of brain size

    1. Microcephaly with normal to thin cortex

    2. Microlissencephaly (extreme microcephaly with thick cortex)

    3. Microcephaly with extensive polymicrogyria

    4. Macrocephalies

  B. Abnormal proliferation (abnormal cell types)

    1. Non-neoplastic

      a. Cortical hamartomas of tuberous sclerosis

      b. Cortical dysplasia with balloon cells

      c. Hemimegalencephaly

    2. Neoplastic (associated with disordered cortex)

      a. Dysembryoplastic neuroepithelial tumor

      b. Ganglioglioma

      c. Gangliocytoma

II. Malformations due to abnormal neuronal migration

  A. Lissencephaly/subcortical band heterotopia spectrum

  B. Cobblestone complex/congenital muscular dystrophy syndromes

  C. Heterotopia

    1. Subependymal (periventricular)

    2. Subcortical (other than band heterotopia)

    3. Marginal glioneuronal

III. Malformations due to abnormal cortical organization (including late neuronal migration)

  A. Polymicrogyria and schizencephaly

    1. Bilateral polymicrogyria syndromes

    2. Schizencephaly (polymicrogyria with clefts)

    3. Polymicrogyria or schizencephaly as part of multiple congenital anomaly/mental retardation syndromes

  B. Cortical dysplasia without balloon cells

  C. Microdysgenesis

IV. Malformations of cortical development, not otherwise classified

  A. Malformations secondary to inborn errors of metabolism

    1. Mitochondrial and pyruvate metabolic disorders

    2. Peroxisomal disorders

  B. Other unclassified malformations

    1. Sublobar dysplasia

    2. Others

FOCAL CORTICAL DYSPLASIA

The term *focal cortical dysplasia* (FCD) designates a spectrum of abnormalities of the laminar structure of the cortex, variably associated with cytopathologic features including giant (or cytomegalic) neurons, dysmorphic neurons, and balloon cells (Palmini et al. 2004; Tassi et al. 2002). Balloon cells are of uncertain lineage and exhibit an abundant pale-staining cytoplasm, peripherally positioned nuclei, no cellular processes, and cell-surface markers for pluripotent stem cells (Ying et al. 2005). Although attempts have been made to classify FCD based on subtle histologic characteristics (Palmini et al. 2004; Tassi et al. 2002), no consistent nomenclature has been reached. In fact, FCD might not represent a single entity (Golden and Harding 2004). According to the prevailing hypothesis, FCD originates from abnormal migration, maturation, and cell apoptosis during ontogenesis (Najm 2007; Ying 2005). In particular, balloon cells and dysplastic neurons are derived from radial progenitors in the telencephalic ventricular zone (Lamparello 2007). Three main histopathologic patterns of FCD are recognized in surgical series (Tassi et al. 2002): (1) architectural dysplasia, featuring abnormal cortical lamination and ectopic neurons in the white matter; (2) cytoarchitectural dysplasia, characterized by giant neurofilament-enriched neurons and altered cortical lamination; and (3) Taylor-type cortical dysplasia, featuring giant dysmorphic neurons and balloon cells as well as cortical laminar disruption. The histologically abnormal area is not sharply defined from the adjacent tissue and may extend well beyond the area of abnormality as visible by MRI or by direct brain inspection (Olivier 1996). In one large surgical series, it was estimated that MRI may be unrevealing in up to 34% of patients, especially in those with architectural dysplasia only (Tassi et al. 2002).

Such abnormalities probably originate at different times in embryogenesis and are difficult to classify uniformly. For example, architectural dysplasia is included in the framework of FCD without there being elements that indicate abnormal neural proliferation. It should therefore be classified as a disorder with abnormal cortical organization (or lamination) (Table 3.1).

Distinctive signal alterations on T2-weighted or FLAIR images are present in most patients with cyto-architectural and Taylor-type dysplasia (Fig. 3.1A), often consisting of abnormal wedge-shaped hyperintense signal on T2, extending from the cortex toward the ventricular wall (transmantle sign, Fig. 3.2) (Bronen 1997), and often associated with focal areas of cortical thickening (Fig. 3.1B), simplified gyration, blurring of the gray–white border, or rectilinear boundaries between gray and white matter. Architectural dysplasia can appear as focal hypoplastic cortex (Tassi 2002) with hypotrophic-like changes (Fig. 3.3). Architectural dysplasia, however, is often missed by imaging. The presence of the transmantle sign is best seen on FLAIR and proton density (PD) images, and might help to distinguish FCD from wedge-like low-grade tumors on MRI (Urbach 2004). Neither mass effect nor enhancement after gadolinium is usually observed. The signal

Table 3.2 Genetic Malformations of Cortical Development Assigned to Known Genes or Loci

Malformation	Gene	Locus	Reference
Malformations from abnormal proliferation			
Tuberous sclerosis	*TSC1*	9q34.13	(Dabora et al. 2001)
Tuberous sclerosis	*TSC2*	16p13.3	(Dabora et al. 2002)
Malformations from abnormal migration			
Lissencephaly (XL, AD)			
X-linked lissencephaly with abnormal genitalia	*ARX*	Xp22.1	(Kato et al. 2004)
Isolated lissencephaly sequence (ILS) or subcortical band heterotopia (SBH)	*DCX*	Xq22.3-q23	(Matsumoto et al. 2001)
ILS	*TUBA1A*	12q13.12	(Poirier et al. 2007)
ILS	*TUBB2B*	6p25.2	(Jaglin et al. 2009)
ILS or SBH	*LIS1*	17p13.3	(Cardoso et al. 2002)
Miller-Dieker syndrome	*LIS1+YWHAE*	17p13.3	(Cardoso et al. 2003)
Lissencephaly (AR)			
Lissencephaly with cerebellar hypoplasia (LCH) group b	*RELN*	7q22.1	(Zaki et al. 2007)
LCH group b	*VLDLR*	9p24.2	(Boycott et al. 2005)
Heterotopia (XL, AD)			
Classical bilateral periventricular nodular heterotopia (PNH)	*FLNA*	Xq28	(Parrini et al. 2006)
Ehlers-Danlos syndrome and PNH	*FLNA*	Xq28	(Parrini et al. 2006)
Facial dysmorphisms, severe constipation, and PNH	*FLNA*	Xq28	(Hehr et al. 2006)
Fragile X syndrome and PNH	*FMR1*	Xq27.3	(Moro et al. 2006)
Williams syndrome and PNH	...	7q11.23	(Ferland et al. 2006)
PNH with syndactyly and developmental delay	...	Xq28	(Fink et al. 1997)
Agenesis of the corpus callosum and PNH	...	1p36.22-pter	(Neal et al. 2006)
Agenesis of the corpus callosum, polymicrogyria, and PNH	...	6q26-qter	(Eash et al. 2005)
PNH with developmental delay and spasticity	...	5p15.1	(Sheen et al. 2003)
PNH, hypotonia, minor dysmorphic features	...	5p15.33	(Sheen et al. 2003)
PNH, developmental delay, dysmorphic features	...	4p15	(Gawlik-Kuklinska et al. 2008)
PNH, facial dysmorphism, developmental delay	...	5q14.3-q15	(Cardoso et al. 2008)
Heterotopia (AR)			
Microcephaly and PNH	*ARFGEF2*	20p13	(Sheen et al. 2004)
Donnai-Barrow syndrome and PNH	*LRP2*	2q24-q31	(Kantarci et al. 2007)
Cobblestone cortical malformations (AR)			
Fukuyama congenital muscular dystrophy or Walker-Warburg syndrome (WWS)	*FCMD*	9q31.2	(Kondo-Iida et al. 1999)
Muscle-eye-brain disease (MEB) or WWS	*FKRP*	19q13.32	(Beltran-Valero de Bernabé et al. 2004)
MEB	*LARGE*	22q12.3	(Longman et al. 2003)
MEB	*POMGnT1*	1p34.1	(Beltran-Valero de Bernabé et al. 2002)
MEB or WWS	*POMT1*	9q34.13	(van Reeuwijk et al. 2006)
MEB or WWS	*POMT2*	14q24.3	(van Reeuwijk et al. 2005)
Bilateral fronto-parietal cobblestone malformation (previously polymicrogyria)	*GPR56*	16q13	(Piao et al. 2005)
CEDNIK syndrome	*SNAP29*	22q11.2	(Sprecher et al. 2005)

(continued)

Table 3.2 Genetic Malformations of Cortical Development Assigned to Known Genes or Loci (*continued*)

Malformation	Gene	Locus	Reference
Malformations from abnormal cortical organization			
Polymicrogyria (XL, AD)			
Rolandic seizures, oromotor dyspraxia	*SRPX2*	Xq22	(Roll et al. 2006)
Agenesis of the corpus callosum, microcephaly, and polymicrogyria (PMG)	*TBR2*	3p21	(Baala et al. 2007)
Aniridia and PMG	*PAX6*	11p13	(Glaser et al. 1994)
PMG	...	1p36.3-pter	(Ribeiro et al. 2007)
Microcephaly, PMG	...	1q44-qter	(Zollino et al. 2003)
Facial dysmorphism and PMG	...	2p16.1-p23	(Dobyns et al. 2008)
Microcephaly, hydrocephalus, and PMG		4q21-q22	(Nowaczyk et al. 1997)
PMG	...	21q2	(Yao et al. 2006)
DiGeorge syndrome and PMG	...	22q11.2	(Robin et al. 2006)
Polymicrogyria (AR)			
Goldberg-Shprintzen syndrome	*KIAA1279*	10q21.3	(Brooks et al. 2005)
Micro syndrome	*RAB3GAP1*	2q21.3	(Aligianis et al. 2005)

AD, autosomal dominant; AR, autosomal recessive; XL, X linked

intensity of FCD varies with the age of the patient. In neonates and young infants, FCD is usually hypointense in T2-weighted images and hyperintense in T1-weighted images. After white matter myelination has reached significant levels (24 months), the hyperintensity is easily seen in FLAIR images. A meta-analysis on 868 patients found that most MRI features of FCD can be detected on FLAIR and T2-weighted images, limiting the usefulness of standard T1-weighted images. However, 3D T1-weighted images with small slice thickness can prove helpful for visualizing small areas of FCD. Spoiled gradient echo techniques (SPGR), with the ability to acquire thin slices (1 mm), are useful to detect subtle cortical dysplasia and particularly subtle areas of T1 shortening in neonates and young infants (Woermann and Vollmar 2009).

FCD has been associated with other brain pathologies ("dual pathology"), including low-grade tumors, infarcts, and hippocampal sclerosis (Fig. 3.3). This association can be particularly misleading when surgery for intractable seizures is planned in patients in whom architectural or cytoarchitectural dysplasia is barely detectable or not detectable at all on imaging while hippocampal sclerosis is easily seen. Standard anterior temporal lobectomy will often fail in such patients if neocortical dysplasia, extending back beyond and above the limits of the resection, is present.

MRI may still be unrevealing in up to 34% of patients, especially in those with architectural dysplasia only (Tassi et al. 2002), and up to 50% of patients with normal MRI at the time of surgery were found to have some form of FCD, especially architectural dysplasia on histopathology (Bautista 2003; Lerner 2009).

Improved capacity of detecting even subtle areas of dysplasia is crucial in a presurgical setting, in which a precise evaluation of the epileptogenic area using a multidisciplinary approach and subsequent complete surgical resection are the main prognostic factors towards seizure freedom (Krsek 2009). Advanced MRI techniques may increase recognition of subtle areas of dysplasia, often missed by more conventional studies. The most promising imaging techniques in this field are diffusion tensor MRI (DTI), voxel-based morphometry (VBM), the combination of MRI and functional imaging such as positron emission tomography (PET), and magnetoencephalography-magnetic source imaging (MEG-MSI). The high-field magnets (3T) that are available in many epilepsy surgery centers can detect small cortical lesions with a high sensitivity rate when compared to 1.5T scanners, particularly if phased array surface coils are used (Knake 2005; Phal 2008). DTI allows a quantitative assessment of connectivity in the subcortical white matter surrounding a lesion. However, the findings are not specific and can be demonstrated in different cortical malformations and in patients with epilepsy and normal MRI (Eriksson 2001; Lee 2004). Other quantitative methods, such as VBM, might be helpful in FCD detection in a presurgical workup, and recent efforts were made to apply this method at the single-subject level (Huppertz 2009; Kassubek 2003). MRI features and in particular blurring of the white–gray matter junction or abnormal distribution of gray matter are revealed with an automated process on 3D T1 images, and these highlighted cortical areas then can be reinspected on the original MR images (Huppertz 2009; Keller 2008).

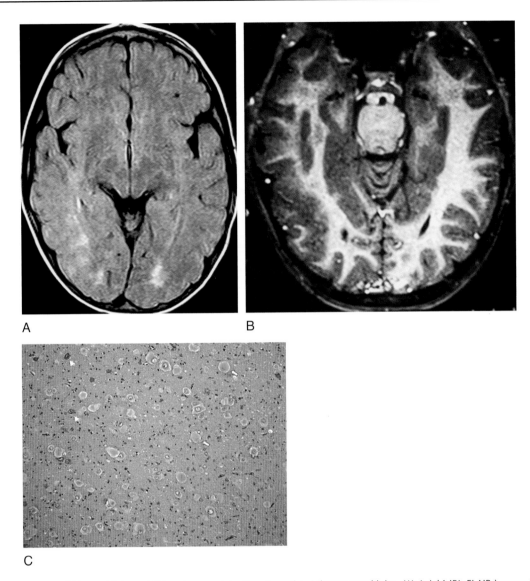

A

B

C

Figure 3.1 Seven-year-old boy with intractable seizures originating from the right temporal lobe. (A) Axial MRI. FLAIR image showing mild white matter hyperintensity of the right posterior temporal lobe, with blurring of gray–white matter junction. (B) T1-weighted inversion recovery (IR) showing thickened and irregularly folded cortex in the same region. (C) Postsurgery histopathology. Hematoxylin-eosin stain showing balloon cells (*white arrows*) and dysmorphic neurons (*arrowheads*), consistent with "Taylor"-type focal cortical dysplasia.

Increased sensitivity using these new MRI methods comes at the cost of an increased rate of false-positive results; therefore, neuroimaging findings should always be incorporated in a complex clinical and neurophysiological setting, with a consequent localizing a priori hypothesis, mostly in the context of surgical decision-making (Woermann and Vollmar 2009). PET/MRI co-registration has been applied for many years (see Chapter 9 for applications and Chapter 15 for methodology) and can also enhance the noninvasive detection and successful surgical treatment of patients with FCD, especially those with architectural dysplasia (Salamon 2008).

Clinical presentation in FCD is typically that of intractable focal epilepsy developing at a variable age, but generally before adulthood. Infantile spasms are frequent (Chugani 1990; Dulac 1996), but no other types of age-related epilepsy syndromes are usually observed. Focal status epilepticus has been frequently reported and location in the precentral gyrus can cause epilepsia partialis continua (Ferrer 1992; Kuzniecky 1988, 1993). Unless the dysplastic area is large, patients do not suffer from severe neurologic deficits. The different histologic subtypes of FCD may carry different chances of seizure freedom after surgery. According to Tassi et al. (2002), who used depth electrodes in most cases, patients with Taylor-type dysplasia had the best outcome, with 75% achieving seizure freedom, compared to 50% in those with cytoarchitectural dysplasia and 43% of those with

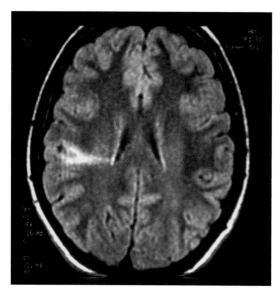

Figure 3.2 Axial fast-FLAIR showing the transmantle sign in a patient with "Taylor"-type focal cortical dysplasia.

architectural dysplasia. In fact, the area of resection could be better defined in patients with Taylor-type dysplasia, possibly due to the distinctive interictal epileptiform discharges and MRI abnormalities. The patients in this series did not undergo PET scanning. Approaching FCD with lesionectomy is accompanied by less satisfactory surgical results in that the epilepto-

genic network is often larger than the area of visible dysplasia on the MRI (Schäuble 2003).

HEMIMEGALENCEPHALY

In this condition one cerebral hemisphere is enlarged and structurally abnormal, with thick cortex, wide convolutions, and reduced sulci. The abnormality is usually unilateral based on gross structure. Laminar organization is absent in the cortex, and the demarcation between gray and white matter is poor. The histopathologic characteristics of hemimegalencephaly are similar to those of FCD, with which differences seem to be more quantitative than qualitative. Hemimegalencephaly is probably a heterogeneous condition. On MRI a spectrum of abnormalities can be found. In the most severe cases one entire hemisphere is involved (Fig. 3.4), with ipsilateral ventricular enlargement, thickened and smooth cortex (Fig. 3.5), shallow and abnormally oriented sylvian fissure, and diffuse white matter hyperintensities on T2. Partial hemispheric involvement without apparent white matter abnormalities represents the milder end of the spectrum (D'Agostino et al. 2002). The lateral ventricles are enlarged with frontal horns that appear straight and pointed anteriorly and superiorly. Calcifications and areas of gray matter heterotopia can be found.

Hemimegalencephaly has been be associated with many different disorders, including epidermal

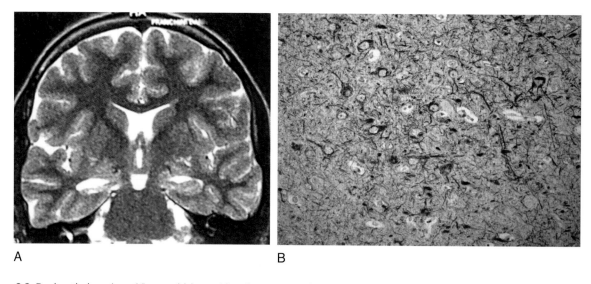

A   B

Figure 3.3 Dual pathology in a 15-year-old boy with refractory complex partial seizures and right hippocampal sclerosis. (A) Coronal T2-weighted MR image showing right hippocampal atrophy with ventricular horn dilatation. Neuropathology showed cytoarchitectural dysplasia in the temporal neocortex, in addition to hippocampal sclerosis. A second intervention with complete removal of the dysplastic tissue in the posterior temporal lobe was necessary to obtain seizure freedom after invasive EEG recording allowed definition of the posterior extent of the epileptogenic dysplastic neocortex (not visible on MRI). (B) Cytoarchitectural dysplasia: immunohistochemistry with antibodies against neurofilaments.

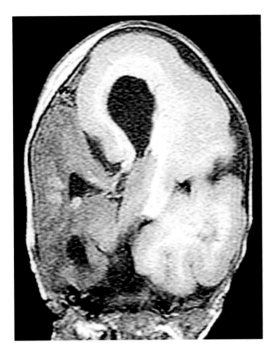

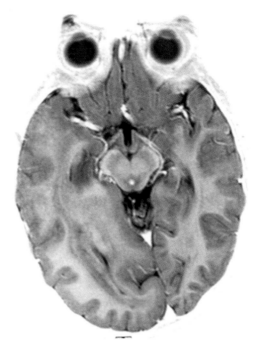

Figure 3.4 A 4-month old boy with neonatal seizures and subsequent infantile spasms in relation to severe left hemimegalencephaly. On T1-weighted MRI coronal section, the skull is asymmetric and the head circumference is at the 90th centile. The left hemisphere is hugely increased in size and occupies most of the intracranial space. The cortex is smooth, with almost complete agyria and lack of cortical–white matter digitations on the convexity. A simplified gyral pattern is detected in the temporal lobe. The lateral ventricle is enlarged and signal intensity of the white matter is increased throughout. The right hemisphere appears to be compressed so that its structure is difficult to assess. There are areas of increased signal intensity in the subcortical and periventricular white matter.

Figure 3.5 Child with hemimegalencephaly involving the right hemisphere. On T1-weighted MRI axial section, increased volume of the right temporo-occipital parenchyma is noted. The occipital cortex bulges across the midline. There is mild increase of the cortical thickness and simplified gyral pattern on the right, with blurring of the cortical–white matter junction in the anterior and mesial aspects of the temporal lobe. An area of abnormal signal intensity is present in the right hippocampus.

nevus syndrome, Proteus syndrome, hypomelanosis of Ito, neurofibromatosis type 1, and tuberous sclerosis (Guerrini 1999), but it occurs most often as an isolated malformation. The clinical appearance of hemimegalencephaly ranges from cases with severe epileptic encephalopathy beginning in the neonatal period, to rare patients who may have a normal cognitive level, with or without epilepsy. However, the most typical presentation is with hemiparesis and hemianopia, cognitive impairment, and early-onset seizures. The most severely affected children have almost continuous focal seizures, accompanied by infantile spasms and a suppression-burst pattern on EEG (Paladin 1989). Early surgery with hemispherectomy often controls the seizures. Hemispherotomy (hemispheric disconnection) is preferred to functional or anatomical hemispherectomy in some centers. Behavioral and cognitive improvement has been reported but is usually moderate (Pulsifer et al. 2004). Potential reasons for a less-than-optimum cognitive outcome are

discussed in Chapter 10. Although pre-existing hemiplegia and visual field defect are worsened or unchanged in most children, hemiplegia might be improved in some (Devlin et al. 2003).

TUBEROUS SCLEROSIS COMPLEX

Tuberous sclerosis complex (TSC) is a multisystemic disorder characterized by multiple hamartomas in the central nervous system, skin, and kidney. TSC is an autosomal dominant disorder, with variable expression. Between 50% and 75% of all cases result from de novo mutations. Two genes, TSC1 and TSC2, have been identified. TSC1 codes for the protein named hamartin; TSC2 codes for a protein named tuberin. Both proteins are thought to act as tumor suppressors. Few phenotypic differences have been noted in individuals carrying either TSC1 or TSC2 mutations, although it has been suggested that TSC1-related disease implies less severe epilepsy and a smaller risk of cognitive impairment (Dabora et al. 2001). The classic clinical triad including mental retardation, epilepsy, and adenoma sebaceum (facial angiofibromas) is recognizable in only one third of patients. Seizures are the most common presenting symptom in infants and children. They usually begin in the first 2 years of life, and infantile spasms are the most common seizure type (Guerrini and Pellacani 2007). Signs of tuberous sclerosis should always be carefully looked for in infants with spasms of recent onset. The course of epilepsy is severe in one third of patients, and development of an early epileptic encephalopathy is accompanied by a high risk of cognitive impairment and autistic features (Curatolo et al. 2008).

The characteristic intracranial lesions of TSC are cortical tubers, subependymal nodules, and subependymal giant cell astrocytomas. On MRI, tubers are relatively circumscribed areas of hypointensity in T1-weighted and increased signal intensity on T2-weighted and FLAIR images with cortical-subcortical distribution (Figs. 3.6 and 3.7). In newborns and small infants, tubers exhibit an opposite appearance due to ongoing myelination; they are hypointense compared to the surrounding unmyelinated white matter on T2-weighted images (Fig. 3.8) and hyperintense on T1-weighted images (Barkovich 2005). Magnetization transfer T1-weighted images are considered more sensitive than FLAIR for detecting white matter lesions and of comparable sensitivity for cortical tubers. Contrast enhancement is visible in about 3% to 4% of cases, usually involving multiple tubers (Pinto Gama 2006). Cortical tubers consist of giant cells, gliosis, disordered myelin sheaths, and balloon cells (Robain 1996). Such histopathologic features

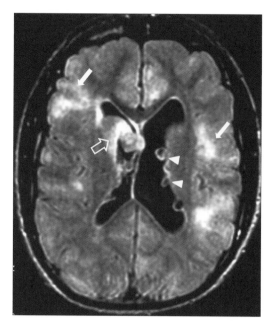

Figure 3.7 A 16-year-old boy with partial epilepsy and tuberous sclerosis. Axial fast-FLAIR sequence showing several large tubers in both hemispheres (*white arrows*), subependymal nodules (*arrowheads*), and a giant cell astrocytoma protruding into the right lateral ventricle (*empty arrow*).

share similarities with Taylor-type cortical dysplasia, or cytoarchitectural dysplasia (Guerrini et al. 2008), from which individual lesions may be impossible to distinguish, both neuroradiologically and histologically. In the past, some investigators had defined FCD as a *forme fruste* of TSC. In one study, mutation analysis in patients with FCD showed a higher frequency of mild and not clearly pathogenic sequence changes in the TSC1 gene compared to controls, as well as loss of heterozygosity of markers surrounding the TSC1 gene in the dysplastic compared to control tissue (Becker et al. 2002). These findings support some role for TSC1 in the pathogenesis of FCD, although this might be small and yet to be confirmed.

Subependymal hamartomas are located along the ventricular surface of the caudate nuclei (Figs. 3.7 and 3.9); less commonly they are observed along the temporal and frontal horns of the lateral ventricles. The imaging appearance of these lesions can vary as the child grows older. Likewise, in the first months of life, cortical tubers appear relatively hypointense in T2-weighted and hyperintense in T1-weighted images. They gradually become isointense with the surrounding white matter during myelination. Calcifications can develop after the first year of life, appearing on MR imaging as irregular nodules that protrude into the ventricles. T2* sequences are optimal for detecting calcified lesions.

Subependymal hamartomas and giant cell tumors exhibit a radiographic and pathologic continuum,

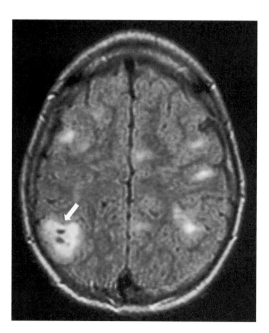

Figure 3.6 A 15-year-old girl with tuberous sclerosis: cortical tubers are hyperintense on FLAIR images. A cortical tuber with microcystic component (*white arrow*) is visible in the right parietal area.

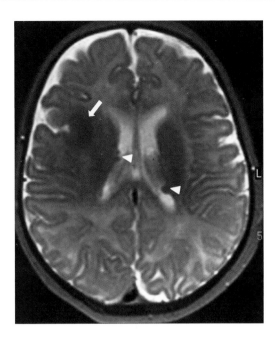

Figure 3.8 Six-month-old girl with tuberous sclerosis. T2-weighted image showing subependymal nodules (*arrowheads*) and a large hypointense lesion in the right frontal lobe (*white arrow*). In the developing unmyelinated brain, cortical tubers appear hypointense in T2 compared to the surrounding white matter.

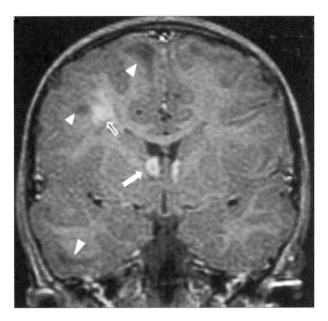

Figure 3.9 A 4-year-old girl with tuberous sclerosis. Coronal post-contrast T1-weighted image. A subependymal giant cell astrocytoma (SEGA) is readily visible in the right lateral ventricle, close to the interventricular foramen (*white arrow*). Hypointense cortical tubers are located in the frontal and temporal cortex and adjacent subcortical white matter (*arrowheads*). A contrast-enhancing tuber is visible in the right frontal lobe (*empty arrow*).

making it difficult to predict progression of the lesion. Subependymal nodules may exhibit a variable degree of contrast enhancement, which per se does not have clinical implications (Fig. 3.9) (Barkovich 2005). However, lesion growth plus contrast enhancement is strongly suggestive of a giant cell tumor (Clarke et al. 2006). Giant cell tumors are usually located in the periventricular zone, close to the foramen of Monro. This characteristic location is responsible for the clinical presentation with hydrocephalus.

Nonconventional MRI techniques such as MR spectroscopy, perfusion MRI, and DTI have been used to define the full extent of TSC pathology, to describe neuropathology in vivo, and to localize epileptogenic areas during presurgical evaluation. Disruption in cortical organization within tubers has been demonstrated using DTI (Karadagh 2005; Piao et al. 2009). High apparent diffusion coefficient (ADC) and low fractional anisotropy (FA) on DTI reflect the presence of gliosis, hypomyelination, and loss of the integrity of tissue within hamartomas. The same alterations have also been found in the normal-appearing supratentorial white matter, distant from tubers, suggesting diffuse white matter disorganization (Makki et al. 2007). Since TSC is the expression of multifocal CNS pathology, an important challenge in this condition is to detect the epileptogenic area using noninvasive methods. Co-registration of different structural and functional imaging methods has been used to combine the complementary information from each tool.

Superimposition of glucose metabolism PET with MRI and DTI data was performed by Chandra et al. (2006). Epileptogenic tubers were characterized by a disproportionate hypometabolism in relation to their size, and by a higher ADC value in the adjacent white matter, but it is unclear how useful this approach is for individual patients. Other methods include the use of the tryptophan analog in PET imaging (Kagawa et al. 2005; see Chapter 12) and magnetoencephalography (Wu et al. 2006). In the latter method, the spatially localized magnetic field produced by electric current flowing within neurons in an epileptogenic area could be co-registered with anatomical imaging information (magnetic source imaging). A consistent finding in these studies is that the epileptogenic area is localized in the cortex *adjacent* to a tuber, and the remaining tubers do not usually exhibit epileptic activity (Jansen et al. 2007). This observation is consistent with the good surgical outcome that follows the resection when a single epileptogenic tuber can be reliably identified (Cross et al. 2006; Kagawa et al. 2005).

LISSENCEPHALIES

Lissencephaly and Subcortical Band Heterotopia

The term *lissencephaly* refers to a paucity of gyral and sulcal development of cerebral cortex. A spectrum of pathologic condition is included, ranging from complete agyria to regional pachygyria, including subcortical band heterotopias (SBH) (Barkovich et al. 2005). Lissencephaly is traditionally classified into a classic type (cLIS or lissencephaly type 1) and cobblestone complex (CBSC or lissencephaly type 2). While the agyria/pachygyria complex in cLIS is mainly the result of incomplete neuronal migration, CBSC is primarily related to overmigration of neurons, many of which pass through gaps in the glia limiting membrane (Guerrini 2009).

To date several genes have been identified as causing or contributing to cLIS, including *LIS1, DCX, RELN, ARX, VLDLR, TUBA1A*, and probably TUBA2B (Guerrini and Parrini 2009; Jaglin et al. 2010). Genetic and neuropathologic features allow the identification of several distinct subtypes of lissencephaly. A first group (i), caused by LIS1 gene mutations, including the Miller-Dieker syndrome, is characterized by a four-layered cortex, with the abnormality most prominent posteriorly (Figs. 3.10 and 3.11), normally layered cerebellar cortex, nodular cerebellar heterotopia, and a small to normal pons. A second group (ii), caused by *DCX* mutations, is again characterized by four-layered cortex but anteriorly predominant abnormality (Fig. 3.12). A third group (iii) is caused by *ARX* mutations, a three-layered cortex, with normal cerebellum and small pons due to hypoplasia of the corticospinal tracts (Fig. 3.13). The fourth group (iv) includes severe, diffuse lissencephaly with two-layered cortex, cerebellar hypoplasia, and brain stem involvement

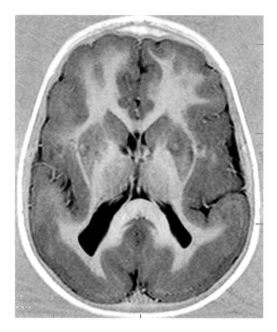

Figure 3.11 A 5-year old boy with mental retardation, developmental delay, and a history of infantile spasms. A T1-weighted IR shows posterior > anterior pachygyria. A *LIS1* gene mutation was demonstrated.

(Hong et al. 2000). The anatomic spectrum caused by mutations of the *TUBA1A* and *TUBA2B* genes is still poorly defined due to the paucity of reported cases and their apparent heterogeneity, but it appears to be wide and includes lissencephaly and polymicrogyria (Fig. 3.14) (Jaglin et al. 2009).

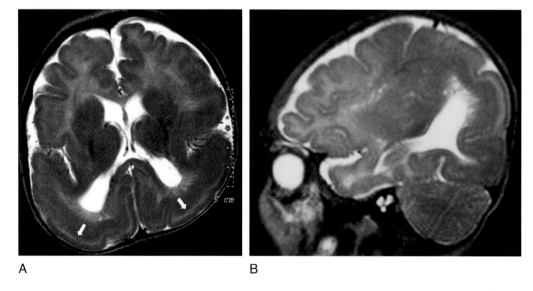

A   B

Figure 3.10 A 5-month-old boy with severe developmental retardation, strabismus, infantile spasms, and a deletion of the LIS1 gene. Axial (A) and sagittal (B) T2-weighted images show posteriorly predominant pachygyria with thickened cortex and shallow sulci. Note the hyperintense line within the thickness of the cortex, indicating the cell sparse layer (*white arrows*). The cell sparse layer should be differentiated from the subcortical white matter that separates the cortex from heterotopic neurons in subcortical band heterotopia.

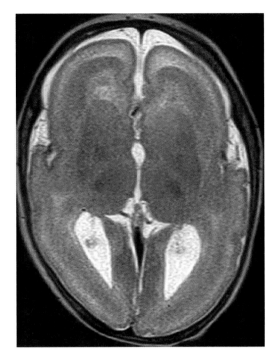

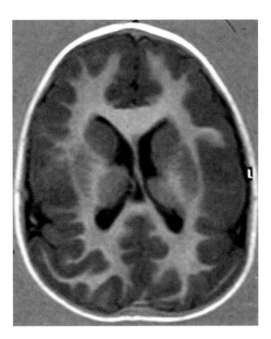

Figure 3.14 A 3-year-old girl with generalized epilepsy and severe developmental delay due to mutation of the TUBB2B gene. Axial T1-weighted IR image showing anteriorly predominant polymicrogyria.

Figure 3.12 Lissencephaly due to *DCX* gene mutation in a 3-year-old boy with infantile spasms and severe developmental delay. Note the anterior > posterior abnormality (T2-weighted image).

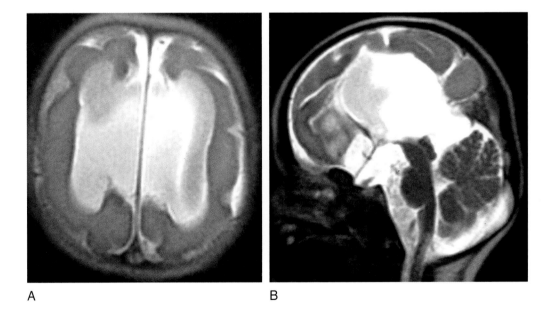

A   B

Figure 3.13 Axial (A) and sagittal (B) T2-weighted images from a 12-month-old boy with corpus callosum agenesis, lissencephaly, and ambiguous genitalia. The syndrome is caused by *ARX* gene mutation and is accompanied by profound developmental delay and very-early-onset seizures with a suppression-burst EEG.

Lissencephaly is characterized by absent (agyria) or decreased (pachygyria) surface convolutions, producing a smooth cerebral surface, and by an abnormally thick cortex, usually measuring 10 to 15 mm. In SBH, which is usually a milder malformation than

lissencephaly (Barkovich 1994), the cerebral convolutions appear either normal or mildly broad, but just beneath the cortical ribbon (Fig. 3.15 and 3.16), a thin band of white matter separates the cortex from the bands of gray matter. Transitional forms of

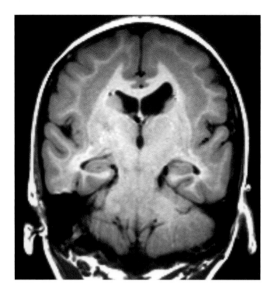

Figure 3.15 Subcortical band heterotopia due to *DCX* gene mutation in a 15-year-old girl with generalized symptomatic epilepsy and moderate mental retardation.

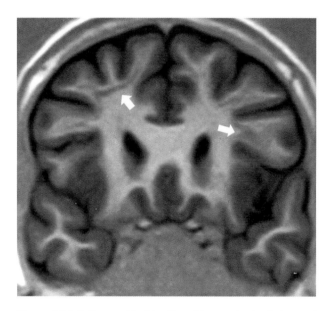

Figure 3.16 A 7-year-old girl with mild mental retardation and intractable focal epilepsy. T1-weighted IR MRI shows subtle laminae of subcortical band heterotopia bilaterally in the frontal lobes. A mutation of the *DCX* gene was demonstrated.

lissencephaly may include anterior pachygyria, which merges with posterior SBH in some patients, and partial frontal or posterior bands (Barkovich et al. 2005). Subtle forms of SBH could go unrecognized on conventional visual MRI examination. A post-process analysis with VBM applied on T1-weighted images allowed small regional SBH to be identified in a recent study (Huppertz 2008). Broad gyri and shallow sulci, without a thickened cortex, a frequent finding in some forms of microcephaly, should not be considered as lissencephaly but, instead, a simplified gyral pattern.

Most cases of lissencephaly occur without any associated malformations outside the brain (isolated lissencephaly sequence [ILS]), but some belong to more complex malformation syndromes. The best known of these is Miller-Dieker syndrome, which also features facial abnormalities and is caused by large deletions of the *LIS1* gene, mapping to chromosome 17p13.3, and contiguous genes. About 80% of cases of ILS are caused by mutations, or deletions-duplications of the *LIS1* gene and mutations of the *DCX* gene (Gleeson et al. 1998; Mei et al. 2007, 2008). *LIS1* lissencephaly occurs in both genders and has until now always been sporadic. X-linked lissencephaly occurs only in boys and may be inherited from females with SBH, carrying *DCX* gene mutations. Children with *DCX* mutations have lissencephaly that is more prominent anteriorly (Fig. 3.11), whereas children with *LIS1* mutations and Miller-Dieker syndrome have lissencephaly that is more severe posteriorly (Fig. 3.12) (Dobyns et al. 1999). Mosaic mutations of the *LIS1* gene cause mild, posterior pachygyria with SBH (Sicca et al. 2003). Mild forms of pachygyria may result from mild mutations of the *LIS1* gene (Leventer et al. 2001), and epilepsy with normal MRI has been reported in *DCX* mutation carriers (Guerrini et al. 2003).

In SBH (also called double cortex syndrome), the band is sometimes continuous and uniform or may be prominent in, or confined to, the anterior or posterior part of the brain. SBH is much more frequent in females since it is mainly transmitted as an X-linked trait. However, sporadic SBH may be genetically heterogeneous, as only approximately 60% of cases carry *DCX* mutations (Gleeson et al. 2000a). Maternal germline or mosaic *DCX* mutations may occur in about 10% of cases of either SBH or X-linked lissencephaly (Gleeson et al. 2000b). The recurrence risk for females carrying *DCX* gene mutations is high: 50% of their sons will have lissencephaly and 50% of their daughters will have SBH.

There is some evidence that heterotopic neurons in SBH can be epileptogenic and are functionally active (Mai et al. 2003; Pinard et al. 2000) (Fig. 3.17). All patients with severe lissencephaly have early developmental delay and eventual profound or severe mental retardation. Rare patients with pachygyria may have moderate mental retardation. Other neurologic manifestations include early hypotonia and later spastic quadriplegia. Seizures occur in over 90% of patients, with onset before 6 months in about 75%. About 80% of children have infantile spasms in the first year of life. Later, most children have various seizure types but usually will continue to manifest epileptic spasms. Characteristic EEG changes (very-high-amplitude rhythmic activity) with high diagnostic specificity but low sensitivity have been described (Quirk et al. 1993).

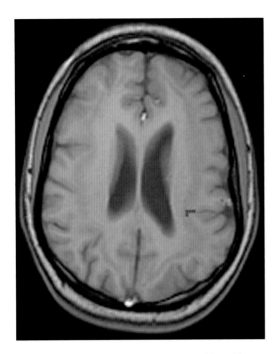

Figure 3.17 A 16-year-old girl with subcortical band heterotopia due to *DCX* gene mutation. Functional MRI reveals a task-dependent increase of blood oxygen level-dependent signal in the primary motor cortex as well as in the underlying heterotopic gray matter in the left hemisphere.

Mental retardation and epilepsy are frequently associated with SBH. Children with gyral abnormalities may have more severe ventricular enlargement and thicker heterotopic bands and a significantly earlier seizure onset (Barkovich et al. 1994). About 90% of reported patients with SBH had epilepsy and about 50% of them a form of generalized epilepsy, often with the characteristics of Lennox-Gastaut syndrome.

Autosomal Recessive Lissencephaly with Cerebellar Hypoplasia due to Mutations of the RELN Gene

This form of lissencephaly was characterized by Hong et al. (2000) in two recessive pedigrees with three affected sibs each, showing moderately severe pachygyria and severe cerebellar hypoplasia. Affected children in one family had congenital lymphedema, hypotonia, severe developmental delay, and generalized seizures. Severe hypotonia, developmental delay, and seizures were observed in both pedigrees.

X-linked Lissencephaly with Callosum Agenesis and Abnormal (or Ambiguous) Genitalia (XLAG)

XLAG is a variant LIS in genotypic males. This malformation is characterized by a more severe migration abnormality in the posterior brain (posterior > anterior gradient) and intermediate (8–10 mm) cortical thickness, usually complete agenesis of the corpus callosum, severe ventricular enlargement, often cavitated or indistinct basal ganglia, severe postnatal microcephaly, and ambiguous or severely hypoplastic genitalia. Affected children have profound mental retardation, hypothalamic dysfunction with poor temperature regulation, intractable epilepsy typically beginning on the first days of life, infancy-onset dyskinesia that may be difficult to distinguish from seizures, and chronic diarrhea (Kato et al. 2004). Early death is frequent. Female relatives, including some mothers, have isolated agenesis of the corpus callosum and, rarely, mild mental retardation and epilepsy (Bonneau et al. 2002).

Brain neuropathology in this condition reveals an abnormally laminated cortex exclusively containing pyramidal neurons, with a pattern suggesting disruption of both tangential and radial migration, dysplastic basal ganglia, hypoplastic olfactory bulbs and optic nerves, abnormal gliotic white matter containing numerous heterotopic neurons, and complete agenesis of the corpus callosum without Probst bundles (Bonneau et al. 2002).

COBBLESTONE BRAIN MALFORMATIONS (COBBLESTONE COMPLEX)

Cobblestone complex (previously called type 2 or cobblestone lissencephaly) is a severe brain malformation consisting of cobblestone cortex, abnormal white matter, enlarged ventricles often with hydrocephalus, small brain stem, and small dysplastic cerebellum (Dobyns et al. 1999; Haltia et al. 1997; Takada et al. 1988). In the most severely affected patients, the brain surface is smooth, which led to the designation as lissencephaly, although less severe cobblestone malformations have an irregular and pebbled rather than smooth surface. Severe expression may include progressive hydrocephalus, large posterior fossa cysts (atypical for Dandy-Walker malformation), and occipital cephalocele. Eye malformations are frequent, and congenital muscular dystrophy is probably always present.

The cobblestone malformation has been observed in three genetic syndromes, although they may clearly overlap: Fukuyama congenital muscular dystrophy, muscle-eye-brain disease, and Walker-Warburg syndrome. All share a clinical course of severe to profound mental retardation, severe hypotonia, mild distal spasticity and, often, poor vision.

Fukuyama congenital muscular dystrophy consists of relatively mild cobblestone complex, moderate to severe mental retardation, epilepsy, and severe congenital muscular dystrophy with progressive weakness, joint contractures, and elevated serum levels of creatine kinase. The causative *FCMD* gene was identified, as well as a common founder mutation of this gene in the Japanese population (Kobayashi et al. 1998).

Muscle-eye-brain disease consists of moderate cobblestone dysplasia with moderate to severe mental retardation, epilepsy, complex eye abnormalities (including retinal and choroidal hypoplasia, optic nerve pallor, high-grade myopia, anterior chamber-angle abnormalities, glaucoma, iris hypoplasia, cataracts, and rare colobomata), and congenital muscular dystrophy or myopathy with weakness, contractures, and elevated serum levels of creatine kinase. Mutations of three genes, *FKRP*, *LARGE*, and *POMGnT1*, have been found.

Walker-Warburg syndrome includes lissencephaly and the most severe brain stem and cerebellar malformations of any of the cobblestone group. Most patients have hydrocephalus, and approximately 25% have occipital cephaloceles. All patients have profound mental retardation, epilepsy, and eye abnormalities similar to those of muscle-eye-brain disease and the same congenital muscular dystrophy or myopathy with elevated serum levels of creatine kinase and contractures. Mutations of *POMGnT1* do not appear to cause Walker-Warburg syndrome (Dobyns et al. 1989). However, mutations of *POMT1* and *FCMD* have been found in a few patients (Beltran-Valero De Bernabé et al. 2003; Silan et al. 2003).

AICARDI SYNDROME

Aicardi syndrome is a complex malformation including irregularly distributed polymicrogyric cortex (Fig. 3.18A) and periventricular and subcortical nodular heterotopia in addition to agenesis or hypoplasia of the corpus callosum (Hopkins et al. 2008). The syndrome is observed only in females, with the exception of two reported males who had two X chromosomes (Aicardi 1996), and is thought to be caused by an X-linked gene with lethality in homozygous males. All reported cases were sporadic, with the exception of two affected sisters (Molina et al. 1989). Clinical features include severe mental retardation, infantile spasms, and chorioretinal lacunae. Additional malformations include choroid plexus cysts, ependymal cysts, especially around the third ventricle, cerebellar dysgenesis, cystic malformations of the posterior fossa (Fig. 3.18B), colobomata, and vertebral and costal abnormalities. Spasms were the only seizure type in 47% of 184 reported patients and were associated with partial seizures in 35% (Aicardi 1996). Seizure patterns change little, if at all, in older children, and seizures are almost always resistant.

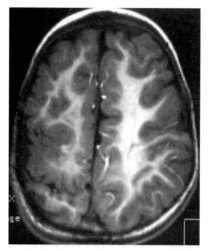

A

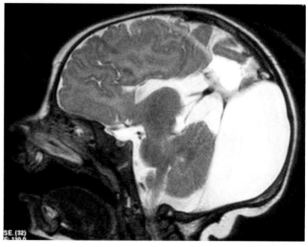

B

Figure 3.18 Aicardi syndrome in a 6-year-old girl. The axial T1-weighted MRI (A) shows abnormal cortical folding and sulcation in the right hemisphere. In the sagittal T2-weighted MRI (B), a large cyst is present in the posterior fossa and several interhemispheric cysts are visible. There is tentorium elevation and corpus callosum agenesis. The patient also exhibits chorioretinal lacunae, epileptic spasms, and asymmetric tonic seizures.

GRAY MATTER HETEROTOPIA

Heterotopia is defined as groups of cells found in an inappropriate location in the correct tissue of origin. There are three main groups of heterotopia: periventricular (usually nodular [PNH]), subcortical (either nodular or laminar), and leptomeningeal; only the first two can be detected by imaging. Periventricular heterotopia (PH) is by far the most common. Subcortical band heterotopia is a mild form of lissencephaly and classified in that group. We will consider here PH, which is the best-known form of nodular heterotopia and subcortical heterotopia.

Periventricular Heterotopia

PH is most often nodular, either unilateral or bilateral. The cerebral cortex is most often normal, but in some patients abnormal cortical folding of the overlying cortex is visible, especially if the heterotopic nodule is close to the depth of a sulcus (Fig. 3.19). The best-known condition featuring PH is bilateral PNH, which consists of confluent and symmetric subependymal nodules of gray matter located along the superolateral walls of the lateral ventricles, extending from the frontal horns to the trigones, particularly along the ventricular body (Fig. 3.20). The malformation is mainly seen in females, often showing familial distribution consistent with an X-linked transmission. Mutations of the *filamin 1* gene (*FLN1*) (Fox et al. 1998) have been observed in almost all X-linked pedigrees and are often associated with epilepsy in females with normal or borderline IQ and prenatal or early postnatal lethality in males. In some individuals with *FLN1* mutations, PH can be unilateral or even manifested as an isolated nodule (Guerrini et al. 2004). Rare male patients with unilateral or bilateral PH and epilepsy due to mild germline or mosaic *FLN1* mutations have been reported (Guerrini et al. 2004). However, many patients of both genders having PH, either unilateral or bilateral, are sporadic and do not have *FLN1* mutations (Parrini et al. 2006). Those with mutations usually have a typical bilateral PH pattern, but most patients with atypical PH do not have *FLN1* mutation (Parrini et al. 2006; Poussaint et al. 2000). The genetic recurrence risk for

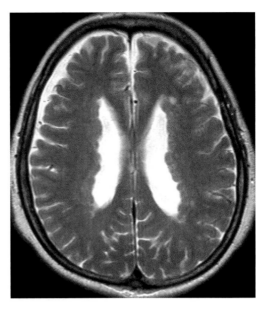

Figure 3.20 Axial T2-weighted MRI in a 20-year-old woman with partial epilepsy symptomatic of bilateral periventricular nodular heterotopia due to *FLN1* mutation. Contiguous nodules of heterotopic gray matter are lining the walls of the lateral ventricles bilaterally and protrude into them.

women with X-linked bilateral PH is 50% for daughters and unknown but presumably much lower for severely affected sons with an increase in the rate of miscarriages. A rare recessive form of bilateral PH, accompanied by microcephaly, severe developmental delay, and early-onset intractable seizures, has been

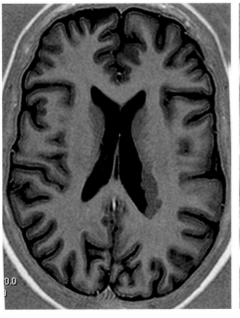

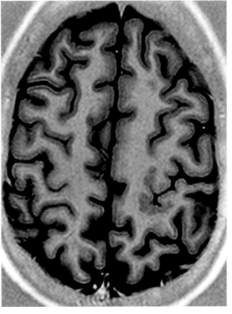

A   B

Figure 3.19 A 9-year-old boy with focal epilepsy. Axial T1-weighted IR. Periventricular nodular heterotopia on the left (A) with ipsilateral perirolandic dysplastic cortex and irregular rolandic sulcation (B).

linked to mutations of the *ARGEF2* gene (Sheen et al. 2004). Numerous other syndromes featuring bilateral PH, mental retardation, and often epilepsy have been described, most often occurring sporadically (Guerrini and Parrini 2010; Parrini et al. 2006). Some of these rare syndromes featuring PH have been associated with recurrent genomic unbalances (Table 3.2).

Applications of advanced MRI techniques can help better characterize PH in dubious cases. MR spectroscopy can confirm the normal appearance, for example in the differential diagnosis of low-grade tumors, and DWI confirms the characteristics of the signal analog to the normal gray matter. PWI in some cases can identify areas of hyperperfusion, and fMRI can show activated areas responding to stimuli as in normal cortex (Lange et al. 2004), suggesting the participation of heterotopic cortex to integrated functional networks (Ferland and Guerrini 2009).

The most common clinical manifestation of PH is epilepsy, occurring in 80% to 90% of patients, with most having intractable focal seizures (Dubeau et al. 1995). Studies using depth electrodes in patients with PH and epilepsy have shown that the nodules are able to generate epileptic activity and are often involved in complex epileptogenic networks with simultaneous ictal onset within the nodule and in normally migrated cortex (Sherer et al. 2005; Tassi et al. 2005).

Subcortical Nodular Heterotopia

Subcortical nodular heterotopia is a relatively common condition and, when of large size, is accompanied by irregular folding of the overlying cortex (Fig. 3.21). Its etiology and genetic basis, if any, remain unknown. This migration abnormality is usually detected when performing brain MRI after seizure onset since, in most cases, it produces no neurologic signs or cognitive impairment. Functional MRI studies have demonstrated functional activation of the heterotopic cortex. Neuropathologic and gene-expression profile studies indicate that subcortical heterotopia has a rudimentary layering pattern (Garbelli et al. 2009) and includes upper cortical neurons. At the same time, correctly targeted neurons appear to have reached the appropriate cortical layers (Ferland and Guerrini 2009; Garbelli et al. 2009). Good results have been reported after surgical treatment of epilepsy, but the use of depth electrodes is advised since the epileptogenic and ictal onset zone may include both the cortex and the heterotopic tissue (Tassi et al. 2005).

POLYMICROGYRIA

The term *polymicrogyria* designates an excessive number of small and prominent convolutions separated by

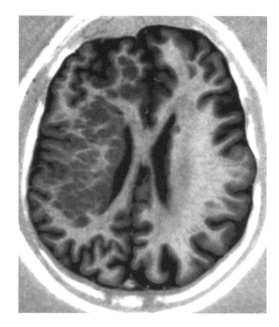

Figure 3.21 Adult man with intractable focal epilepsy and normal cognitive level. Axial T1-weighted IR image. Large macronodular heterotopia involving the right frontal and anterior parietal lobes is seen. The heterotopia extends from the ventricular wall to the cortex, which is irregularly folded. A small, isolated periventricular heterotopic nodule is also visible on the left.

shallow and enlarged sulci, giving the cortical surface a lumpy aspect. Polymicrogyria is probably one of the most common of the MCD. It is often difficult, both on direct brain inspection and MRI, to recognize polymicrogyria or to differentiate it from pachygyria because the microconvolutions are packed and their molecular layers are fused (Guerrini et al. 1992). However, the associated irregular cortical folding often produces secondary alterations of the gyral pattern that are macroscopically recognizable. The imaging appearance of polymicrogyria varies with the patient's age (Takanashi and Barkovich 2003). In newborns and young infants, the malformed cortex is very thin, with multiple, very small undulations. After myelination, polymicrogyria appears as thickened cortex with irregular cortex–white matter junction. Morphologic abnormalities in the fine interdigitations between gray and white matter, typical of polymicrogyria, can be properly investigated using phase array surface coils. Brain pathology demonstrates abnormal development or loss of neurons in the middle and deep cortical layers (Englund et al. 2005), variably associated with an unlayered cortical structure (Harding and Copp 1997). Polymicrogyria is a common cortical malformation and is associated with a wide number of patterns and syndromes and with mutations in several genes (Table 3.2). Its pathogenesis is not well understood.

Polymicrogyria can be localized to a single gyrus, can involve portions of a hemisphere, and can be bilateral and asymmetrical, bilateral and symmetrical, or diffuse. Sometimes it is associated with deep clefts that might extend through the entire cerebral mantle to communicate with the lateral ventricle (schizencephaly). The clinical sequelae of polymicrogyria are highly variable depending on its extent and location, the presence of other brain malformations, and the influence of complications such as epilepsy. In addition, polymicrogyria is reported as an occasional component in multiple different syndromes or disorders including metabolic disorders, congenital cytomegalovirus infection, chromosome deletion syndromes, and multiple congenital anomaly syndromes. These patients may have a wide spectrum of clinical problems other than those attributable to the polymicrogyria. Clinical manifestations associated with polymicrogyria vary in relation to the extent of the cortical abnormality and range from severe encephalopathies with spastic quadriparesis, profound mental retardation, and intractable epilepsy to normal individuals with selective impairment of higher-order neurologic functions (Guerrini et al. 2008). Various polymicrogyria syndromes have been identified using MRI, and these are discussed next.

Bilateral perisylvian polymicrogyria involves bilaterally the gray matter bordering the lateral fissure, which in typical cases is shallow and almost vertical and in continuity with the central or postcentral sulcus (Fig. 3.22). The cortical abnormality is most often symmetrical, but of variable extent. Familial cases have been reported with possible autosomal recessive,

X-linked dominant and X-linked recessive inheritance, indicating genetic heterogeneity (Guerreiro et al. 2000). A locus for X-linked bilateral perisylvian polymicrogyria maps to Xq28 (Villard et al. 2002). Since some patients with extensive perisylvian polymicrogyria have associated chromosome 22q11.2 deletions, FISH analysis for 22q11.2 is an essential investigation in patients with this malformation (Robin et al. 2006). Bilateral perisylvian polymicrogyria has also been reported following twin-to-twin transfusion syndrome, with death of the co-twin between the 10th and 18th week of gestation (Van Bogaert et al. 1996).

The clinical features of bilateral perisylvian polymicrogyria are often distinctive, consisting of oromotor, facial, and pharyngeal motor dysfunction resulting in problems with sucking and swallowing, excessive drooling, and facial diplegia (Guerrini et al. 1992b; Kuzniecky et al. 1993). Speech production impairment ranges from mild dysarthria to complete absence of speech. Motor dysfunction may include limb spasticity, although this is rarely severe if present. Almost all patients have intellectual disability and most have epilepsy. Seizures, often atypical absence, tonic, or atonic drop attacks, and tonic-clonic seizures, often present with features of the Lennox-Gastaut syndrome. A minority of patients (26%) have partial seizures, predominantly involving the perioral or facial muscles. Most of these patients have severe epilepsies whose characteristics are similar to those of the bilateral perisylvian syndrome or may have partial epilepsies with seizure onset in the occipital or parietal lobes. It is

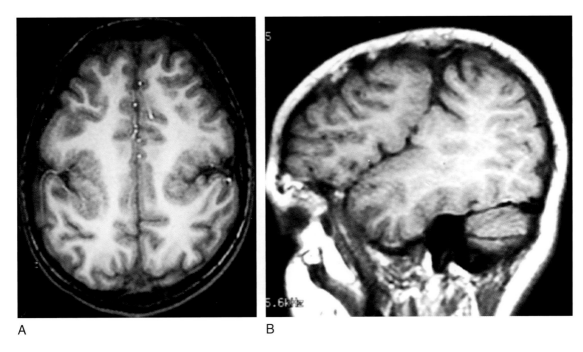

A   B

Figure 3.22 A 9-year-old girl with generalized epilepsy and severe developmental delay. Axial (A) T1-weighted and sagittal (B) images showing bilateral perisylvian polymicrogyria with verticalized sylvian fissures, merging with the rolandic sulci. There is apparent cortical thickening and pronounced infolding of the malformed cortex.

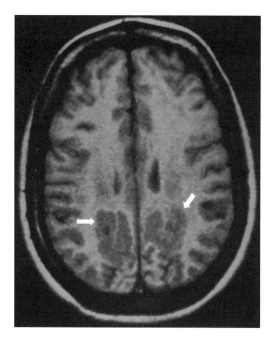

Figure 3.23 Patient with complex partial seizures and normal cognitive level. Axial T1-weighted MRI reveals bilateral parieto-occipital polymicrogyria, visible as thickened and abnormally folded cortex at the parieto-occipital junction (*arrows*).

unclear whether this form is distinct from the classical bilateral perisylvian polymicrogyria.

Bilateral parasagittal parieto-occipital polymicrogyria (Fig. 3.23) has been demonstrated on MRI in

unrelated patients with partial epilepsy (Guerrini et al. 1997). There is no genetic mechanism known for this abnormality. In some patients perisylvian polymicrogyria extends posteriorly to involve the parieto-occipital cortex, the sylvian fissure being prolonged across the entire hemispheric convexity and up to the mesial surface. Bilateral frontal polymicrogyria was described in children with developmental delay, mild spastic quadriparesis, and epilepsy (Guerrini et al. 2000). Bilateral frontoparietal polymicrogyria has been reported in consanguineous and non-consanguineous families with recessive pedigrees and has been associated with mutations of the *GPR56* gene (Piao et al. 2004). The topography of the cortical abnormality, as well as the pattern of expression of mouse Gpr56, suggests that *GPR56* regulates cortical patterning. The imaging characteristics of bilateral frontoparietal polymicrogyria (myelination defects, cerebellar cortical dysplasia with cysts, frequent involvement of the medial aspects of the cerebral hemispheres; Fig. 3.24) resemble those of the cobblestone malformation spectrum (muscle-eye-brain disease and Fukuyama congenital muscular dystrophy) that are also associated with N-glycosylation defects in the developing brain (Jin et al. 2007). Therefore, it has been suggested that this disorder might be best classified as a cobblestone malformation (Guerrini et al. 2008).

Polymicrogyria involving a discrete region of one hemisphere is usually detected on brain MRI, prompted by onset of focal seizures in school-age, otherwise

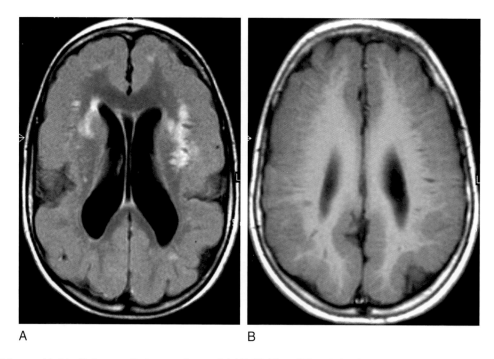

A   B

Figure 3.24 A 15-year old girl with Lennox-Gastaut syndrome. Axial FLAIR (A) and T1-weighted (B) MRI. There is increased cortical thickness, a simplified gyral pattern, and multiple patchy areas of increased signal intensity seen in the white matter (A). Abnormal radial migration is visible on the T1-weighted image (B).

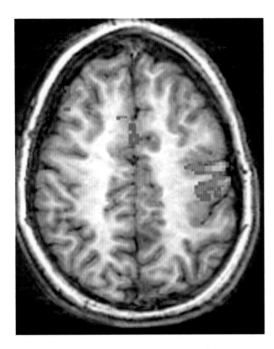

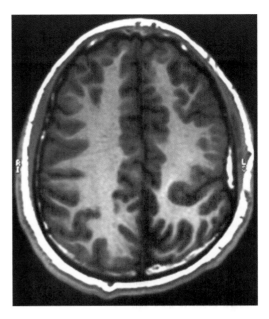

Figure 3.26 Young man with mild right hemiparesis and a history of focal seizures and atypical absences. Axial T1-weighted MRI. Polymicrogyria affecting the left hemisphere with verticalized sylvian fissure and irregular cortical folding in the perisylvian and rolandic cortex.

Figure 3.25 Adult man with focal epilepsy and left perisylvian and rolandic polymicrogyria. FMRI task-dependent (motor) increase of blood oxygen level-dependent signal in the motor cortex, indicating functional integrity of the polymicrogyric area.

healthy individuals. Functional MRI in such patients show that the polymicrogyric cortex tends to preserve functionality in the expected sites (Araujo et al. 2006) (Fig. 3.25). Large areas of polymicrogyric cortex, involving a whole hemisphere or a major portion of one hemisphere (unilateral hemispheric polymicrogyria), usually in the perisylvian region, are often associated with hypoplasia of the affected hemisphere (Fig. 3.26) and cerebral peduncle together with enlargement of the ipsilateral ventricle. This malformation may be associated with a specific clinical syndrome including seizures, hemiparesis, and mild to moderate cognitive impairment (Guerrini et al. 1998). Patients have continuous generalized EEG discharges during slow-wave sleep and suffer from partial motor, atonic, and atypical absence seizures with cognitive deterioration. The condition is usually detected between ages 2 and 10 years and may last for months to years.

Recently, different types of polymicrogyria as part of complex syndromes have been associated with pathogenic copy number variants in at least five new chromosomal loci (Table 3.2).

SCHIZENCEPHALY

Schizencephaly (cleft brain) consists of a full-thickness unilateral or bilateral cleft of the cerebral hemispheres with communication between the ventricle(s) and pericerebral subarachnoid space. The cortex surrounding

the cleft and the lips of the fissure is polymicrogyric (Ferrer 1984). The walls of the clefts may be widely separated (open-lip schizencephaly) (Fig. 3.27) or closely apposed (closed-lip schizencephaly). The clefts may be located in any region of the hemispheres, but are by far most common in the perisylvian area (Barkovich and Kjos 1992). Bilateral clefts are usually symmetrical in location but not necessarily in size. Unilateral clefts, especially if large, may be associated with a localized cortical abnormality in the contralateral hemisphere. It is difficult to establish at which time during embryonic development schizencephaly originates. There is no agreement as to whether it should be classified as a defect originating early, with localized errors in neuronal proliferation. The presence of polymicrogyric cortex, however, is the hallmark of a disorder of cortical layering that extends through late cortical organization. Although schizencephaly is usually sporadic, familial occurrence has been reported and a specific genetic origin is possible in some cases. Several sporadic patients and two siblings of both sexes harboring germline mutations in the homeobox gene *EMX2* have been described, but involvement of this gene has not been confirmed in large series (Merello et al. 2008). The possible pattern(s) of inheritance and the practical usefulness of *EMX2* mutation detection in an individual with schizencephaly are still unclear.

Clinical findings in schizencephaly include focal seizures, which are present in most patients (81% of cases in one large review), usually beginning before

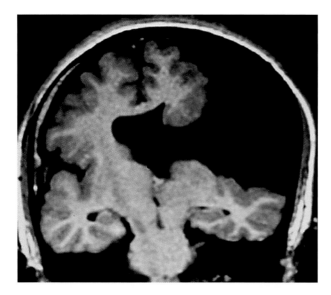

Figure 3.27 A 12-year-old boy with focal epilepsy and spastic quadriparesis, more severe on the right. Left-sided open-lip schizencephaly, lined by polymicrogyric cortex. Note the absence of the corticopontine tract on the left.

age 3 years if bilateral clefts are present. Bilateral clefts are usually associated with severe neurologic abnormalities, whereas unilateral schizencephaly is usually accompanied by hemiparesis or just detected after seizure onset in otherwise neurologically normal individuals.

Selected patients with unilateral schizencephaly have been treated with surgery for intractable epilepsy (Leblanc et al. 1996). Identifying anatomical landmarks of eloquent areas for planning surgical treatment can be particularly complex. Functional MRI studies and intracranial recordings are almost always necessary.

REFERENCES

Aicardi, J. 1996. Aicardi syndrome. In R. Guerrini, F. Andermann, R. Canapicchi, et al., eds. *Dysplasias of cerebral cortex and epilepsy*. Philadelphia/New York: Lippincott-Raven, 211–6.

Aligianis, I. A., C. A. Johnson, P. Gissen, et al. 2005. Mutations of the catalytic subunit of RAB3GAP cause Warburg Micro syndrome. *Nature Genetics* 37: 221–3.

Araujo, D., D. B. de Araujo, O. M. Pontes-Neto, et al. 2006. Language and motor fMRI activation in polymicrogyric cortex. *Epilepsia* 47: 589–92.

Ashburner, J., and K. J. Friston. 2000. Voxel-based morphometry: the methods. *Neuroimage* 11: 805–21.

Baala, L., S. Briault, H. C. Etchevers, et al. 2007. Homozygous silencing of T-box transcription factor EOMES leads to microcephaly with polymicrogyria and corpus callosum agenesis. *Nature Genetics* 39: 454–6.

Barkovich, A. J., and B. O. Kjos. 1992. Schizencephaly: correlation of clinical findings with MR characteristics. *AJNR American Journal of Neuroradiology* 13: 85–94.

Barkovich, A. J., R. Guerrini, G. Battaglia, et al. 1994. Band heterotopia: correlation of outcome with magnetic resonance imaging parameters. *Annals of Neurology* 36: 609–617.

Barkovich, A. J., R. I. Kuzniecky, G. D. Jackson, et al. 2001. Classification system for malformations of cortical development. *Neurology* 57: 2168–78.

Barkovich, A. J., R. I. Kuzniecky, G. D. Jackson, et al. 2005. A developmental and genetic classification for malformations of cortical development. *Neurology* 65: 1873–87.

Bast, T., G. Ramantani, A. Seitz, et al. 2006. Focal cortical dysplasia: prevalence, clinical presentation and epilepsy in children and adults. *Acta Neurologica Scandinavica* 113: 72–81.

Bastos, A. C., R. M. Comeau, F. Andermann, et al. 1999. Diagnosis of subtle focal dysplastic lesions: curvilinear reformatting from three-dimensional magnetic resonance imaging. *Annals of Neurology* 46: 88–94.

Baulac, M., N. De Grissac, D. Hasboun, et al. 1998. Hippocampal developmental changes in patients with partial epilepsy: magnetic resonance imaging and clinical aspects. *Annals of Neurology* 44: 223–33.

Bautista, J. F., N. Foldvary-Schaefer, W. E. Bingaman, et al. 2003. Focal cortical dysplasia and intractable epilepsy in adults: clinical, EEG, imaging and surgical features. *Epilepsy Research* 55: 131–6.

Becker, A. J., H. Urbach, B. Scheffler, et al. 2002. Focal cortical dysplasia of Taylor's balloon cell type: mutational analysis of the TSC1 gene indicates a pathogenic relationship to tuberous sclerosis. *Annals of Neurology* 52: 29–37.

Beltran-Valero de Bernabè, D., S. Currier, A. Steinbrecher, et al. 2002. Mutations in the O-mannosyltransferase gene POMT1 give rise to the severe neuronal migration disorder Walker-Warburg syndrome. *American Journal of Human Genetics* 71: 1033–43.

Beltran-Valero De Bernabe, D., H. van Bokhoven, E. van Beusekom, et al. 2003. A homozygous nonsense mutation in the Fukutin gene causes a Walker-Warburg syndrome phenotype. *Journal of Medical Genetics* 40: 845–8.

Beltran-Valero de Bernabè, D., T. Voit, C. Longman, et al. 2004. Mutations in the FKRP gene can cause muscle-eye-brain disease and Walker-Warburg syndrome. *Journal of Medical Genetics* 41: e61.

Bergin, P. S., Fish, D. R., Shorvon, S. D. et al. 1995. Magnetic resonance imaging in partial epilepsy: additional abnormalities shown with the fluid attenuated inversion recovery (FLAIR) pulse sequence. *Journal of Neurology Neurosurgery Psychiatry* 58: 439–43.

Bonneau, D., A. Toutain, A. Laquerriere, et al. 2002. X-linked lissencephaly with absent corpus callosum and ambiguous genitalia (XLAG): clinical, magnetic resonance imaging, and neuropathological findings. *Annals of Neurology* 51: 340–9.

Boycott, K. M., S. Flavelle, A. Bureau, et al. 2005. Homozygous deletion of the very low density lipoprotein receptor gene causes autosomal recessive cerebellar hypoplasia with cerebral gyral simplification. *American Journal of Human Genetics* 77: 477–83.

Bronen, R. A., K. P. Vives, I. H. Kim, et al. 1997. Focal cortical dysplasia of Taylor, balloon cell subtype: MR differentiation from low-grade tumors. *AJNR American Journal of Neuroradiology* 18: 1141–51.

Brooks, A. S., A. M. Bertoli-Avella, G. M. Burzynski, et al. 2005. Homozygous nonsense mutations in KIAA1279 are associated with malformations of the central and enteric nervous systems. *American Journal of Human Genetics* 77: 120–6.

Cardoso, C., R. J. Leventer, J. J. Dowling, et al. 2002. Clinical and molecular basis of classical lissencephaly: mutations in the LIS1 gene (PAFAH1B1). *Human Mutation* 19: 4–15.

Cardoso, C., R. J. Leventer, H. L. Ward, et al. 2003. Refinement of a 400-kb critical region allows genotypic differentiation between isolated lissencephaly, Miller- Dieker syndrome, and other phenotypes secondary to deletions of 17p13.3. *American Journal of Human Genetics* 72: 918–30.

Cardoso, C., A. Boys, E. Parrini, et al. 2008. Periventricular heterotopia, mental retardation, and epilepsy associated with 5q14.3–q15 deletion. *Neurology* 3: 784–92.

Chandra, P. S., N. Salamon, J. Huang, et al. 2006. FDG-PET/MRI coregistration and diffusion-tensor imaging distinguish epileptogenic tubers and cortex in patients with tuberous sclerosis complex: a preliminary report. *Epilepsia* 47: 1543–9.

Chugani, H. T., W. D. Shields, D. A. Shewmon, et al. 1990. Infantile spasms: I. PET identifies focal cortical dysgenesis in cryptogenic cases for surgical treatment. *Annals of Neurology* 27: 406–413.

Clarke, M. J., A. B. Foy, N. Wetjen, et al. 2006. Imaging characteristics and growth of subependymal giant cell astrocytomas. *Neurosurgery Focus* 20: E5.

Cohen, M., R. Campbell, and F. Yaghmai. 1989b. Neuropathological abnormalities in developmental dysphasia. *Annals of Neurology* 25: 567–70.

Cross, J. H., P. Jayakar, D. Nordli, et al. 2006. Proposed criteria for referral and evaluation of children for epilepsy surgery: recommendations of the submission for pediatric epilepsy surgery. *Epilepsia* 47: 952–9.

Curatolo, P., R. Bombardieri, and S. Jozwiak. 2008. Tuberous sclerosis. *Lancet* 372: 657–68.

Dabora, S. L., S. Jozwiak, D. N. Franz, et al. 2001. Mutational analysis in a cohort of 224 tuberous sclerosis patients indicates increased severity of TSC2, compared with TSC1, disease in multiple organs. *American Journal of Human Genetics* 68: 64–80.

Dabora, S. L., P. Roberts, A. Nieto, et al. 2002. Association between a high-expressing interferon-gamma allele and a lower frequency of kidney angiomyolipomas in TSC2 patients. *American Journal of Human Genetics* 71: 750–8.

D'agostino, M. D., A. Bastos, C. Piras, et al. 2004. Posterior quadrantic dysplasia of hemi-hemimegalencephaly: a characteristic brain malformation. *Neurology* 62: 2214–20.

Desbiens, R., S. F. Berkovic, F. Dubeau, et al. 1993. Life-threatening focal status epilepticus due to occult cortical dysplasia. *Archives of Neurology* 50: 695–700.

Devlin, A. M., J. H. Cross, W. Harkness, et al. 2003. Clinical outcome of hemispherectomy for epilepsy in childhood and adolescence. *Brain* 126: 556–66.

Di Rocco, C. 1996. Surgical treatment of hemimegalencephaly. In R. Guerrini, F. Andermann, R. Canapicchi, et al., eds. *Dysplasias of cerebral cortex and epilepsy.* Philadelphia/New York: Lippincott-Raven, 295–304.

Dobyns, W. B., R. A. Pagon, D. Armstrong, et al. 1989. Diagnostic criteria for Walker-Warburg syndrome. *American Journal of Medical Genetics* 32: 195–210.

Dobyns, W. B., C. L. Truwit, M. E. Ross, et al. 1999. Differences in gyral pattern distinguish chromosome 17-linked and X-linked lissencephaly. *Neurology* 53: 270–7.

Dobyns, W. B., G. Mirzaa, S. L. Christian, et al. 2008. Consistent chromosome abnormalities identify novel polymicrogyria loci in 1p36.3, 2p16.1–p23.1, 4q21.21–q22.1, 6q26–q27, and 21q2. *American Journal of Medical Genetics A* 146A: 1637–54.

Dubeau, F., D. Tampieri, N. Lee, et al. 1995. Periventricular and subcortical nodular heterotopia. A study of 33 patients. *Brain* 118: 1273–87.

Dulac, O., J-M. Pinard, and P. Plouin. 1996. Infantile spasms associated with cortical dysplasia and tuberous sclerosis. In R. Guerrini, F. Andermann, R. Canapicchi, et al., eds. *Dysplasias of cerebral cortex and epilepsy.* Philadelphia/New York: Lippincott-Raven, 217–25.

Eash, D., D. Waggoner, J. Chung, et al. 2005. Calibration of 6q subtelomere deletions to define genotype/phenotype correlations. *Clinical Genetics* 67: 396–403.

Englund, C., R. D. Folkerth, D. Born, et al. 2005. Aberrant neuronal-glial differentiation in Taylor-type focal cortical dysplasia (type IIA/B). *Acta Neuropathologica* 109(5): 519–33.

Eriksson, S. H., F. J. Rugg-Gunn, M. R. Symms, et al. 2001. Diffusion tensor imaging in patients with epilepsy and malformation of cortical development. *Brain* 124: 617–26.

Fauser, S., and A. Schulze-Bonhage. 2006. Epileptogenicity of cortical dysplasia in temporal lobe dual pathology: an electrophysiological study with invasive recordings. *Brain* 129: 82–95.

Ferland, R. J., J. N. Gaitanis, K. Apse, et al. 2006. Periventricular nodular heterotopia and Williams syndrome. *American Journal of Medical Genetics A* 140: 1305–11.

Ferland, R. J., and R. Guerrini. 2009. Nodular heterotopia is built upon layers. *Neurology* 73: 742–3.

Ferrer, I. 1984. A Golgi analysis of unlayered polymicrogyria. *Acta Neuropathologica* 65: 69–76.

Ferrer, I., M. Pineda, M. Tallada, et al. 1992. Abnormal local circuit neurons in epilepsia partialis continua associated with focal cortical dysplasia. *Acta Neuropathologica* 83: 647–52.

Fink, J. M., W. B. Dobyns, R. Guerrini, et al. 1997. Identification of a duplication of Xq28 associated with bilateral periventricular nodular heterotopia. *American Journal of Human Genetics* 61: 379–87.

Fox, J. W., E. D. Lamperti, Y. Z. Eksioglu, et al. 1998. Mutations in filamin 1 prevent migration of cerebral cortical neurons in human periventricular heterotopia. *Neuron* 21: 1315–25.

Fusco, L., S. Ferracuti, G. Fariello, et al. 1992. Hemimegalencephaly and normal intellectual development. *Journal of Neurology Neurosurgery & Psychiatry* 55: 720–722.

Garbelli, R., L. Rossini, R. F. Moroni, et al. 2009. Layer-specific genes reveal a rudimentary laminar pattern in human nodular heterotopia. *Neurology* 73: 746–53.

Gawlik-Kuklinska, K., J. Wierzba, A. Wozniak, et al. 2008. Periventricular heterotopia in a boy with interstitial deletion of chromosome 4p. *European Journal of Medical Genetics* 51: 165–171.

Gleeson, J. G., K. A. Allen, J. W. Fox, et al. 1998. Doublecortin, a brain-specific gene mutated in human X-linked lissencephaly and double cortex syndrome, encodes a putative signaling protein. *Cell* 92: 63–72.

Gleeson, J. G., R. F. Luo, P. E. Grant, et al. 2000a. Genetic and neuroradiological heterogeneity of double cortex syndrome. *Annals of Neurology* 47: 265–9.

Gleeson, J. G., S. Minnerath, R. I. Kuzniecky, et al. 2000b. Somatic and germline mosaic mutations in the doublecortin gene are associated with variable phenotypes. *American Journal of Human Genetics* 67: 574–81.

Glaser, T., L. Jepeal, J. G. Edwards, et al. 1994. PAX6 gene dosage effect in a family with congenital cataracts, aniridia, anophthalmia and central nervous system defects. *Nature Genetics* 7: 463–71.

Golden, J. A., and B. N. Harding. 2004. *Pathology & genetics developmental neuropathology.* Basel: ISN Neuropath Press.

Granata, T., E. Freri, C. Caccia, et al. 2005. Schizencephaly: clinical spectrum, epilepsy and pathogenesis. *Journal of Child Neurology* 20: 313–8.

Guerreiro, M. M., E. Andermann, R. Guerrini, et al. 2000. Familial perisylvian polymicrogyria: a new familial syndrome of cortical maldevelopment. *Annals of Neurology* 48: 39–48.

Guerrini, R., C. Dravet, C. Raybaud, et al. 1992a. Epilepsy and focal gyral anomalies detected by MRI: electroclinico-morphological correlations and follow-up. *Developmental Medicine & Child Neurology* 34: 706–18.

Guerrini, R., C. Dravet, C. Raybaud, et al. 1992b. Neurological findings and seizure outcome in children with bilateral opercular macrogyric-like changes detected by MRI. *Developmental Medicine & Child Neurology* 34: 694–705.

Guerrini, R., C. Dravet, M. Bureau, et al. 1996d. Diffuse and localised dysplasias of cerebral cortex: clinical presentation, outcome and proposal for a morphologic MRI classification based on a study of 90 patients. In R. Guerrini, F. Andermann, R. Canapicchi, et al., eds. *Dysplasias of cerebral cortex and epilepsy.* Philadephia/New York: Lippincott-Raven, 255–69.

Guerrini, R., F. Dubeau, O. Dulac, et al. 1997b. Bilateral parasagittal parietooccipital polymicrogyria and epilepsy. *Annals of Neurology* 41: 65–73.

Guerrini, R., P. Genton, M. Bureau, et al. 1998. Multilobar polymicrogyria, intractable drop attack seizures, and sleep-related electrical status epilepticus. *Neurology* 51: 504–12.

Guerrini, R., E. Anderman, M. Avoli, et al. 1999. Cortical dysplasias, genetics and epileptogenesis. *Advances in Neurology* 79: 95–121.

Guerrini, R., A. J. Barkovich, L. Sztriha, et al. 2000. Bilateral frontal polymicrogyria: a newly recognized brain malformation syndrome. *Neurology* 54: 909–13.

Guerrini, R., F. Moro, E. Andermann, et al. 2003. Nonsyndromic mental retardation and cryptogenic epilepsy in women with DCX mutations. *Annals of Neurology* 54: 30–7.

Guerrini, R., D. Mei, S. Sisodiya, et al. 2004. Germline and mosaic mutations of FLN1 in men with periventricular heterotopia. *Neurology* 63: 51–56.

Guerrini, R., and S. Pellacani. 2007. Infantile spasms and West syndrome: anatomo-electroclinical patterns and etiology. In F. Guzzetta, B. Dalla Bernardina, and R. Guerrini. *Progress in epileptic spasms and West syndrome.* John Libbey Eurotex, 23–41.

Guerrini, R., W. B, Dobyns, and J. A. Barkovich. 2008. Abnormal development of the human cerebral cortex: genetics, functional consequences and treatment options. *Trends in Neuroscience* 31: 153–6.

Guerrini, R., and E. Parrini. 2010. Neuronal migration disorders. *Neurobiology of Disease.* 38: 154–66.

Good, C. D., C. J. Price, K. J. Friston, et al. 2001. Voxel-based morphometric study of aeging in 465 normal adult humans brains. *Neuroimage* 14: 21–36.

Haltia, M., I. Leivo, H. Somer, et al. 1997. Muscle-eye-brain disease: a neuropathological study. *Annals of Neurology* 41: 173–80.

Hammers, A., M. J. Koepp, M. P. Richardson et al. 2001. Central benzodiazepine receptors in malformations of cortical development: a quantitative study. *Brain* 124: 1555–65.

Harding, B., and A. Copp. 1997. Malformations of the nervous system. In J. Graham and P. L. Lantons, eds, *Greenfield's neuropathology.* London-Melbourne-Auckland: Edward Arnold, 521–38.

Hehr, U., A. Hehr, G. Uyanik, et al. 2006. A filamin A splice mutation resulting in a syndrome of facial dysmorphism, periventricular nodular heterotopia, and severe constipation reminiscent of cerebro-fronto-facial syndrome. *Journal of Medical Genetics* 43: 541–4.

Hong, S. E., Y. Y. Shugart, D. T. Huang, et al. 2000. Autosomal recessive lissencephaly with cerebellar hypoplasia is associated with human RELN mutations. *Nature Genetics* 26: 93–96.

Hopkins, V., R. Sutton, R. A. Lewis, et al. 2008. Neuroimaging aspects of Aicardi syndrome. *American Journal of Medical Genetics A* 146: 2871–8.

Hosey, T., G. Williams, and R. Ansorge. 2005. Inference of multiple fiber orientations in high angular resolution diffusion imaging. *Magnetic Resonance in Medicine* 54: 1480–9.

Huppertz, H. J., C. Grim, S. Fauser, et al. 2005. Enhanced visualization of blurred grey-white matter junctions in focal cortical dysplasia by voxel-based 3D MRI analysis. *Epilepsy Research* 67: 35–40.

Huppertz, H. J., J. Wellmer, A. M. Staack, et al. 2008. Voxel-based 3D MRI analysis helps to detect subtle forms of subcortical band heterotopia. *Epilepsia* 49: 772–85.

Huppertz, H. J., M. Kurthen, J. Kassubek, et al. 2009. Voxel-based 3D MRI analysis for the detection of epileptogenic lesion at single subject level. *Epilepsia* 50: 155–6.

Jaglin, X. H., K. Poirier, Y. Saillour, et al. 2009. Mutations in the beta-tubulin gene TUBB2B result in asymmetrical polymicrogyria. *Nature Genetics* May 24.

Jansen, F. E., A. C. van Huffelen, A. Algra, et al. 2007. Epilepsy surgery in tuberous sclerosis: a systematic review. *Epilepsia* 48: 1477–84.

Jin, Z., I. Tietjen, L. Bu, et al. 2007. Disease-associated mutations affect GPR56 protein trafficking and cell surface expression. *Human Molecular Genetics* 16: 1972–85.

Kagawa, K., D. C. Chugani, E. Asano, et al. 2005. Epilepsy surgery outcome in children with tuberous sclerosis complex evaluated with alpha-[11C]methyl-L-tryptophan positron emission tomography (PET). *Journal of Child Neurology* 20: 429–38.

Kantarci, S., L. Al-Gazali, R. S. Hill, et al. 2007. Mutations in LRP2, which encodes the multiligand receptor megalin, cause Donnai–Barrow and facio-oculo-acoustico-renal syndromes. *Nature Genetics* 39: 957–9.

Karadag, D., H. J. Mentzel, D. Güllmar, et al. 2005. Diffusion tensor imaging in children and adolescents with tuberous sclerosis. *Pediatric Radiology* 35: 980–3.

Kassubek, W. M., S. Ziyeh, a. Schulze-Bonhage, et al. 2003. Automated detection of grey matter malformations using optimized voxel-based morphometry: a systematic approach. *Neuroimage* 20: 330–43.

Kato, M., S. Das, K. Petras, et al. 2004. Mutations of ARX are associated with striking pleiotropy and consistent genotype-phenotype correlation. *Human Mutation* 23: 147–59.

Keller, S. S., and N. Roberts. 2008. Voxel-based morphometry of temporal lobe epilepsy: an introduction and review of the literature. *Epilepsia* 49: 741–57.

King, M., J. B. P. Stephenson, M. Ziervogel, et al. 1985. Hemimegalencephaly A case for hemispherectomy. *Neuropediatrics* 16: 46–55.

Knake, S., C. Trianatfyllou, L. I. Wald, et al. 2005. 3T phased array MRI improves the presurgical evaluation in focal epilepsies: a prospective study. *Neurology* 65: 1026–31.

Kobayashi, K., Y. Nakahori, M. Miyake et al. 1998. An ancient retrotransposal insertion causes Fukuyama type congenital muscular dystrophy. *Nature* 394: 388–392.

Kondo-Iida, E., K. Kobayashi, M. Watanabe, et al. 1999. Novel mutations and genotypephenotype relationships in 107 families with Fukuyama-type congenital muscular dystrophy (FCMD). *Hum Mol Genet* 8: 2303–9.

Krsek, P., B. Maton, P. Jayakar, et al. 2009. Incomplete resection of cortical dysplasia is the main predictor of poor postsurgical outcome. *Neurology* 72: 217–23.

Kuzniecky, R., F. Andermann, D. Melanson, et al. 1988. Focal cortical myoclonus and rolandic cortical dysplasia: Clarification by magnetic resonance imaging. *Annals of Neurology* 23: 317–25.

Kuzniecky, R., and R. Powers. 1993. Epilepsia partialis continua due to cortical dysplasia. *Journal of Child Neurology* 8: 386–388.

Kuzniecky, R., F. Andermann, and R. Guerrini. 1993. Congenital bilateral perisylvian syndrome: study of 31 patients. The CBPS Multicenter Collaborative Study. *Lancet* 341: 608–12.

Kuzniecky, R. I. 1996. MRI in focal cortical dysplasia. In R. Guerrini, F. Andermann, R. Canapicchi, et al., eds. *Dysplasias of cerebral cortex and epilepsy.* Philadelphia/New York: Lippincott-Raven, 145–50.

Lamparello, P., M. Baybis, J. Pollard, et al. 2007. Developmental lineage of cell types in cortical dysplasia with balloon cells. *Brain* 130: 2267–76.

Lange, M., B. Winner, J. L. Müller, et al. 2004. Functional imaging in periventricular nodule heterotopy caused by a new FilaminA mutation. *Neurology* 62: 151–2.

Leblanc, R., E. Meyer, R. Zatorre, et al. 1996. Functional imaging of cerebral arteriovenous malformations with a comment on cortical reorganization. *Neurosurgery Focus* 1: e4.

Lee, S. K., D. I. Kim, S. Mori, et al. 2004. Diffusion tensor MRI visualizes decreased subcortical fiber connectivity in focal cortical dysplasia. *Neuroimage* 22: 1826–9.

Lerner, J. T., N. Salamon, J. S. Hauptman, et al. 2009. Assessment and surgical outcomes for mild type I and severe type II cortical dysplasia: a critical review and the UCLA experience. *Epilepsia* Jan 19.

Leventer, R. J., C. Cardoso, D. H. Ledbetter, et al. 2001. LIS1 missense mutations cause milder lissencephaly phenotypes including a child with normal IQ. *Neurology* 57: 416–22.

Longman, C., M. Brockington, S. Torelli, et al. 2003. Mutations in the human LARGE gene cause MDC1D, a novel form of congenital muscular dystrophy with severe mental retardation and abnormal glycosylation of a-dystroglycan. *Human Molecular Genetics* 12: 2853–61.

Mai, R., L. Tassi, M. Cossu, et al. 2003. A neuropathological, stereo-EEG, and MRI study of subcortical band heterotopia. *Neurology* 60: 1834–8.

Makki, M. I., D. C. Chugani, J. Janisse, et al. 2007. Characteristics of abnormal diffusivity in normal-appearing white matter investigated with diffusion tensor MR imaging in tuberous sclerosis complex. *AJNR American Journal of Neuroradiology* 28: 1662–7.

Matsumoto, N., R. J. Leventer, J. A. Kuc, et al. 2001. Mutation analysis of the DCX gene and genotype/phenotype correlation in subcortical band heterotopia. *European Journal of Human Genetics* 9: 5–12.

Mattia, D., A. Olivier, and M. Avoli. 1995. Seizure-like discharges recorded in the human dysplastic neocortex maintained in vitro. *Neurology* 45: 1391–5.

Mei, D., E. Parrini, M. Pasqualetti, et al. 2007. Multiplex ligation-dependent probe amplification detects DCX gene deletions in band heterotopia. *Neurology* 68: 446–50.

Mei, D., R. Lewis, E. Parrini, et al. 2008. High frequency of genomic deletions—and a duplication—in the LIS1 gene in lissencephaly: implications for molecular diagnosis. *Journal of Medical Genetics* 45: 355–61.

Merello, E., E. Swanson, P. De Marco, et al. 2008. No major role for the EMX2 gene in schizencephaly. *American Journal of Medical Genetics A* 146A: 1142–50.

Minassian, B. A., H. Otsubo, S. Weiss, et al. 1999. Magnetoencephalographic localization in pediatric epilepsy surgery: comparison of noninvasive intracranial electroencephalography. *Annals of Neurology* 46: 627–33.

Molina, J. A., F. Mateos, M. Merino, et al. 1989. Aicardi syndrome in two sisters. *Journal of Pediatrics* 115: 282–283.

Moro, F., T. Pisano, B. D. Bernardina, et al. 2006. Periventricular heterotopia in fragile X syndrome. *Neurology* 67: 713–5.

Munari, C., S. Francione, P. Kahane, et al. 1996. Usefulness of stereo EEG investigations in partial epilepsy associated with cortical dysplastic lesions and gray matter heterotopia. In R. Guerrini, F. Andermann, R. Canapicchi, et al., eds. *Dysplasias of cerebral cortex and epilepsy.* Philadelphia/New York: Lippincott-Raven, 383–94.

Najm, I. M., C. Tilelli, and R. Oghlakian. 2007. Pathophysiological mechanisms of focal cortical dysplasia: a critical review of human tissue studies and animal models. *Epilepsia* 48: 21–32.

Neal, J., K. Apse, M. Sahin, et al. 2006. Deletion of chromosome 1p36 is associated with periventricular nodular heterotopia. *American Journal of Medical Genetics A* 140: 1692–5.

Nowaczyk, M. J., I. E. Teshima, J. Siegel-Bartelt, et al. 1997. Deletion 4q21/4q22 syndrome: two patients with de novo 4q21.3q23 and 4q13.2q23 deletions. *American Journal of Medical Genetics* 69: 400–5.

Olivier, A., F. Andermann, A. Palmini, et al. 1996. Surgical treatment of the cortical dysplasias. In R. Guerrini, F. Andermann, R. Canapicchi, et al., eds. *Dysplasias of cerebral cortex and epilepsy.* Philadelphia/New York: Lippincott-Raven, 351–66.

Otsubo, H., A. Ochi, I. Elliot, et al. 2001. MEG predicts epileptic zone in lesional extrahippocampal epilepsy: 12 pediatric surgery cases. *Epilepsia* 42: 1523–30.

Paladin, F., C. Chiron, O. Dulac, et al. 1989. Electro-encephalographic aspects of hemimegalencephaly. *Developmental Medicine & Child Neurology* 31: 377–383.

Palmini, A., F. Andermann, A. Olivier, et al. 1991b. Focal neuronal migration disorders and intractable partial epilepsy: Results of surgical treatment. *Annals of Neurology* 30: 750–7.

Palmini, A., F. Andermann, A. Olivier, et al. 1991c. Focal neuronal migration disorders and intractable partial epilepsy: A study of 30 patients. *Annals of Neurology* 30: 741–9.

Palmini, A., A. Gambardella, F. Andermann, et al. 1995. Intrinsic epileptogenicity of human dysplastic cortex as suggested by corticography and surgical results. *Annals of Neurology* 37: 476–87.

Palmini, A., I. Najm, G. Avanzini, et al. 2004. Terminology and classification of the cortical dysplasias. *Neurology* 62: S2–8.

Papanicolaou, A. C., E. Pataraia, R. Billingsley-Marshall, et al. 2005. Toward the substitution of invasive electro-encephalography in epilepsy surgery. *Journal of Clinical Neurophysiology* 22: 231–7.

Perrin, M., C. Poupon, B. Rieul, et al. 2005. Validation of q-ball imaging with a diffusion fibre-crossing phantom on a clinical scanner. *Philosophical Transactions of the Royal Society of London B Biological Sciences* 360: 881–91.

Parrini, E., A. Ramazzotti, W. B. Dobyns, et al. 2006. Periventricular heterotopia: phenotypic heterogeneity and correlation with Filamin A mutations. *Brain* 129: 1892–906.

Phal, P. M., A. Usmanov, G. M. Nesbit, et al. 2008. Qualitative comparison of 3-T and 1.5-T MRI in the evaluation of epilepsy. *AJR American Journal of Roentgenology* 191: 890–5.

Piao, C., A. Yu, K. Li, et al. 2009. Cerebral diffusion tensor imaging in tuberous sclerosis. *European Journal of Radiology* 71: 249–52.

Piao, X., R. S. Hill, A. Bodell, et al. 2004. G protein-coupled receptor dependent development of human frontal cortex. *Science* 303: 2033–6.

Piao, X., B. S. Chang, A. Bodell, et al. 2005. Genotype-phenotype analysis of human frontoparietal polymicrogyria syndromes. *Annals of Neurology* 58: 680–7.

Pinard, J. M., A. Feydy, R. Carlier, et al. 2000. Functional MRI in double cortex: Functionality of heterotopia. *Neurology* 54: 1531–3.

Pinto-Gama, H. P., A. J. da Rocha, F. T. Braga, et al. 2006. Comparative analysis of MRI sequences to detect structural brain lesions in tuberous sclerosis. *Pediatric Radiology* 36: 119–25.

Poirier, K., D. A. Keays, F. Francis, et al. 2007. Large spectrum of lissencephaly and pachygyria phenotypes resulting from de novo missense mutations in tubulin a 1A (TUBA1A). *Human Mutation* 28: 1055–64.

Poussaint, T. Y., J. W. Fox, W. B. Dobyns, et al. 2000. Periventricular nodular heterotopia in patients with filamin-1 gene mutations: neuroimaging findings. *Pediatric Radiology* 30: 748–55.

Pulsifer, M. D., J. Brandt, C. F. Salorio, et al. 2004. The cognitive outcome of hemispherectomy in 71 children. *Epilepsia* 45: 243–54.

Quirk, J. A., B. Kendall, D. P. E. Kingsley, et al. 1993. EEG features of cortical dysplasia in children. *Neuropediatrics* 24: 193–9.

Ribeiro Mdo, C., S. Gama de Sousa, M. M. Freitas, et al. 2007. Bilateral perisylvian polymicrogyria and chromosome 1 anomaly. *Pediatric Neurology* 36: 418–20.

Robain, O., C. Floquet, H. Heldt, et al. 1988. Hemimegalencephaly: A clinicopathological study of four cases. *Neuropathology & Applied Neurobiology* 14: 125–35.

Robain, O., and A. Gelot. 1996. Neuropathology of hemimegalencephaly. In R. Guerrini, F. Andermann, R. Canapicchi, et al., eds. *Dysplasias of cerebral cortex and epilepsy.* Philadelphia/New York: Lippincott-Raven, 89–92.

Robain, O. 1996b. Introduction to the pathology of cerebral cortical dysplasia. In R. Guerrini, F. Andermann, R. Canapicchi, et al., eds. *Dysplasias of cerebral cortex and epilepsy.* Philadelphia/New York: Lippincott-Raven, 1–9.

Robin, N. H., C. J. Taylor, D. M. McDonald-McGinn, et al. 2006. Polymicrogyria and deletion 22q11.2 syndrome: window to the etiology of a common cortical malformation. *American Journal of Medical Genetics A* 140: 2416–25.

Roll, P., G. Rudolf, S. Pereira, et al. 2006. SRPX2 mutations in disorders of language cortex and cognition. *Human Molecular Genetics* 15: 1195–207.

Salamon, N., B. A. Kung, S. J. Shaw, et al. 2008. FDG-PET/MRI coregistration improves detection of cortical dysplasia in patients with epilepsy. *Neurology* 71: 1594–601.

Salmenpera, T. M., M. R. Symms, F. J. Rugg-Gunn, et al. 2007. Evaluation of quantitative magneting resonance imaging contrast in MRI-negative refractory focal epilepsy. *Epilepsia* 48: 229–37.

Schäuble, B., and G. D. Cascino. 2003. Advances in neuroimaging: management of partial epileptic syndromes. *Neurosurgical Review* 26: 233–46.

Scherer, C., S. Schuele, L. Minotti, et al. 2005. Intrinsic epileptogenicity of an isolated periventricular nodular heterotopia. *Neurology* 65: 495–6.

Sheen, V. L., J. W. Wheless, A. Bodell, et al. 2003. Periventricular heterotopia associated with chromosome 5p anomalies. *Neurology* 60: 1033–6.

Sheen, V. L., V. S. Ganesh, M. Topcu, et al. 2004. Mutations in ARFGEF2 implicate vesicle trafficking in neural progenitor proliferation and migration in the human cerebral cortex. *Nature Genetics* 36: 69–76.

Sicca, F., A. Kelemen, P. Genton, et al. 2003. Mosaic mutations of the LIS1 gene cause subcortical band heterotopia. *Neurology* 61: 1042–6.

Silan, F., M. Yoshioka, K. Kobayashi, et al. 2003. A new mutation of the Fukutin gene in a non-Japanese patient. *Annals of Neurology* 53: 392–396.

Sisodiya, S. M., S. Free, D. R. Fish, et al. 1999. Novel magnetic resonance imaging methods for quantifying changes in the cortical ribbon in patients with epilepsy. *Advances in Neurology* 81: 81–7.

Sisodiya, S. M., S. L. Free, J. M. Stevens, et al. 1995. Widespread cerebral structural changes in patients with cortical dysgenesis and epilepsy. *Brain* 118: 1039–50.

Spreafico, R., G. Battaglia, P. Arcelli, et al. 1998. Cortical dysplasia: an immunocytochemical study of three patients. *Neurology* 50: 27–36.

Sprecher, E., A. Ishida-Yamamoto, M. Mizrahi-Koren, et al. 2005. A mutation in SNAP29, coding for a SNARE protein involved in intracellular trafficking, causes a novel neurocutaneous syndrome characterized by cerebral dysgenesis, neuropathy, ichthyosis, and palmoplantar keratoderma. *American Journal of Human Genetics* 77: 242–51.

Takada, K., L. E. Becker, and F. Chan. 1988. Aberrant dendritic development in the human agyric cortex: a quantitative and qualitative Golgi study of two cases. *Clinical Neuropathology* 7: 111–9.

Takanashi, J., and A. J. Barkovich. 2003. The changing MR imaging appearance of polymicrogyria: a consequence of myelination. *AJNR American Journal of Neuroradiology* 24: 788–93.

Tassi, L., N. Colombo, R. Garbelli, et al. 2002. Focal cortical dysplasia: neuropathological subtypes, EEG, neuroimaging and surgical outcome. *Brain* 125: 1719–32.

Tassi, L., N. Colombo, M. Cossu, et al. 2005. Electroclinical, MRI and neuropathological study of 10 patients with nodular heterotopia, with surgical outcomes. *Brain* 128: 321–37.

Taylor, D. C., and B. D. Bower. 1971. Prevention in epileptic disorders. *Lancet* 2: 1136–8.

ten Donkelaar, H. J. 2006. Development and developmental disorders of the human cerebellum. In H. J. ten Donkelaar, et al., eds. *Clinical neuroembryology*. Springer, 309–44.

Tietjen, I., A. Bodell, K. Apse, et al. 2007. Comprehensive EMX2 genotyping of a large schizencephaly case series. *American Journal of Medical Genetics A* 143: 1313–6.

Tijam, A. T., S. Stefenko, V. W. D. Schenk, et al. 1978. Infantile spasms associated with hemihypsarrhythmia and hemimegalencephaly. *Developmental Medicine & Child Neurology* 20: 779–98.

Trounce, J. Q., N. Rutter, and D. H. Mellor. 1991. Hemimegalencephaly: diagnosis and treatment. *Developmental Medicine & Child Neurology* 33: 257–66.

Urbach, H., J. Hattingen, J. von Oertzen, et al. 2004. MR imaging in the presurgical workup of patients with drug-resistant epilepsy. *AJNR American Journal of Neuroradiology* 25: 919–26.

Van Bogaert, P., C. Donner, P. David, et al. 1996. Congenital bilateral perisylvian syndrome in a monozygotic twin with intra-uterine death of the co-twin. *Developmental Medicine & Child Neurology* 38: 166–71.

van Reeuwijk, J., M. Janssen, C. van den Elzen, et al. 2005. POMT2 mutations cause a-dystroglycan hypoglycosylation and Walker-Warburg syndrome. *Journal of Medical Genetics* 42: 907–12.

van Reeuwijk, J., S. Maugenre, C. van den Elzen, et al. 2006. The expanding phenotype of POMT1 mutations: from Walker-Warburg syndrome to congenital muscular dystrophy, microcephaly, and mental retardation. *Human Mutation* 27: 453–9.

Vigevano, F., E. Bertini, R. Boldrini, et al. 1989a. Hemimegalencephaly and intractable epilepsy: benefits of hemispherectomy. *Epilepsia* 30: 833–43.

Vigevano, F., L. Fusco, T. Granata, et al. 1996. Hemimegalencephaly: clinical and EEG characteristics. In R. Guerrini, F. Andermann, R. Canapicchi, et al., eds. *Dysplasias of cerebral cortex and epilepsy*. Philadelphia/New York: Lippincott-Raven, 285–294.

Villard, L., K. Nguyen, C. Cardoso, et al. 2002. A locus for bilateral perisylvian polymicrogyria maps to Xq28. *American Journal of Human Genetics* 70: 1003–8.

Villemure, J. G., and C. R. Mascon. 1995. Peri-insular hemispherotomy: surgical principles and anatomy. *Neurosurgery* 37: 975–81.

Wilke, M., J. Kassubek, S. Ziyeh, et al. 2003. Automated detection of gray matter malformations using optimised voxel-based morphometry: a systematic approach. *Neuroimage* 20: 330–43.

Widjaja, E., H. Otsubo, C. Raybaud, et al. 2008. Characteristics of MEG and MRI between Taylor's focal cortical dysplasia (type II) and other cortical dysplasia: surgical outcome after complete resection of MEG spike source and MR lesion in paediatric cortical dysplasia. *Epilepsy Research* 82: 147–55.

Widjaja, E., S. Z. Mahmoodabadi, H. Otsubo, et al. 2009. Subcortical alteration in tissue microstructure adjacent to focal cortical dysplasia: detection at diffusion-tensor MR imaging by using magnetoencephalographic dipole cluster localization. *Radiology* 251: 206–15.

Woermann, F. G., and C. Vollmar. 2009. Clinical MRI in children and adults with focal epilepsy: a critical review. *Epilepsy & Behaviour* 15: 40–9.

Wu, J. Y., W. W. Sutherling, S. Koh, et al. 2006. Magnetic source imaging localizes epileptogenic zone in children with tuberous sclerosis complex. *Neurology* 25: 1270–2.

Yao, G., X. N. Chen, L. Flores-Sarnat, et al. 2006. Deletion of chromosome 21 disturbs human brain morphogenesis. *Genet Med* 8: 1–7.

Ying, Z., J. Gonzales-Martinez, C. Tilelli C, et al. 2005. Expression of neuroal stem cell surface marker CD133 in balloon cells of human focal cortical dysplasia. *Epilepsia* 46: 1716–23.

Zaki, M., M. Shehab, A. A. El-Aleem, et al. 2007. Identification of a novel recessive RELN mutation using a homozygous balanced reciprocal translocation. *American Journal of Medical Genetics A* 143: 939–44.

Zollino, M., C. Colosimo, O. Zuffardi, et al. 2003. Cryptic t(1;12)(q44;p13.3) translocation in a previously described syndrome with polymicrogyria, segregating as an apparently X-linked trait. *American Journal of Medical Genetics A* 117: 65–71.

Chapter *4*

MAGNETIC RESONANCE SPECTROSCOPY
Hoby Hetherington

INTRODUCTION

Unlike standard magnetic resonance imaging (MRI) studies, which are based on the amount of water and differences in the cellular environment of the water, magnetic resonance spectroscopy (MRS) focuses on providing measures of small low-concentration mobile metabolites. In the presence of a magnetic field, molecules with nuclei that have non-zero nuclear spin (such as ^{1}H or ^{31}P) absorb and emit radiofrequency signals. These signals have varying frequencies, depending upon the nucleus (^{1}H or ^{31}P) and the type of chemical bonds present. Thus, MRS allows different chemical compounds to be identified by their unique fingerprint of frequencies. In the field of organic chemistry, MRS is routinely used to determine the presence, purity, and structure of the sample of interest. In biochemistry, the interaction of adjacent amino acid residues is used to help identify the structure of different proteins. With the development of wide-bore magnets capable of accommodating humans, MRS has been extended to studies of a variety of organs in the body, including the brain.

To date, most clinical ^{1}H spectroscopy studies applied in evaluating epilepsy have focused on *decreases* in N-acetyl aspartate (NAA), a compound synthesized only in neuronal mitochondria, to identify regions of neuronal loss and injury (Cendes et al. 1994; Connelly et al. 1994; Constantinidis et al. 1996; Hetherington et al. 1995; Hugg et al. 1993; Ng et al. 1994). *Increases* in total creatine (both phosphorylated and non-phosphorylated forms) and choline have been interpreted as reflecting gliosis and altered membrane turnover. In temporal lobe epilepsy (TLE), where neuronal loss and reactive gliosis are common findings, decreases in NAA and/or increases in creatine and choline have been shown to have lateralization sensitivities as high as 97% (Kuzniecky et al. 1998). ^{31}P spectroscopic measurements provide in vivo concentrations of phosphocreatine (PCr), ATP, and inorganic phosphate along with intracellular pH to yield a measure of bioenergetic status. In patients with mesial TLE, PCr levels are reduced (Chu et al. 1996, 1998; Pan et al. 2005) and correlate with the degree of injury as reflected by the degree of gliosis. Finally, using more sophisticated acquisition methods, intracellular levels of glutamate and GABA can be measured, providing a window into neurotransmitter metabolism.

In this chapter, we review the role of MRS as a clinical tool in identifying and characterizing epileptic foci and monitoring the response to antiepileptic medications and resective surgery. We then discuss the biological and clinical significance of these findings and their relevance to the pathophysiology of seizure disorders. We will also identify and discuss some of the technical hurdles that must be accounted for in acquiring and accurately interpreting in vivo MRS data. Finally, we will discuss the potential advantages of new technologies in extending the utility of MRS in epilepsy and their unique hurdles.

¹H MRS AND SPECTROSCOPIC IMAGING

Unlike MRS studies of small aqueous samples as carried out by biochemists and chemists, in vivo measurements of the human brain require some form of spatial localization so as to link a metabolic profile with a specific anatomical structure. Depending upon the methods and hardware used, the spatial resolution of these measurements range from a few tens of cubic centimeters (cc) to several hundred microliters. To achieve spatial localization of the signal, a variety of techniques based on the concepts used in MRI have been developed to select specific regions of the brain. Most of these utilize spatially selective excitation and refocusing pulses to acquire a single three-dimensional volume, typically 1 to 8 cc. More recently, spectroscopic imaging methods have been developed that allow spectra from multiple locations to be acquired simultaneously (i.e., imaged), thus displaying metabolic images (Fig. 4.1). These methods provide a highly efficient method for probing focal changes in metabolism that are characteristic of epileptogenic brain regions.

¹H SPECTROSCOPY AND TLE

In the mid-1990s a number of investigators from different laboratories demonstrated the sensitivity of MRS measurements of NAA for the lateralization of the epileptogenic region in patients with TLE (Cendes et al. 1994; Connelly et al. 1994; Constantinidis et al. 1996; Hetherington et al. 1995; Hugg et al. 1993; Ng et al. 1994). Specifically, changes in NAA content (Hugg et al. 1993) and its ratio to other metabolites such as creatine, NAA/Cr (Cendes et al. 1994; Constantinidis et al. 1996; Hetherington et al. 1995); choline, NAA/Ch (Ng et al. 1994); and the sum of creatine and choline, NAA/(Cr+Ch) (Connelly et al. 1994), were used to lateralize the seizure focus in patients with intractable TLE (Fig. 4.2). As a lateralization and localization tool, the reported sensitivities have ranged from 60% (Connelly et al. 1994) to 97% (Kuzniecky et al. 1998), somewhat higher than the 70% to 80% typically reported for conventional MRI studies. For example, Chu et al. (2000) reported that MR spectroscopic imaging when combined with tissue segmentation correctly lateralized the epileptogenic hippocampus in patients without MRI detectable volumetric loss. The ability of MRS to attain higher sensitivities in comparison to standard imaging is most likely the result of the following factors: (1) the metabolic perturbation seen in TLE is widespread, affecting not only the hippocampus (3 to 4 cc in volume)

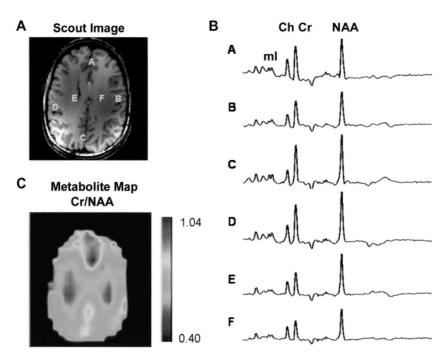

Figure 4.1 (A) Scout image acquired at 7T of a human brain with six loci identified (A–F). (B) Spectra from these six loci, including the resonances of myoinositol (mI), choline (Ch), creatine (Cr), and N-acetyl aspartate (NAA). (C) Map of the ratio of Cr/NAA.

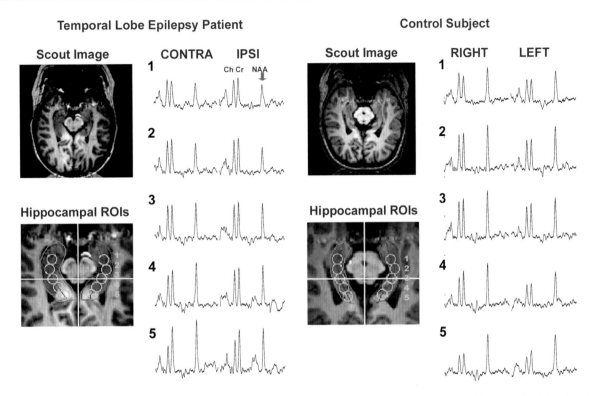

Figure 4.2 Data acquired at 4T from the hippocampi of a patient with temporal lobe epilepsy (left) and a healthy control subject (right). The locations of five spectra along each hippocampus are identified by yellow circles. The spectra from these loci are displayed. Note the substantial declines in NAA/Cr from the ipsilateral hippocampus in the epilepsy patient in comparison to the control subject.

but also surrounding temporal gray and white matter, and (2) detectable decreases in hippocampal volume by conventional MRI may require neuronal losses of up to 50%. Thus, for TLE, where the effects of the disease are macroscopic and sub-millimeter spatial resolution is not required, the biochemical specificity afforded by spectroscopy can provide significant advantages over higher spatial resolution measurements of tissue water.

In addition to providing a highly sensitive method for lateralizing the seizure focus, spectroscopic imaging studies may also provide some predictive insight as to surgical outcome. Notably, among the patients classified as having unilateral TLE, based on EEG measurements, some 40% to 50% have significant decreases in NAA in the contralateral hemisphere (Chu et al. 2000; Connelly et al. 1994; Ende et al. 1997; Hetherington et al. 1995; Ng et al. 1994). These data indicate that although the seizures may emanate from one hippocampus, the effects are clearly manifesting themselves in the contralateral hemisphere. In one study (Kuzniecky et al. 1999), the severity of NAA/Cr alterations in the ipsilateral and contralateral hippocampi were compared with surgical outcome. Although the severity of NAA/Cr abnormality in the ipsilateral hippocampus did not appear to have a significant impact on surgical outcome, more severe

alterations in the contralateral hippocampus were associated with poorer surgical outcomes (i.e., continuing seizures). Similarly, another study (Suhy et al. 2002) reported that in MRI-negative patients, the presence of more severe reductions in NAA in the contralateral hippocampus also correlated with worse outcomes following surgery. Finally, in patients with bilateral disease, poorer surgical outcomes were again associated with the presence of more severe reductions in the contralateral hippocampus (Li et al. 2000). Thus, the presence of MRS abnormalities in the presence or absence of MRI defects in the contralateral temporal lobe is predictive of poorer surgical outcomes.

NAA AND NEOCORTICAL EPILEPSY

The finding of decreased NAA is not solely restricted to TLE. In particular, reduced NAA levels have been reported in a variety of epileptic subtypes, including frontal lobe epilepsy (Garcia et al. 1997; Lundbom et al. 2001) as well as malformations of cortical development (Kuzniecky et al. 1997; Li et al. 1998). Unlike subjects with TLE, who often have well-defined foci, patients with neocortical epilepsy often have poorly defined epileptogenic regions and may have no accompanying MRI abnormality. This poses significant additional demands with regard to data acquisition and analysis. In addition to evaluating the observed ratios of NAA, Cr, and Ch in hundreds (or thousands) of locations, natural tissue-specific alterations must also be considered. For example, as seen in Figure 4.1, white matter concentrations of Cr have been reported to be ~6 mM (Hetherington et al. 1996; Michaelis et al. 1993), while gray matter values are ~8 to 9 mM. Also, variations in the content of these same compounds have been reported between different lobes (Wiedermann et al. 2001). Thus, depending upon the location of the region of interest and its mixture of gray and white matter, the "normal" levels of these metabolites will vary and complicate the detection of "abnormal" regions.

To overcome the effects of tissue heterogeneity, some investigators have used linear regression analyses to compensate for the inclusion of varying levels of gray and white matter. Although these methods are most commonly used in global pathologies to identify specific alterations of gray or white matter in comparison to control subjects, they can also be used on a voxel-by-voxel basis within subjects (Chu et al. 2000). Using segmented anatomical images, the gray and white matter content of each spectroscopic imaging voxel can be determined. From these data a regression analysis can be performed in healthy volunteers to obtain the "pure" gray and white matter metabolite contents and ratios (Fig. 4.3). Using the population statistics of these data, the probability that any voxel of specific gray and white matter content in a patient is abnormal can be calculated (Chu et al. 2000). Voxels that are statistically abnormal ($p < 0.05$) can then be color-coded according to p value and superimposed on the anatomical images for easy evaluation and interpretation (Fig. 4.3). Chu et al. (2000) have demonstrated that when this regression-based statistical method with image segmentation is used in patients with TLE, false-negative findings and incorrect lateralizations are reduced in comparison to simple left–right voxel comparisons.

NAA AND EPILEPTOGENIC NETWORKS

The presence of decreased NAA in patients with TLE is also not restricted to the temporal lobe, and reductions in NAA have been reported in the frontal and parietal lobes (Vermathen et al. 2003). Using corrections for tissue content, Mueller et al. (2004) identified increased numbers of metabolically abnormal pixels in the parietal and frontal lobes of patients with mesial TLE. Further, ~28% of the pixels from the ipsilateral insula were metabolically abnormal (Mueller et al. 2004). Notably, hippocampal abnormalities are

also frequently seen in patients with neocortical epilepsy (Mueller et al. 2006). These abnormalities may arise due to true pathology or may reflect the distributed nature of injury in epilepsy. Using positron emission tomography (PET), a number of investigators have reported that the thalamus may show decreased glucose metabolism in TLE (Benedek et al. 2004; Dlugos et al. 1999). This suggested the possibility of a network of metabolic disturbances associated with temporal lobe seizures, involving the thalamus. To evaluate the relationship between various components of the macroscopic network, individual loci within the hippocampus, thalamus, and basal ganglia were averaged and a correlation analysis was then performed to evaluate relationships between the ipsilateral and contralateral hippocampi with the other structures (Hetherington et al. 2007) (Fig. 4.4). This analysis identified highly significant correlations in decrements in NAA/Cr between the ipsilateral hippocampus and the bilateral thalami and basal ganglia. An exceptionally strong correlation was detected between the ipsilateral hippocampus and the anterior thalamus ($R = +0.76$, $p < 1 \times 10^{-5}$). The contralateral hippocampus showed generally weaker correlations and primarily with ipsilateral structures (ipsilateral hippocampus, ipsilateral anterior thalamus, and ipsilateral putamen). The only significant correlation within the same hemisphere for the contralateral hippocampus was the correlation with the contralateral anterior thalamus ($p < 0.03$). In contrast to the very strong correlations between the hippocampi, thalami, and putamen in patients, no significant correlations were observed in controls between the hippocampi and thalamus within the same hemisphere or across hemispheres. Similar correlations have been reported in patients with juvenile myoclonic epilepsy, where reductions in NAA/Cr in the prefrontal motor cortex and insula were found to be strongly correlated (Lin et al. 2009). Thus, it is clear that decreases in NAA not only reflect neuronal injury and the processes that give rise to epileptogenic foci, but also reflect injury/dysfunction in regions that are involved in the propagation of seizures.

INTERPRETATION OF DECREASED NAA LEVELS

Despite the obvious linkage between neuronal loss in epilepsy and decreases in NAA, there have been few correlative in vivo studies. In epilepsy patients with malformations of cortical development, significant reductions were also observed in NAA/Cr in the epileptogenic region (Kuzniecky et al. 1997; Li et al. 1998). In these patients, NAA alterations were seen in the absence of neuronal loss (Kuzniecky et al. 1997).

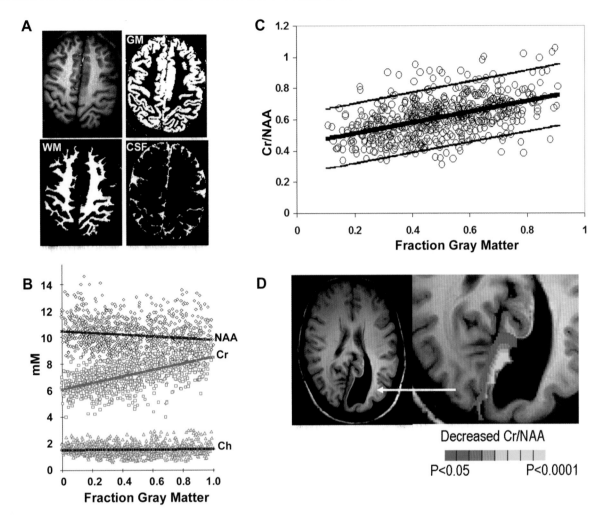

Figure 4.3 Data acquired at 4.1T. (A) Scout image and tissue segmented images for gray matter (GM), white matter (WM), and cerebrospinal fluid (CSF). (B) Plots of concentration of NAA (blue), Cr (red), and Ch (green) as a function of gray matter content for 10 subjects (~100 pixels each). (C) Regression analysis for Cr/NAA as a function of gray matter content from the data in B. The 95% confidence intervals for a single additional pixel (*thin lines*) are displayed along with the regression line (*thick line*). (D) An example from a patient with a developmental malformation, where pixels with abnormal Cr/NAA levels have been identified, color-coded according to *p* value and superimposed on the scout image for identification.

Specifically, the resected tissue showed normal or elevated numbers of neurons, although morphologically the neurons were abnormal (Kuzniecky et al. 1997). Subsequently, it was demonstrated that NAA losses in patients with TLE were also not significantly correlated with neuronal densities (Kuzniecky et al. 2001). To further probe the histologic basis for the alterations in NAA, in vivo measurements of NAA from the hippocampi of patients with intractable TLE were compared with quantitative measurement of neuronal loss and reactive astrocyte proliferation in the resected tissue (Cohen Gadol et al. 2004). Proliferation of reactive astrocytes, as expressed by the presence of glial fibrillary acidic protein (GFAP), has been associated with recent or ongoing neuronal injury. Regression analyses of NAA/Cr measured in vivo with quantitative neuronal counting across CA1-CA4 and the dentate gyrus revealed statistically significant correlations only in the CA2 sector. Interestingly, a similar correlation between GFAP staining with neuronal number revealed statistically significant correlations again only in the CA2 sector of the hippocampus. However, statistically significant correlations were found between NAA/Cr and GFAP staining across all four sectors. This suggests that in TLE, reductions in NAA/Cr more closely correlate with the presence of reactive astrocytes than alterations in neuronal density. The presence of reactive astrocytes is largely interpreted as a marker for recent or ongoing neuronal injury. Neuronal loss in the CA1, CA3, and dentate gyrus is typically believed to be largely due to the initial precipitating insult in TLE, while neuronal loss in the CA2 is more generally believed to correlate with the progression of the disease.

A   **Significant correlations between the ipsilateral hippocampus and other structures**

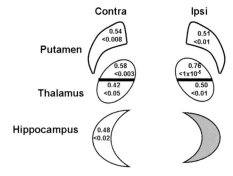

B   **Significant correlationsbetween the contralateral hippocampus and other structures**

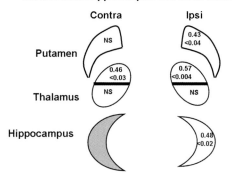

Figure 4.4 Correlation analysis showing statistically significant correlations in NAA/Cr between the ipsilateral (top) and contralateral hippocampus (bottom) for patients with temporal lobe epilepsy. (From Hetherington, H. P., R. I. Kuzniecky, et al. 2007. A subcortical network of dysfunction in TLE measured by magnetic resonance spectroscopy. *Neurology* 69(24): 2256–65.)

Given the lack of correlation between NAA levels and degree of neuronal loss in TLE and malformations of cortical development, the biochemical changes underlying the reductions in NAA are of significant interest. NAA has been reported to act as a source of acetate transfer from the mitochondria to the cytoplasm for lipid synthesis. NAA has also been proposed to act as a transporter of amino nitrogen from the mitochondria to the cytoplasm, and as an osmotic agent, based on its redistribution between extracellular/intracellular compartments in response to osmotic stress (see Moffett et al. 2007 for review). Indeed, agents that perturb mitochondrial function have been demonstrated to affect NAA levels and production rates. For example, studies using mitochondrial poisons in isolated rat brain mitochondria have demonstrated that ATP production, oxygen consumption, and NAA production are strongly correlated and significantly decreased in response to these agents (Heales et al. 1995, Bates et al. 1996).

These in vitro findings identifying a linkage between NAA and bioenergetics have also found support from in vivo studies. In a study of healthy control subjects, a highly significant correlation between hippocampal NAA levels and ADP was identified (Pan and Takahashi 2005). Surprisingly, this relationship displayed a positive slope, with higher NAA levels associated with higher ADP levels. This implies that in the healthy human brain, NAA levels, reflecting neuronal function, are responsive to demand as reflected by ADP. This is also consistent with the finding that in epilepsy patients with cortical malformations of development who are well controlled (less than four seizures per year), NAA levels are not altered despite the presence of structural abnormalities (Kuzniecky et al. 1997). Therefore, in epilepsy patients with intractable seizures, the decreased NAA levels often seen may reflect an inability to respond to energetic demand due to mitochondrial injury. This would suggest that bioenergetic deficits (decreased PCr/ATP) should be present in the hippocampi of patients with TLE and that upon successful treatment the decrement in NAA from affected loci could normalize.

The reversibility of the NAA changes in TLE was first reported by Hugg et al. (1996), who found that NAA recovered in the contralateral hippocampus in patients with bilateral abnormalities one year after successful surgery. This finding was confirmed by other investigators (Cendes et al. 1997; Vermathen et al., 2002). In a follow-up study, on average 50% of the metabolic recovery occurred over a period of less than 6 months, demonstrating a slow but responsive nature of neuronal NAA levels (Serles et al. 2001). The reversibility of decreased NAA in the contralateral hippocampus with successful surgical outcome (i.e., cessation of seizures) suggests that the recovering NAA levels reflect a "healing" or "normalization" of cellular process in the contralateral hippocampus. The fact that NAA normalization is associated with "normalization" of neuronal function (i.e., cessation of seizures) suggests that the processes that link the balance between NAA synthesis (correlated with ATP production) and degradation directly reflect the dysfunction seen in epilepsy. However, it is not yet clear whether the impairment in bioenergetics as reflected by decreased NAA is merely a secondary effect of the presence (reduced NAA) or absence (normalization of NAA) of seizures.

31P SPECTROSCOPIC MEASUREMENTS OF BIOENERGETICS IN HUMAN EPILEPSY

Prior to the widespread availability of ^{1}H spectroscopy on clinical MR systems, the use of ^{31}P spectroscopy for the lateralization of epileptogenic regions had been evaluated by some investigators (Laxer et al 1992, Hugg et al 1992). In these initial studies at 2.0T,

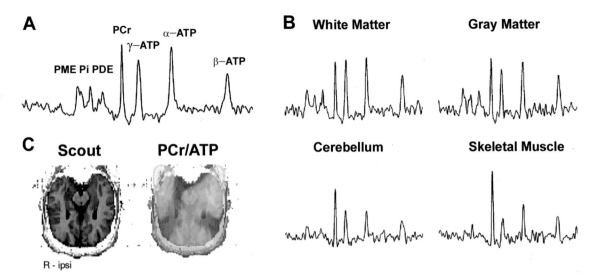

Figure 4.5 ^{31}P MRSI data acquired at 4T. (A) Example spectrum from human brain (~9 cc). (B) Representative spectra from white matter, gray matter, the cerebellum, and skeletal muscle. Due to the small thickness of the temporalis muscle, which fills only a small fraction of the voxel, the intensities in the skeletal muscle spectrum are markedly decreased. (C) Map of PCr/ATP from a patient with temporal lobe epilepsy overlaid on the scout image. Red-yellow colors indicate high PCr/ATP ratios, while blue represents a low PCr/ATP ratio.

significant increases in inorganic phosphate were reported (Fig. 4.5). Other investigators, using a 1.5T MR system, reported that PCr/Pi was reduced by 50% in the temporal lobe ipsilateral to seizure onset, whereas it was reduced by 24% in the contralateral temporal lobe (Kuzniecky et al. 1992). At 4.1T, PCr/Pi was significantly decreased in both the ipsilateral (32%) and contralateral (19%) temporal lobes. Within this group, 73% of the patients were correctly lateralized using the PCr/Pi ratio. Similar to those seen in the ^{1}H spectrum, these effects are also seen throughout the network involving the thalamus (Pan et al. 2005). Since patients with recent seizures (less than 24 hours prior to MRS procedure) were excluded, these effects are believed not to be an acute effect of seizures, but rather to reflect a chronic impairment of energy metabolism, consistent with a mitochondria-based deficit leading to NAA reductions.

Declines in bioenergetics are also seen in a variety of other forms of epilepsy, including children with Lennox-Gastaut syndrome, in patients with absence seizures, and in adults with frontal lobe epilepsy (Garcia et al. 1994; Pan et al. 1999). In children with Lennox-Gastaut syndrome and in patients with absence seizures, PCr/ATP was decreased in the cortical gray matter in comparison to control subjects. Notably, no such change was seen in white matter, reflecting the specificity to neuronal bodies and their high energetic demands. In patients with frontal lobe epilepsy, elevations of inorganic phosphate were reported, consistent with a decrease in overall energy charge (Garcia et al. 1994). Therefore, it appears that the finding of bioenergetic impairment is not restricted to TLE but may reflect a basic mechanism underlying epilepsy as a whole.

FACTORS AFFECTING THE INTERPRETATION OF ^{31}P DATA

Although ^{31}P studies have shown that abnormalities in bioenergetics are present, their use to date has been limited. Part of the limited use of ^{31}P spectroscopy can be attributed to the large range of normal values for cerebral PCr (3 to 5 mM) and ATP (2 to 4 mM) in low field studies, and the resulting perception that ^{31}P spectroscopy is highly inaccurate. These initial reports used large volumes (25 to 100 cc) and did not attempt to account for tissue or regional heterogeneity. Although spatial resolution for ^{31}P studies is limited by the signal-to-noise ratio, recent studies at high field have identified clear regional heterogeneities in ^{31}P metabolites using regression analyses (Hetherington et al. 2001). Depending upon tissue type (cerebral, cerebellar, or skeletal muscle), the concentrations of PCr (3 to 25 mM) and ATP (2 to 8 mM) vary (Fig. 5.5B). Similarly, depending upon the content of gray matter in the tissue, the ratio of PCr/ATP in cerebral structures varies by ~40%. In Figure 5.5C, a map of PCr/ATP shows very high PCr/ATP ratios (yellow-red) overlying the temporalis muscle, while low PCr/ATP ratios (purple) are seen from cerebral white matter. In this case, the decreased PCr/ATP from the ipsilateral hippocampus has PCr/ATP ratios that are similar to that of white matter, and that are significantly decreased in comparison to the contralateral hippocampus.

Importantly, failure to account for these differences can result in substantial variability that is reflective not of underlying pathology, but rather normal heterogeneity based on tissue composition.

INTERPRETATION OF ALTERATIONS IN ³¹P METABOLISM IN EPILEPSY

In pediatric epilepsy patients being treated with the ketogenic diet, bioenergetic impairments present prior to initiation of the diet are reversed as the seizures are brought under control (Pan et al. 1999). Specifically, after 4 months of the ketogenic diet therapy, the PCr/Pi and PCr/ATP ratios had improved by 22% and 14%, respectively. It seems that both reductions in NAA and impairments in bioenergetics appear to be tightly linked with seizure activity and can be reversed with successful treatment. This indicated that the alterations in ³¹P metabolites were also not solely due to neuronal death, but reflected a dynamic and reversible process. Although the exact mechanism for the antiseizure effect of the ketogenic diet remains controversial, it is known that ketones can supplement or replace glucose as a fuel source for oxidation, thereby potentially modulating bioenergetics. Notably, decreased PCr/ATP in the hippocampi, as is the case for NAA, is not correlated with neuronal loss (Pan et al. 2005). To determine the extent to which decreased PCr/ATP levels might be associated with electrophysiologic properties, Williamson et al. (2005) correlated in vivo hippocampal PCr/ATP levels with membrane repolarization times ($p < 0.01$, positive correlation) following stimulation and hyperexcitability (the ability to fire multiple spikes in response to a single stimulus, $p < 0.03$, negative correlation). In both cases, decreased PCr/ATP was associated with impaired electrophysiologic responses, consistent with epileptic behavior. Although these findings strongly suggest that there is a significant bioenergetic component to the etiology of seizure disorders, it remains unclear whether this reflects the general damage associated with seizures or is a causative factor.

GLUTAMATE AND GABA: INTRACELLULAR ALTERATIONS IN NEUROTRANSMITTERS

As alluded to so far in this chapter, most measurements using MR spectroscopy and spectroscopic imaging have focused on measurements of NAA, creatine, choline, and to a lesser extent ³¹P metabolites. Together, these measurements have suggested a strong role for metabolism and bioenergetics in the pathophysiology of epilepsy. However, these measurements do not directly assess the neurotransmitter changes that occur in epilepsy. Using ¹H MRS and specialized methods, it is possible to measure both glutamate and GABA in vivo.

Glutamate is the primary excitatory neurotransmitter in human brain. The finding of elevated extracellular glutamate and decreased rates of glutamate uptake in epileptogenic hippocampi (During and Spencer 1993) have sparked substantial interest in measuring in vivo glutamate levels in patients with epilepsy. However, unlike the main resonances of NAA and Cr, which are singlet resonances, glutamate's primary resonances represent two equivalent protons (CH₂ group) as opposed to three equivalent protons (CH₃ group) and are triplets or higher-order multiplets (Fig. 4.6). Thus, despite a concentration similar to that of Cr (5 to 9 mM), their resonance is smaller and distributed over a broader range of frequencies, making detection more difficult. Further, unlike NAA and other singlet resonances, the appearance of these multiplets is strongly dependent upon the exact timings of the acquisition method used. As such, specialized sequences and timings are required for their detection, making routine measurement more demanding. Further, due to spectral overlap with glutamine, low field measurements (1.5T) are exceptionally difficult to interpret. However, with increasing field strength (3T, 4T, and most recently 7T) these hurdles can be overcome.

Although much less commonly acquired than measurements of NAA, a number of investigators have evaluated glutamate content in patients with TLE.

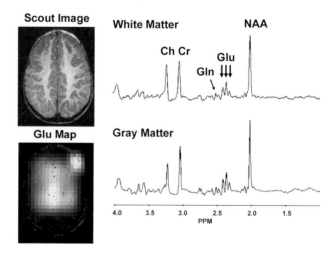

Figure 4.6 Spectroscopic imaging data acquired at 4.1T. Top left shows a scout image. On the right are representative spectra from white matter (top) and gray matter (bottom), including the glutamate triplet (*three arrows*, 2.34 ppm) and glutamine. Bottom left is a map of glutamate. An in-plane localization was used, resulting in a rectangular shape. Note the elevation of glutamate in gray-matter–rich locations.

Pfund et al. (2000) reported that the combined resonance of glutamate and glutamine (the signals were not resolvable at 1.5T) were decreased in EEG-defined neocortical epileptogenic regions in comparison to the corresponding contralateral location. Others (Simister et al 2002, Woermann et al. 1999) have reported that the combined resonance of glutamate and glutamine was alternately elevated in the ipsilateral or contralateral hippocampus of MRI-negative TLE patients. At 4T, where the resonances of glutamate and glutamine can be better resolved, Pan et al. (2006) evaluated a group of TLE patients and reported that ipsilateral glutamate and NAA were significantly decreased (5.1 ± 1.2 mM and 8.0 ± 1.1 mM) in comparison to controls (6.7 ± 1.5 mM and 9.5 ± 1.0 mM), respectively, yielding declines of ~25% in glutamate and ~16% in NAA (Fig. 4.7). Notably, the measurement of glutamate reflects total tissue glutamate levels where the intracellular levels dominate the micromolar extracellular levels. The presence of large elevations in extracellular glutamate combined with the relatively small volume cannot overcome even small losses in cytosolic glutamate or numbers of glutamatergic neurons. Thus, the finding of decreased total glutamate levels by Pan et al (2006) most likely reflects the loss of glutamatergic neurons. The greater fractional decline in glutamate as opposed to NAA suggests that measurements of glutamate may be a more sensitive indicator of neuronal loss. However, this advantage is likely to be realized only at very high field strengths (7T) where signal-to-noise ratio and spectral resolution are less limiting.

As the primary inhibitory neurotransmitter for mammalian brain, GABA and its receptor systems have been an area of intense study in epilepsy, including MRS application. Due to its low concentration (~1 mM) and spectral overlap with glutamate, glutamine, and creatine, the measurement of GABA requires the use of specialized methods, commonly referred to as "spectral editing" (Hetherington et al. 1998; Rothman et al. 1984). These methods typically utilize the unique frequencies of the ^{1}H resonances of GABA to selectively perturb the GABA resonance in alternating scans and through that interaction modulate the appearance of the adjacent ^{1}H resonance on the GABA molecule through its chemical bond. Since other resonances are not affected by the selective perturbation, subtraction of the two measurements results in an "edited" spectrum displaying the GABA resonance free of spectral overlap (Fig. 4.8). More recently, a variety of methods using multiple quantum coherence (Simister et al., 2003, 2007) have been used to provide immunity to artifacts associated with patient movement during the subtraction-based spectral editing. Although these methods provide single-shot resolution of GABA from overlapping resonances, their decreased sensitivity

and increased vulnerability to transmitter coil homogeneity limit their widespread use.

Given the difficulties of low signal-to-noise ratio, the majority of MRS studies of GABA have evaluated the occipital lobe, where small highly sensitive surface coils can be placed in close proximity to the tissue. For example, Petroff et al.(1996a) studied the resting levels of intracellular occipital GABA in patients with complex partial seizures and juvenile myoclonic epilepsy. In the complex partial seizures group, low GABA was associated with poor seizure control, while juvenile myoclonic epilepsy patients showed low GABA independent of seizure control. These findings of reduced in vivo GABA are similar to those reported by the same investigators in various other forms of epilepsy (Petroff et al. 1999, 2001). Notably, the occipital lobe represents a site distant from the presumed epileptogenic region, predisposing the patients to seizure spread as opposed to seizure initiation. To evaluate the concentrations of GABA in the actual seizure focus, Simister et al. (2003) acquired data from patients with occipital lobe seizures. Although these investigators failed to identify a decrease in occipital lobe GABA, the study used a volume coil (lower sensitivity), and the test–retest accuracy for GABA in controls was only 38%. Thus, whether GABA is increased or decreased in the epileptogenic region remains an open issue.

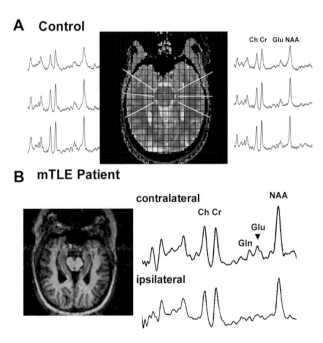

Figure 4.7 ^{1}H spectroscopic imaging data of glutamate from the temporal lobe of a healthy control (A) and a patient with temporal lobe epilepsy (B). In (A) the locations of the spectra are identified on the scout image. In (B) the mid-body spectra from the hippocampi contralateral and ipsilateral to the seizure focus are displayed. Note the substantial decrement in glutamate in the ipsilateral hippocampus.

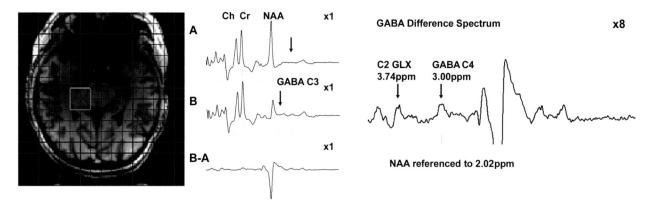

Figure 4.8 Spectroscopic imaging data of GABA from the temporal lobe acquired at 7T. At far left is a scout image showing the spectroscopic imaging grid (blue) and block of 4 voxels (green) that were averaged to produce the data shown to the right. In the middle are data acquired using a spectral editing sequence with the inversion pulse applied (A) at the GABA C-3 resonance 1.9 ppm and (B) at 1.3 ppm; the difference of the two spectra is shown below (B-A). A magnified (×8) trace of the spectrum (B-A) is shown to the far right. The edited GABA resonance at 3.00 ppm is labeled. Due to the proximity of the glutamate and glutamine C-3 resonances at 2–2.1 ppm, there is a partially edited resonance at 3.74 ppm from the sum of glutamate and glutamine (GLX) C2 resonance.

Despite this uncertainty of the status of GABA in the seizure focus, in vivo measurements of GABA have become quite useful in assessing the GABA response to various antiepileptic medications. For example, Petroff et al. (1996b) established an in vivo dose–response curve for vigabatrin, an inhibitor of GABA transaminase that catabolizes GABA. A dose-escalation study revealed increases in cerebral GABA as a function of vigabatrin dose up to 3 g/day. Above 3 g/day, brain GABA levels remained constant and did not rise further, indicating that a maximal inhibitory effect on brain GABA transaminase had been reached. Although the mechanism for the elevation of GABA in response to vigabatrin is clear, other common antiepileptic drugs have also been shown to result in an elevation of GABA (Kuzniecky et al. 2002; Petroff et al. 2000, 2001). For example, topiramate, gabapentin, and lamotrigine can all raise brain GABA levels in control subjects under acute (topiramate and gabapentin) and chronic (lamotrigine) conditions (Kuzniecky et al. 2002). Conversely, levetiracetam had no effect on brain GABA levels. One limitation of this work is that due to the low sensitivity of the GABA measurements because of its low concentration in human brain (~1 mM), the majority of studies of brain GABA have been performed in the occipital lobe, so that the measurements reflect a global response of the brain to seizures and pharmaceutical interventions rather than regional responses.

Finally, the findings of increased GABA in response to gabapentin and topiramate were contrary to those described in the rodent literature (Leach et al. 1997; Sills et al. 2003). In subsequent studies, Errante and Petroff (2003) and Errante et al. (2002) showed that the differential effect of gabapentin was due to species differences. In a slice preparation of normal rats and tissue from epilepsy patients, gabapentin had no effect on the rat brain slices but significantly increased GABA levels in the human slices. Similarly, no effects of gabapentin on GABA were seen in the in vivo rat brain as assessed by tissue extracts. Thus, when investigating the effects of various drugs or interventions with the potential to affect the GABAergic system in experimental models of epilepsy, it is important to take into account species differences between humans and rodents.

HIGH FIELD MRI

As described earlier, ^{1}H and ^{31}P MRS imaging provides the ability to monitor a variety of processes that are highly relevant in the pathophysiology of epilepsy. However, spectroscopic studies are inherently limited by the signal-to-noise ratio achievable, due to the low concentrations of most cerebral metabolites. Further, the measurement of glutamate and GABA is challenging due to spectral overlap with other compounds. With recent advances in magnet technology, ultrahigh field magnets (7T and higher) with bore sizes capable of accommodating the adult human head have become available from a variety of research and clinical vendors. The increased field strength confers the intrinsic advantages of increased signal-to-noise ratio and, for spectroscopic studies, increased spectral resolution and spectral simplification for J-coupled resonances. Thus, spectroscopic imaging at 7T should provide an ideal platform for evaluating these compounds.

Despite the use of 7T and 8T systems dating from the late 1990s (Robitaille et al. 1998; Vaughan et al.

2001), there have been few reports of their use in spectroscopic imaging studies. This limitation is largely due to the inherent disadvantages of high field, which include (1) a dramatic increase in detector inhomogeneity (up to ±50%) due to high-frequency effects governing the interaction of tissue with magnetic fields in conventional volume head coils; (2) a field-dependent linear decrease in excitation field strength for equivalent applied power; and (3) a field-dependent linear increase in static magnetic field inhomogeneity. The first two effects decrease homogeneity and efficiency for generation of excitation fields and significantly limit the use of conventional volume localization sequences for spectroscopy, resulting in the misregistration of volumes from different metabolites and excessive power deposition, exceeding FDA guidelines. The last effect, overall poorer magnetic field homogeneity, reduces spectral quality, increasing resonance overlap, and thus negating some of the advantages of high field.

Based on the issues of radiofrequency (RF) inhomogeneity and power deposition, there has been intense interest in developing alternative designs to conventional volume head coils for efficient and homogeneous coverage of substantial portions of the human brain at 7T. One design, the transceiver array (Adriany et al. 2008; Avdievich et al. 2009), consists of an array of surface coils circumscribing the head and can be used for reception and transmission. By varying the amplitude and phase of the RF delivered to each coil simultaneously during transmission ("RF shimming"), the spatial distribution of the RF can be optimized to provide improved homogeneity and efficiency (Avdievich et al. 2009). For example, for superior brain regions, homogeneities of approximately ±10% can be

achieved, similar to that seen in conventional head coils at 3T. Further, these multichannel transmission systems can be used to "sculpt" the excitation fields spatially so as to provide volume localization at dramatically lower power deposition levels (Hetherington et al. 2010). Figure 4.9 shows data acquired from the hippocampi of a healthy control subject and a patient with TLE at 7T using a transceiver array. NAA/Cr from the ipsilateral hippocampus is reduced in comparison to the contralateral hippocampus and both hippocampi show decreased NAA/CR in comparison to the control subject. Notably, the 7T data show a signal-to-noise ratio increase of more than 2 in comparison to the 4T data (Fig. 4.2) despite identical volume sizes and a decreased acquisition time (15 minutes vs. 19 minutes).

The increased inhomogeneity at higher field strengths is due to the linear dependence of susceptibility effects arising from air–tissue interfaces such as in the sinuses and ear canals. Both theoretical models and measurements show dramatic shifts (~ppm over cm distances) near the sinuses and ear canals (Li et al. 1995, 1996). These large susceptibility shifts are the origin of signal dropout and distortions seen in gradient echo imaging, echo-planar imaging, susceptibility weighted imaging, and spectroscopic imaging. These shifts generate complex spatial dependencies in the main magnetic field, with overall spatial dependencies ranging from the third to the sixth power. Although these higher-order terms decay with distance away from the origin of the susceptibility shift, their effects can be seen throughout the brain. Thus, what may seem to be moderate effects at 1.5T become limiting at 3T and problematic at 7T. Unfortunately, to date, most MRI systems at 1.5, 3, and 7T are typically only

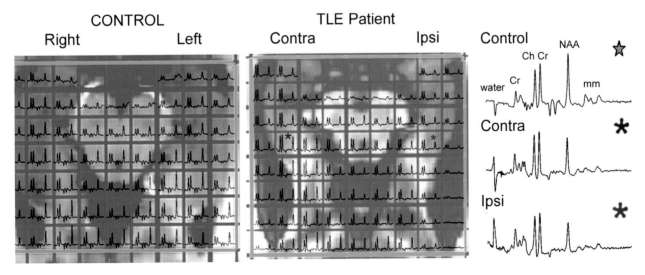

Figure 4.9 Spectroscopic imaging data acquired at 7T from the temporal lobe in a healthy control subject and a patient with temporal lobe epilepsy. Representative spectral data are shown to the far right and demarcated on the images.

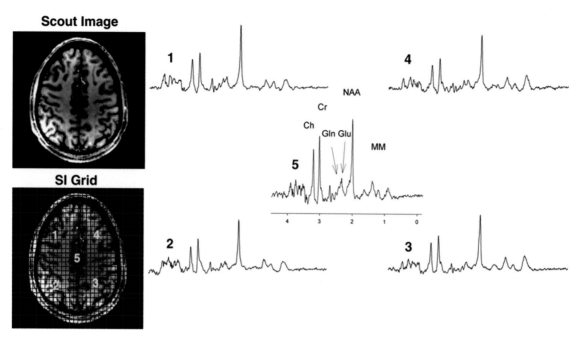

Figure 4.10 Spectroscopic imaging data of glutamate acquired at 7T acquired with a spatial resolution of 0.36 cc. Top left shows a scout image and bottom left shows the scout image with the spectroscopic imaging grid superimposed. To the right are five representative spectra, which are demarcated on the scout image (bottom left).

equipped with hardware capable of producing correction terms with first- and second-order spatial dependencies (first- and second-order shims), such that cancellation of these effects globally is not possible. However, with additional hardware (third-order shims) capable of producing more complex patterns, these effects can be overcome and excellent spectral quality can be obtained for large regions of the human brain, including the temporal lobe (Fig. 4.9). Figure 4.10 shows spectroscopic imaging data acquired at 0.36 cc resolution at 7T. In these examples, the improved signal-to-noise ratio at 7T allows for substantially higher spatial resolution.

CONCLUSION

Although the challenges for performing spectroscopic imaging at 7T are substantial, the technology to overcome these limitations is now becoming available. With the increased field strength, improved signal-to-noise ratios and spectral resolution can be achieved. These improvements should significantly enhance the utility of spectroscopic imaging in the evaluation of patients with epilepsy.

REFERENCES

Adriany, G., P. F. Van de Moortele, et al. 2008. A geometrically adjustable 16-channel transmit/receive transmission line array for improved RF efficiency and parallel imaging performance at 7 Tesla. *Magnetic Resonance in Medicine* 59(3): 590–7.

Avdievich, N. I., J. W. Pan, et al. 2009. Short echo spectroscopic imaging of the human brain at 7T using transceiver arrays. *Magnetic Resonance in Medicine* 62: 17–25.

Bates TE, M Strangward st al. 1996. Inhibition of N-acetylaspartate production: implications for 1H MRS studies in vivo. *Neuroreport* 1996;7(8):1397-1400.

Benedek, K., C. Juhasz, et al. 2004. Metabolic changes of subcortical structures in intractable focal epilepsy. *Epilepsia* 45(9): 1100–5.

Cendes, F., F. Andermann, et al. 1997. Normalization of neuronal metabolic dysfunction after surgery for temporal lobe epilepsy. Evidence from proton MR spectroscopic imaging. *Neurology* 49(6): 1525–33.

Cendes, F., F. Andermann, et al. 1994. Lateralization of temporal lobe epilepsy based on regional metabolic abnormalities in proton magnetic resonance spectroscopic images. *Annals of Neurology* 35(2): 211–6.

Chu, W. J., H. P. Hetherington, et al. 1998. Lateralization of human temporal lobe epilepsy by 31P NMR spectroscopic imaging at 4.1 T. *Neurology* 51(2): 472–9.

Chu, W. J., H. P. Hetherington, et al. 1996. Is the intracellular pH different from normal in the epileptic focus of patients with temporal lobe epilepsy? A 31P NMR study. *Neurology* 47(3): 756–60.

Chu, W. J., R. I. Kuzniecky, et al. 2000. Statistically driven identification of focal metabolic abnormalities in temporal lobe epilepsy with corrections for tissue heterogeneity using 1H spectroscopic imaging. *Magnetic Resonance in Medicine* 43(3): 359–67.

Cohen-Gadol AA, JW Pan et al 2004. Mesial temporal lobe epilepsy: a proton magnetic resonance spectroscopy study and a histopathological analysis. *J Neurosurg.* 101(4): 613–620.

Connelly, A., G. D. Jackson, et al. 1994. Magnetic resonance spectroscopy in temporal lobe epilepsy. *Neurology* 44(8): 1411–7.

Constantinidis, I., J. A. Malko, et al. 1996. Evaluation of 1H magnetic resonance spectroscopic imaging as a diagnostic tool for the lateralization of epileptogenic seizure foci. *British Journal of Radiology* 69(817): 15–24.

Dlugos, D. J., J. Jaggi, et al. 1999. Hippocampal cell density and subcortical metabolism in temporal lobe epilepsy. *Epilepsia* 40(4): 408–13.

During, M. J., and D. D. Spencer. 1993. Extracellular hippocampal glutamate and spontaneous seizure in the conscious human brain. *Lancet* 341(8861): 1607–10.

Ende, G. R., K. D. Laxer, et al. 1997. Temporal lobe epilepsy: bilateral hippocampal metabolite changes revealed at proton MR spectroscopic imaging. *Radiology* 202(3): 809–17.

Errante LD, Petroff OA 2003. Acute effects of gabapentin and pregabalin on rat forebrain cellular GABA, glutamate, and glutamine concentrations. *Seizure* 12(5): 300-306.

Errante LD et al. 2002. Gabapentin and vigabatrin increase GABA in the human neocortical slice. *Epilepsy Research* 49(3): 203–210.

Garcia, P. A., K. D. Laxer, et al. 1994. Phosphorus magnetic resonance spectroscopic imaging in patients with frontal lobe epilepsy. *Annals of Neurology* 35(2): 217–21.

Garcia, P. A., K. D. Laxer, et al. 1997. Correlation of seizure frequency with N-acetyl-aspartate levels determined by 1H magnetic resonance spectroscopic imaging. *Magnetic Resonance Imaging* 15(4): 475–8.

Heales SJ, SE Davies et al. 1995. Depletion of brain glutathione is accompanied by impaired mitochondrial function and decreased N-acetyl aspartate concentration. *Neurochem Res* 20(1): 31–38.

Hetherington, H., R. Kuzniecky, et al. 1995. Proton nuclear magnetic resonance spectroscopic imaging of human temporal lobe epilepsy at 4.1 T. *Annals of Neurology* 38(3): 396–404.

Hetherington, H. P., N. I. Avdievich, et al. 2010. RF shimming for spectroscopic localization in the human brain at 7 T. *Magnetic Resonance in Medicine* 63(1): 9–19.

Hetherington, H. P., R. I. Kuzniecky, et al. 2007. A subcortical network of dysfunction in TLE measured by magnetic resonance spectroscopy. *Neurology* 69(24): 2256–65.

Hetherington, H. P., B. R. Newcomer, et al. 1998. Measurements of human cerebral GABA at 4.1 T using numerically optimized editing pulses. *Magnetic Resonance in Medicine* 39(1): 6–10.

Hetherington, H. P., J. W. Pan, et al. 1996. Quantitative 1H spectroscopic imaging of human brain at 4.1 T using image segmentation. *Magnetic Resonance in Medicine* 36(1): 21–9.

Hetherington, H. P., D. D. Spencer, et al. 2001. Quantitative (31)P spectroscopic imaging of human brain at 4 Tesla: assessment of gray and white matter differences of phosphocreatine and ATP. *Magnetic Resonance in Medicine* 45(1): 46–52.

Hugg, J. W., R. I. Kuzniecky, et al. 1996. Normalization of contralateral metabolic function following temporal lobectomy demonstrated by 1H magnetic resonance spectroscopic imaging. *Annals of Neurology* 40(2): 236–9.

Hugg JW, KD Laxer et al. 1992. Lateralization of human focal epilepsy by 31P magnetic resonance spectroscopic imaging. *Neurology* 42(10):2011-2018.

Hugg, J. W., K. D. Laxer, et al. 1993. Neuron loss localizes human temporal lobe epilepsy by in vivo proton magnetic resonance spectroscopic imaging. *Annals of Neurology* 34(6): 788–94.

Kuzniecky, R., G. A. Elgavish, et al. 1992. In vivo 31P nuclear magnetic resonance spectroscopy of human temporal lobe epilepsy. *Neurology* 42(8): 1586–90.

Kuzniecky, R., H. Hetherington, et al. 1997. Proton spectroscopic imaging at 4.1 tesla in patients with malformations of cortical development and epilepsy. *Neurology* 48(4): 1018–24.

Kuzniecky, R., S. Ho, et al. 2002. Modulation of cerebral GABA by topiramate, lamotrigine, and gabapentin in healthy adults. *Neurology* 58(3): 368–72.

Kuzniecky, R., J. Hugg, et al. 1999. Predictive value of 1H MRSI for outcome in temporal lobectomy. *Neurology* 53(4): 694–8.

Kuzniecky, R., J. W. Hugg, et al. 1998. Relative utility of 1H spectroscopic imaging and hippocampal volumetry in the lateralization of mesial temporal lobe epilepsy. *Neurology* 51(1): 66–71.

Kuzniecky R, C. Palmer, et al. 2001. Magnetic resonance spectroscopic imaging in temporal lobe epilepsy: neuronal dysfunction or cell loss? *Archives of Neurology* 58(12):2048-2053.

Laxer KD, B Hubesch et al. 1992. Increased pH and inorganic phosphate in temporal seizure foci demonstrated by [31P]MRS. *Epilepsia* 33(4):618-623.

Leach, J. P., G. J. Sills, et al. 1997. Neurochemical actions of gabapentin in mouse brain. *Epilepsy Research* 27(3): 175–80.

Li, L. M., F. Cendes, et al. 2000. Prognostic value of proton magnetic resonance spectroscopic imaging for surgical outcome in patients with intractable temporal lobe epilepsy and bilateral hippocampal atrophy. *Annals of Neurology* 47(2): 195–200.

Li, L. M., F. Cendes, et al. 1998. Neuronal metabolic dysfunction in patients with cortical developmental malformations: a proton magnetic resonance spectroscopic imaging study. *Neurology* 50(3): 755–9.

Li, S., B. J. Dardzinski, et al. 1996. Three-dimensional mapping of the static magnetic field inside the human head. *Magnetic Resonance in Medicine* 36(5): 705–14.

Li, S., G. D. Williams, et al. 1995. A computer simulation of the static magnetic field distribution in the human head. *Magnetic Resonance in Medicine* 34(2): 268–75.

Lin, K., H. Carrete, Jr., et al. 2009. Magnetic resonance spectroscopy reveals an epileptic network in juvenile myoclonic epilepsy. *Epilepsia* 50(5): 1191–200.

Lundbom, N., E. Gaily, et al. 2001. Proton spectroscopic imaging shows abnormalities in glial and neuronal cell pools in frontal lobe epilepsy. *Epilepsia* 42(12): 1507–14.

Michaelis, T., K. D. Merboldt, et al. 1993. Absolute concentrations of metabolites in the adult human brain in vivo: quantification of localized proton MR spectra. *Radiology* 187(1): 219–27.

Moffett, J. R., B. Ross, et al. 2007. N-Acetylaspartate in the CNS: from neurodiagnostics to neurobiology. *Progress in Neurobiology* 81(2): 89–131.

Mueller, S. G., K. D. Laxer, et al. 2004. Identification of abnormal neuronal metabolism outside the seizure focus in temporal lobe epilepsy. *Epilepsia* 45(4): 355–66.

Mueller, S. G., K. D. Laxer, et al. 2006. Spectroscopic evidence of hippocampal abnormalities in neocortical epilepsy. *European Journal of Neurology* 13(3): 256–60.

Ng, T. C., Y. G. Comair, et al. 1994. Temporal lobe epilepsy: presurgical localization with proton chemical shift imaging. *Radiology* 193(2): 465–72.

Pan, J. W., E. M. Bebin, et al. 1999. Ketosis and epilepsy: 31P spectroscopic imaging at 4.1 T. *Epilepsia* 40(6): 703–7.

Pan, J. W., J. H. Kim, et al. 2005. Regional energetic dysfunction in hippocampal epilepsy. *Acta Neurologica Scandinavica* 111(4): 218–24.

Pan JW, K Takahashi 2005. Interdependence of N-acetyl aspartate and high-energy phosphates in healthy human brain. *Annals of Neurology* 57(1):92-97.

Pan, J. W., T. Venkatraman, et al. 2006. Quantitative glutamate spectroscopic imaging of the human hippocampus. *NMR Biomedicine* 19(2): 209–16.

Petroff, O. A., F. Hyder, et al. 2000. Effects of gabapentin on brain GABA, homocarnosine, and pyrrolidinone in epilepsy patients. *Epilepsia* 41(6): 675–80.

Petroff, O. A., F. Hyder, et al. 2001. Homocarnosine and seizure control in juvenile myoclonic epilepsy and complex partial seizures. *Neurology* 56(6): 709–15.

Petroff, O. A., F. Hyder, et al. 2001. Topiramate rapidly raises brain GABA in epilepsy patients. *Epilepsia* 42(4): 543–8.

Petroff OA, D.L. Rothman et al. 1996a. Low brain GABA level is associated with poor seizure control. *Annals of Neurology* 40(6):908-911.

Petroff, O. A., D. L. Rothman, et al. 1996b. Human brain GABA levels rise rapidly after initiation of vigabatrin therapy. *Neurology* 47(6): 1567–71.

Petroff, O. A., D. L. Rothman, et al. 1999. Effects of valproate and other antiepileptic drugs on brain glutamate, glutamine, and GABA in patients with refractory complex partial seizures. *Seizure* 8(2): 120–7.

Pfund, Z., D. C. Chugani, et al. 2000. Evidence for coupling between glucose metabolism and glutamate cycling using FDG PET and 1H magnetic resonance spectroscopy in patients with epilepsy. *Journal of Cerebral Blood Flow Metabolism* 20(5): 871–8.

Robitaille, P. M., A. M. Abduljalil, et al. 1998. Human magnetic resonance imaging at 8 T. *NMR Biomedicine* 11(6): 263–5.

Rothman, D. L., K. L. Behar, et al. 1984. Homonuclear 1H double-resonance difference spectroscopy of the rat brain in vivo. *Proceedings of the National Academy of Sciences U S A* 81(20): 6330–4.

Serles, W., L. M. Li, et al. 2001. Time course of postoperative recovery of N-acetyl-aspartate in temporal lobe epilepsy. *Epilepsia* 42(2): 190–7.

Sills, G. J., E. Butler, et al. 2003. Vigabatrin, but not gabapentin or topiramate, produces concentration-related effects on enzymes and intermediates of the GABA shunt in rat brain and retina. *Epilepsia* 44(7): 886–92.

Simister, R. J., M. A. McLean, et al. 2003. A proton magnetic resonance spectroscopy study of metabolites in the occipital lobes in epilepsy. *Epilepsia* 44(4): 550–8.

Simister, R. J., M. A. McLean, et al. 2007. Proton magnetic resonance spectroscopy of malformations of cortical development causing epilepsy. *Epilepsy Research* 74(2-3): 107–15.

Simister RJ, FG, Woermann et al. 2002. A short-echo-time proton magnetic resonance spectroscopic imaging study of temporal lobe epilepsy. *Epilepsia* 43(9): 1021-1031.

Suhy, J., K. D. Laxer, et al. 2002. 1H MRSI predicts surgical outcome in MRI-negative temporal lobe epilepsy. *Neurology* 58(5): 821–3.

Vaughan, J. T., M. Garwood, et al. 2001. 7T vs. 4T: RF power, homogeneity, and signal-to-noise comparison in head images. *Magnetic Resonance in Medicine* 46(1): 24–30.

Vermathen, P., G. Ende, et al. 2002. Temporal lobectomy for epilepsy: recovery of the contralateral hippocampus measured by (1)H MRS. *Neurology* 59(4): 633–6.

Vermathen, P., K. D. Laxer, et al. 2003. Evidence of neuronal injury outside the medial temporal lobe in temporal lobe epilepsy: N-acetylaspartate concentration reductions detected with multisection proton MR spectroscopic imaging—initial experience. *Radiology* 226(1): 195–202.

Wiedermann, D., N. Schuff, et al. 2001. Short echo time multislice proton magnetic resonance spectroscopic imaging in human brain: metabolite distributions and reliability. *Magnetic Resonance Imaging* 19(8): 1073–80.

Williamson, A., P. R. Patrylo, et al. 2005. Correlations between granule cell physiology and bioenergetics in human temporal lobe epilepsy. *Brain* 128(Pt 5): 1199–208.

Woermann FG, MA McLean et al. 1999. Short echo time single-voxel 1H magnetic resonance spectroscopy in magnetic resonance imaging-negative temporal lobe epilepsy: different biochemical profile compared with hippocampal sclerosis. *Annals of Neurology* 45(3): 369-376.

Chapter 5

FUNCTIONAL MRI
William Davis Gaillard

The advent of functional MRI (fMRI) has had a significant impact on the management of epilepsy, and its clinical applications continue to grow. fMRI has provided an increasingly available means to reliably identify eloquent cortex to be spared in planning epilepsy surgery and to improve outcomes by minimizing postoperative deficits. In addition, fMRI provides a means of mapping the epileptogenic zone, although this has not yet entered clinical practice. Finally, fMRI provides a means of exploring the neurobiology of epilepsy and its effect on brain networks and brain function.

PRINCIPLES

The fMRI method is based on the observations of Roy and Sherington (1890) that increased brain activity is associated with an increase in cerebral blood flow (CBF). This observation was confirmed by ^{15}O-water positron emission tomography (PET) studies in the 1980s, as was the observation of a paradoxical increase in oxygen in activated cortex, and provides the basis for blood flow-based brain mapping techniques. Further investigations suggested that the signal assessed by CBF techniques reflects synaptic activity (Fox and Raichle 1986; Logothetis 2003). Fast imaging techniques allow measurement of signal change induced by alterations in blood flow and binding of hemoglobin to oxygen. In the activated, compared to the resting, state there is a regionally specific and tightly regulated increase in blood flow associated with a seemingly paradoxical increase in the ratio of oxygenated to deoxyhemoglobin. It is the change in hemoglobin moieties and ratio that leads to the T2* signal change detected by the fMRI blood oxygen-labeled dependent (BOLD) technique (Moonen and Bandettini 2000). There is a delay of 4 to 6 seconds in the hemodynamic response and a similar decay when the stimulus ceases. The spatial resolution attainable by fMRI is less than 1 mm, although in clinical practice voxel sizes are 3 to 4 mm, and the data are typically smoothed to 6 to 8 mm. The delay in the hemodynamic response means that the temporal resolution, while superior to ^{15}O-water PET, does not match the real-time physiologic measures of electroencephalography (EEG) or magnetoencephalography (MEG). Networks can be identified, but not the interplay between or serial processing that occurs in distributed networks. To be effective, the hemodynamic response needs to be triggered, dictated by the contrast between conditions described below; it is an epiphenomenon and only an indirect and relative measure of cerebral activity. BOLD techniques primarily measure signal in the venous side of the capillary bed; direct measures of CBF from the capillary bed can be accomplished with ^{15}O-water PET. More direct measures of blood flow can be made by using MRI with arterial spin labeling techniques. With this method, water in the carotid is tagged by a magnetic signature, and its signal can then be traced until the signature decays. Most of the discussion that follows in this chapter is based on BOLD methods. The signal change detected ranges between 0.8% (for cognitive tasks) and 3% (for sensorimotor tasks).

To identify cerebral areas that participate (i.e., that are active) during a given brain-based activity, a task or paradigm is designed that targets the specific endeavor. That task consists of an experimental condition and a control condition; as fMRI is assessing relative changes in MRI signal, two conditions are necessary: a control condition is needed to which the targeted activity is compared. For a motor task this simply may be tapping fingers compared to rest; for a language task this may be listening to words compared to listening to the same words but presented as reverse speech. In the second example the reverse speech condition controls for first- and second-order auditory processing common to both tasks and helps to isolate the features that are specific for language comprehension inherent in the experimental condition only. Typically, the conditions are presented in blocks of 20 to 40 seconds (20 being the minimal time) run over three to six cycles of alternating experimental and control conditions (four is considered optimal); this is called a "block" design. Image analysis programs then search the image data sets to detect a change in signal between conditions on a voxel-by-voxel basis; those voxels that meet the statistical criteria are deemed "activated" and labeled in a color that denotes the degree of statistical difference. These activated voxels are associated with the task, but they may not be critical to the task. Sometimes there is a decrease in signal, or "deactivation," but this is not the converse, in physiologic terms, of activation, as it may reflect decreased CBF, decreased cerebral activity, or that activity outstrips CBF. There are several statistical approaches to the signal analysis, most using parametric strategies (some differences in signal between tasks correcting for multiple comparisons, or using correlation analysis with a model response function), others using nonparametric tests. The results of these several approaches are comparable.

Some cognitive processes are better identified using event-related designs. Rather than in a block, which often yields a robust and sustained response, brief individual events—for example, the encoding or response to a single word—can be ascertained as the BOLD response will peak 5 seconds after the elicited response (hemodynamic response function). In this way, data can be interrogated based on behavioral response to individual events. This is important for two reasons; first, block design may not yield a signal when some individual events do not result in a correct behavioral response (i.e., the positive signal gets averaged out and lost in null responses). For example, studies on memory work best when the signal from only those items successfully encoded is measured. The second reason is that cognitive studies are more amenable to experimental manipulation with an event-related design. Usually 27 to 30 individual events

(in relation to baseline or control condition) are necessary for proper data interpretation.

Most functional imaging studies are presented in group maps usually transformed into a common anatomical space such as from the Talairach and Tournoux atlas or the Montreal Neurological Institute (MNI) atlas. Early PET studies that employed fixed effect models required this approach to separate signal from noise. Most group studies employ a random effects design that allows statistical extrapolation of findings from the study population to broader populations. While the latter is now accepted as the norm, in practice there is little difference in experimental findings between the two approaches. These approaches, which presume homogeneity in study populations, then generate maps that show the expected pattern of activation for a given task. A current limitation of many patient studies is the penchant to present data in group maps—but heterogeneity within patient populations, especially in epilepsy populations for the study of language and memory, makes such presentation problematic. The advantage of fMRI is the ability to generate individual activation maps in native space that can be used on an individual basis. The healthy control group maps are helpful for interpretation of individual studies. To be useful on an individual basis to improve patient care, tasks need to be robust, and patients need to be able to perform the tasks. There are also threshold effects, with lower thresholds showing more extensive brain areas to be activated. The individual maps may be interpreted visually or using a region-of-interest (ROI) approach (see below) (Fernandez et al. 2001; Gaillard et al. 2002). Activation maps can be co-registered to high-resolution MRI for intraoperative navigation.

APPLICATIONS FOR LOCALIZATION OF ELOQUENT CORTEX

The fMRI method may be used to identify eloquent cortex in planning surgery. Indeed, motor, sensory, and language systems have been relatively well studied and are being applied in the clinical setting. However, fMRI studies of memory remain problematic.

Motor and Sensory

The motor control system can be readily identified by fMRI tasks involving finger tapping, tongue wiggling, or foot tapping compared to rest. Finger tapping results in the least motion artifact. Such activity provides a robust and reproducible signal in primary motor cortex contralateral to the limb moved (Fig. 5.1). In addition, thalamus, basal ganglia, and ipsilateral cerebellum

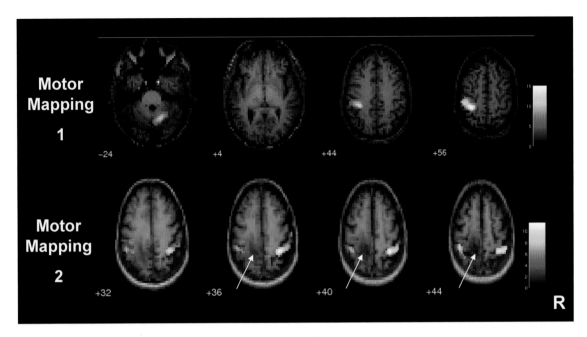

Figure 5.1 Motor mapping studies using fMRI. Left image is left brain. (1) Tapping of right index finger to thumb compared to rest in a 23-year-old right-handed man with left frontal seizure focus and normal MRI. Note activation in ipsilateral deep cerebellum and contralateral primary motor cortex. (2) Tapping of right and left index finger to thumb compared to rest in a 46-year-old man with simple partial seizures. *White arrow* denotes a left-sided mass lesion (astrocytoma). The task identifies bilateral primary motor cortex. The signal on the left motor strip is diminished compared to right activation; the tumor involved motor cortex.

(deep nuclei) are also identified (Jack et al. 1994; Kim et al. 1993; Rao et al. 1993). There is usually some activation in ipsilateral motor cortex. Supplementary cortex may be identified by more complex motor movement (Nelson et al. 2002). Passive movement in younger children or those cognitively delayed or lightly sedated may also be effective, unless sedation is very deep (Altman and Bernal 2001; Souweidane et al. 1999; Wilke et al. 2003). Sensory proprioceptive cortex may be identified by brushing the face, hand, or foot compared to rest (Hammeke et al. 1994; Kwong et al. 1992). Motor and sensory paradigms are used when planning frontal or parietal surgical resections. Auditory cortex may be identified by presenting tones to the individual, and the visual cortex may be identified by presenting a flashing checkerboard pattern. These paradigms are robust, and three cycles of 20 seconds per condition may be all that is necessary. Comparison with evoked potentials or electrocortical stimulation (ECS) finds agreement to within 1 cm (Lehericy et al. 2000).

Language

The greatest experience in applications to epilepsy patients has been with language, primarily as a noninvasive replacement for the intracarotid amobarbital test (IAT). fMRI may be used to lateralize and localize speech functions. Language fMRI alters surgical planning (Medina et al. 2005) and predicts postoperative outcome for the Boston Naming Test in adults (Sabsevitz et al. 2003). Over 20 studies involving more than 250 patients demonstrate excellent but not complete agreement with the IAT for lateralization of language/speech (Adcock et al. 2003; Bahn et al. 1997; Benke et al. 2006; Binder et al. 1996; Desmond et al. 1995; Gaillard et al. 2002; Hertz-Pannier et al. 1997; Lehericy et al. 2000; Medina et al. 2007; Rutten et al. 2002; Sabbah et al. 2003; Spreer et al. 2002; Woermann et al. 2003; Worthington et al. 1997; Yetkin et al. 1998). There is approximately 10% to 15% partial discordance between the IAT and fMRI, but complete disagreement is rare (Gaillard et al. 2002; Ramsey et al. 2001); rather, one test may be lateralized and the other bilateral. Both methods have their limitations, and when disagreement has been reported there are instances where one or the other has proven to be correct (Hunter et al. 1999; Kho et al. 2005; Lanzenberger et al. 2005; Pardo and Fox 1993). There are some strategies that may increase assurance of findings—such as using repeated or similar paradigms, or a panel of tasks targeted at different language functions—but they have only a small effect on increasing agreement between fMRI and IAT (Gaillard et al. 2004; Ramsey et al. 2001). Although IAT provides a sense of what may happen with a resection by disrupting function, IAT involves the use of radiation, has limited sampling time, is more difficult to repeat, carries the risk of stroke and hematoma, and is limited when vascular supply is aberrant. IAT procedures are not standardized and normative data are not available. On the other hand, fMRI can only be performed on patients safe for the MR scanner, and those who are cooperative and not claustrophobic. However, fMRI is more amenable to experimental manipulation and is easier to repeat than the IAT. While fMRI paradigms are not standardized, there is a growing consensus of tasks. Furthermore, fMRI allows acquisition of normal data and can be performed in children as young as 4 to 5 years of age (Byars et al. 2002; Yerys et al. 2009). The discrepancies with IAT may be attributable in part to choice of testing measures. The IAT relies heavily on object naming, a strategy that has not been successful with fMRI, at least in temporal areas; frontal activation can be elicited when a decision based on attributes of the viewed picture is forced. Comparisons of fMRI with IAT predominantly rely on comparisons with tasks that employ verbal fluency and those that identify anterior but not necessarily posterior language areas (Gaillard 2004).

Several language paradigms have been used in fMRI (Fig. 5.2). The most commonly used paradigms utilize some form of verbal fluency. While special techniques may be used to allow overt response, most studies have relied on a covert and unmonitored approach. Fluency may be free or it may be paced. In the former, a subject is asked to generate a list of words that fall into given categories (food, animals, furniture; these are semantic tasks) or letters (C, L, F; these

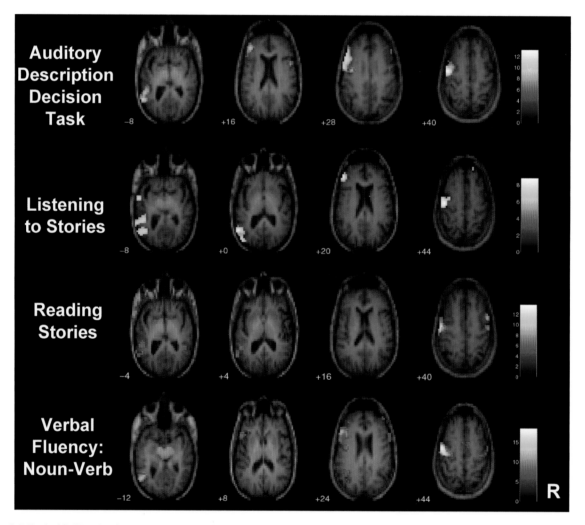

Figure 5.2 Typical fMRI activation patterns in a 38-year-old left-handed woman with right temporal lobe epilepsy. Four tasks are shown. Top row is an auditory description decision task—a word definition decision task (e.g., "A long yellow fruit is a banana; press response button if true") compared to reverse speech (push response button if hear subsequent tone). Second row is listening to stories with reverse speech control. Third row is reading stories with viewing a string of open and filled squares for the control condition. The fourth row is an auditory task of generating verbs to a series of nouns presented every 3 seconds (e.g., ball—hit, pitch, throw, kick) with silent rest and visual fixation control. Activation elicited by tasks identify Wernicke's region in left temporal cortex and Broca's region in left inferior frontal cortex. Additional activation is seen in left midfrontal cortex and premotor cortex. The consistent activation patterns across all tasks demonstrate that this patient is left dominant for language.

are phonemic tasks) over a block of time; results are usually compared to rest (Gaillard et al. 2001; Hertz-Pannier et al. 1997; Lehericy et al. 2000; Pujol et al. 1999; Woermann et al. 2003; Yetkin et al. 1998). Paced fluency happens when a word (a noun) is presented and the subject is asked to generate a verb or verbs in response; nouns are presented every 2 to 4 seconds, with rest or visual fixation for control (Petersen et al. 1988; Wise et al. 1991; Wood et al. 2004). The noun–verb task is a test of semantic fluency, but one can ask for words that rhyme (phonemic) or are antonyms, and so forth (Brown et al. 2005; Schlaggar et al. 2002). Fluency tasks are the simplest but in many ways the most robust, are the easiest to implement, and are consistently replicable despite the absence of behavioral monitoring. The free fluency tasks yield activation in inferior frontal gyrus (IFG), Brodman area (BA) 44-45, as well as middle frontal gyrus (BA 46/9) and premotor areas, with little individual activation in temporal areas. Phonological tasks give more activation in posterior Broca's area, whereas semantic tasks yield more activation in the anterior and superior portions of Broca's region. The paced paradigms give somewhat more temporal activation because of greater demand on word processing and the greater number of stimuli.

The next most commonly used language paradigm in fMRI requires a decision based on presented words, typically whether a word matches a condition or a category. These paradigms have the strength of allowing behavioral monitoring, accuracy, and reaction time, although effort is usually more important than performance, unless unable to do (Binder et al. 1996; Springer et al. 1999). However, this strategy changes the nature of the task and results in greater activation in BA 47. The bulk of the activation is found in anterior brain regions.

The tasks discussed so far primarily target anterior, "expressive" language systems. To target posterior, temporal "receptive" systems, paradigms that stress comprehension need to be used. Several strategies may be employed: stories may be read, or subjects may listen to stories (Ahmad et al. 2003; Holland et al. 2007; Lehericy et al. 1998; Schlosser et al. 1998). More grammatically complex tasks and tasks that require reading tend to yield more bilateral activation (Carpentier et al. 2001; Gaillard et al. 2001; Just et al. 1996). Reading declarative sentences and deciding on a word definition or whether a phrase is grammatically or syntactically correct show robust lateralized activation (Gaillard et al. 2001, 2002). These tasks activate cortex along the posterior two thirds of the superior temporal sulcus extending to the supramarginal and angular gyrus (BA 21, 22, 39, 40). Activation of BA 37 is also seen when reading text or imagining an object is required (Balsamo et al. 2006; Gaillard et al. 2007).

When a decision is required of the presented phrase or sentence, then activation of the inferior frontal gyrus and middle frontal gyrus is seen in the dominant hemisphere (Gaillard et al. 2007).

The presentation of items may be visual or auditory. For the later, using reverse speech, or listening to a foreign and unfamiliar language (Schlosser 1998), for the control condition will account for primary and secondary auditory processing and will isolate speech functions, although the former will present the same range, duration, pitch, and sounds of the experimental condition. Listening to tones may also be used but does not isolate language processing as reverse speech controls. For reading a visual control is needed. Simple strategies, viewing filled or open circles, do not eliminate occipital activation; the use of pseudo-words and false fonts may be too close to reading for unskilled subjects to sustain significant contrast across conditions.

Dominance can be established by visual rating (Fernandez et al. 2001; Gaillard et al. 2002), although for clinical rating images may need to be viewed at several thresholds, or by applying quantitative methods using an ROI approach. ROIs may be hemispheric (Binder et al. 1996) or regional—i.e., Broca's and Wernicke's areas (Gaillard et al. 2002; Spreer et al. 2002; Weber et al. 2006). The narrower regional approaches yield higher asymmetry indices, as areas not involved in language areas are excluded. Several patterns of activation may be identified. Left dominance is characterized by activation in inferior frontal gyrus extending into adjacent middle frontal gyrus and premotor cortex, as well as activation along superior temporal sulcus, fusiform gyrus, and BA 37. When an ROI approach is used, a laterality index (LI = the number of activated voxels in the left region minus the number of activated voxels in the right regions divided by the sum of activated voxels in left and right regions) of 0.15 to 0.25 is the range of thresholds used to define left dominance; most studies use an LI of 0.20—that is, when more than 60% activation occurs on the left (Binder et al. 1996; Gaillard et al. 2002; Pujol et al. 1999; Thivard et al. 2005). Some degree of activation is nearly always seen in right homologues; strong left dominance is characterized by an LI exceeding 0.6 or 0.7. Right dominance occurs when activation is seen in right homologues and LI is less than −0.20.

Several patterns of activation can be seen besides right or left dominance. Bilateral activation takes several forms; true bilateral activation occurs when the activation is similar in both right and left regions ($|LI| < 0.20$). Some patients will exhibit crossed dominance between temporal and frontal areas, others will exhibit task-dependent dominance (e.g., auditory comprehension on the left, reading comprehension on the right), and still others will be bilateral in one region and lateralized in another (Baciu et al. 2003;

Gaillard 2004; Lee et al. 2008; Ries et al. 2004) (Fig. 5.3). When activation is truly bilateral, it is difficult to know which side, if any, is critical for language. Activation shows areas associated with the task, but these areas may not be essential for speech functions. In such cases, more invasive diagnostic methods, such as the IAT or ECS, are necessary to resolve these issues.

To be assured of the reliability of findings, a panel of tasks may be helpful (Gaillard et al. 2004; Ramsey et al. 2001). Tasks that target different aspects of language may be used to map the entire network (Figs. 5.2 and 5.3). While temporal areas usually follow frontal activation, the target of most surgery in adults is one temporal lobe; therefore, tasks that stress comprehension are important for planning temporal lobe epilepsy surgery. The neocortical epilepsy patients with normal MRI are the most challenging, and complete agreement with IAT in this group may be less than for other groups, especially when atypical language is

found (Benke et al. 2006; Brazdil et al. 2005; Woermann et al. 2003).

Few studies have examined the relationship between fMRI and ECS. Indeed, there is only one study, using ^{15}O-water PET, that directly compared the same tasks with functional mapping and ECS (Bookheimer et al. 1997). This study found good but not complete agreement. Nevertheless, it is an important study since it confirms that activation induced by blood flow methods is comparable to disruption induced by stimulation and validates fMRI methods. Other studies that primarily compare object naming with verbal fluency have reported a sensitivity of over 90% and specificity of 65% (FitzGerald et al. 1997; Pouratian et al. 2002; Roux et al. 2003; Rutten et al. 2002). These studies are problematic as there is a different distribution of activation and ECS based on task (Hamberger 2007; Hamberger et al. 2001, 2007; Malow et al. 1996). ECS cannot assess all areas identified by fMRI, including depths of a sulcus (Rutten et al. 2002), and one must

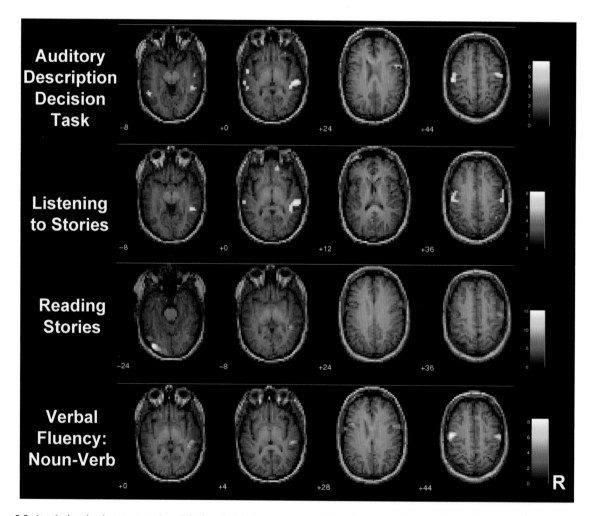

Figure 5.3 Atypical activation patterns in a right-handed 30-year-old man with right temporal lobe epilepsy. The same four tasks are shown as in **Figure 5.2**. The activation patterns across all tasks demonstrate that this patient is right dominant for language in temporal areas, with R > L activation in frontal regions.

make assumptions about threshold to be used with penumbra and distance from cortical stimulation. However, ECS studies do suggest that fMRI-negative areas are generally safe to resect (but only when there are other areas that are activated), whereas areas activated may not always be critical to language functions.

There are four circumstances that disrupt the physiologic basis upon which the BOLD response is based (Gaillard 2004): (1) critical carotid stenosis (Rother et al. 2002), where increased blood flow due to increased physiologic demand cannot occur; in this circumstance a "deactivation" may be seen because there is reduced MR signal from increased oxygen extraction, a decrease in oxyhemoglobin, and an increase in deoxyhemoglobin; (2) a vascular steal that occurs adjacent to arteriovenous malformations; in this case, either the tissue is chronically short of oxyhemoglobin or the blood flow with abundant oxyhemoglobin and mixing due to the malformation overwhelms small signal changes seen with the task (Lehericy et al. 2002); (3) large gliomas with marked mass effect (Gaillard, Bookheimer, et al. 2000); and (4) a postictal state (Jayakar et al. 2002) may alter blood flow or blood flow coupling and yield null activation. In these four circumstances, the roughly 30% of activation seen in homologous regions may be misinterpreted as the primary response and misidentify language dominance. For purposes of epilepsy surgery planning, the observation by Jayakar et al. (2002) of diminished BOLD response in the postictal state is important. Consideration should be given to postpone an fMRI study after a flurry of seizures or in the postictal state. There are no extensive data on the effect of antiepileptic medications on the BOLD response or on activation patterns. There may be an effect of topiramate, which seems to diminish activation, but this may be from a primary effect on cognition (Jansen et al. 2006).

Experience with fMRI also provides insights into patients who may be at risk for atypical language representation in addition to the constraining neurobiological and developmental features that guide atypical language. Using verbal fluency and semantic decision paradigms, 4% to 6% of right-handed normal volunteers exhibit atypical, mostly bilateral, language representation (Pujol et al. 1999; Springer et al. 1999). Normal left-handed volunteers show atypical language 32% to 34% of the time (Pujol et al. 1999; Szaflarski et al. 2002), whereas 30% of localization-related epilepsy patients have some form of atypical language representation (Adcock et al. 2003; Gaillard et al. 2007; Springer et al. 1999; Thivard et al. 2005; Woermann et al. 2003). Those who are left-handed will have approximately 60% atypical language, beyond what might be expected for the normal left-handed population (Gaillard et al. 2007). It is not surprising

that verbal patients with dominant hemisphere stroke all have atypical language representation. However, it is surprising that those with normal MRI are at high risk for atypical language. Patients with tumors and developmental lesions have rates of altered language networks that vary with size and location of the lesion (Briellmann et al. 2006; Hadac et al. 2007; Liegeois et al. 2004). While there is evidence that malformations of cortical development can sustain activation for task when well circumscribed (Vitali et al. 2008) or when diffuse and extensive (Briellmann et al. 2006), most evidence suggests activation is more likely to occur at the margin or in homologous areas for lesions that rest within Broca's or Wernicke's territories. When the malformation is substantial, activation is seen in right homologues (Liegeois et al. 2004; Smith et al. 2004). It is interesting that lesions in mesial structures, such as mesial temporal sclerosis, or foci remote from language neocortex that are not primary language areas are associated with atypical language (Weber et al. 2006); this suggests that verbal memory capacity is linked to the establishment of language dominance. Indeed, one quarter of patients with mesial temporal sclerosis have atypical language dominance that extends beyond temporal regions to affect frontal systems (Gaillard et al. 2002, 2007; Thivard et al. 2005).

Atypical language networks are most closely linked to patients with a history of early brain injury before age 6 years, developmental lesion (e.g., dysplasia, tumor), or seizure onset before the age of 6 years (Gaillard et al. 2007; Springer et al. 1999; Woermann et al. 2003). These observations suggest that atypical language most likely represents the persistence of immature language systems. In this view, typical language development occurs with consolidation of systems in the left (or typically dominant) hemisphere in conjunction with suppression or harnessing of contralateral homologous regions. Consolidation of hemisphere dominance may be mediated by interhemispheric fibers passing through the corpus callosum by the dominant hemisphere and may reflect maturing myelination of these systems. When the left hemisphere is injured before the age of 6 years, then the nondominant systems are not suppressed, and they mature to assume and sustain language functions that are effectively normal (Gaillard et al. 2007). Evidence to support reorganization that is normal after these ages is scant. Some children with chronic focal encephalitis of Rasmussen may make significant recovery following resection of dominant hemispheres after age 9 years, but the language is never normal in such cases (Boatman et al. 1999; Hertz-Pannier et al. 2002; Liegeois et al. 2008; Telfeian et al. 2002; Vargha-Khadem et al. 1991, 1997). It is unclear whether these are patients who had some capacity for language in the nondominant hemisphere before onset of illness (but see Hertz-Pannier et al. 2002). Other investigators have found that the likelihood of atypical dominance is proportional to interictal spike frequency in the left temporal lobe (Janszky et al. 2006). The rare instances of reversed language "dominance" activation patterns following left temporal lobectomy may also support this view (Helmstaedter et al. 2006), as does an ^{15}O-water PET study that demonstrates reversal of the asymmetry index in a verbal fluency task during transcranial magnetic stimulation (Thiel et al. 2006). This raises the possibility that ongoing, smoldering epileptogenic activity may in part drive reorganization, although it is also possible that interictal activity is evidence for more impaired substrate.

The interpretation above is informed by normal data in children and adults. The activation patterns for children are fundamentally the same as they are for adults, at least down to ages 4 to 6 years (Ahmad et al. 2003; Balsamo et al. 2002, 2006; Gaillard et al. 2000; Gaillard et al. 2003; Liegeois et al. 2002; Wood et al. 2004). Still, there are some mild developmental differences. For example, there is slightly more bilateral activation in the youngest children, especially in anterior head regions (Gaillard et al. 2000; Holland et al. 2001, 2007). The findings in pediatric epilepsy are similar to those in adult epilepsy; this is not surprising, as most young adults evaluated at epilepsy centers have childhood-onset epilepsy (Anderson et al. 2006; Gaillard et al. 2002, 2007; Liegeois et al. 2004; Yuan et al. 2006).

There is evidence that altered activation maps represent successful compensation within a distributed network. This may occur as a result of injury to either cortex or to deep white matter tracts (Gaillard et al. 2007; Staudt et al. 2001). When atypical language is seen, except in subjects with stroke, those with atypical language often have preserved language measures (Gaillard et al. 2007; Thivard et al. 2005). Preliminary evaluation of functional connectivity in patients with normal and atypical language networks does not reveal any changes in functional connectivity (unpublished observations). There is also evidence that remote effects of epilepsy may affect anterior language systems despite a posterior focus (Berl et al. 2005; Billingsley et al. 2001; Janszky et al. 2006; Weber et al. 2006). Furthermore, language representation in patients with a right seizure focus may not be as strongly lateralized as in normal populations, especially in temporal areas, and systems implicated in working memory may be independent of the seizure focus (Berl et al. 2005).

The networks that support language are discrete and readily identified to areas in the left hemisphere and homologues in the right. While there is clear evidence for reorganization of language to the right, when this occurs it is restricted to right homologues of Broca's and Wernicke's territories (Mbwana et al.

2009; Rosenberger et al. 2009; Staudt et al. 2001, 2002). Evidence for "intra-hemispheric" reorganization or compensation is hard to find. The few studies that examine this phenomenon find activation on margins of traditional regions known to sustain language (Mbwana et al. 2009; Rosenberger et al. 2009; Voets et al. 2006). In other circumstances, there may be a different weighting of activation within the distributed network for language that may reflect alternative strategies to process different aspects of language (Berl et al. 2005, 2006; Billingsley et al. 2001).

Increasingly, identification of language networks is being informed by imaging of white matter tracts using diffusion tensor imaging (DTI; see also Chapter 6). There are two principal methods: one involves identifying the arcuate fasciculus in centrum semiovale and following the directionality of these fibers (Catani et al. 2005, 2007), and the other is to follow tracts from cortical regions, preferably guided by fMRI activation maps (Powell et al. 2008; Yogarajah et al. 2008). Detailed studies of monkey and human cortex identify three principal pathways from receptive to expressive cortex, the arcuate fasciculus, the superior longitudinal fasciculus, and uncinate fasciculus/extreme capsular fiber system (Frey et al. 2008). The specificity of regional connections remains unsettled, but increasingly sophisticated methods of tractography will likely resolve these matters. However, identification of these fibers may be important in avoiding these tracts when planning surgery.

Memory

In addition to language, memory systems need to be spared in pursuing epilepsy surgery. The goal of imaging endeavors for memory should be to identify patients who will suffer irreparable harm to memory following surgery on hippocampal structures (Powell et al. 2004). These studies are more difficult to perform than imaging motor or language systems. Imaging mesial structures for memory is challenging due to artifacts from the petrous ridge and sphenoid sinus adjacent to the hippocampus. Furthermore, it is difficult to elicit a signal in a structure that is always "on line" or active.

Several aspects to memory can be assessed. Most studies have examined encoding rather than recall, but it is likely that both need to be assessed. Also, the advent of event-related designs (see above) has allowed analysis of imaging runs based on items that have been successfully encoded as ascertained by post-scanning recognition testing (Brewer et al. 1998; Stern et al. 1996). Items not successfully encoded do not elicit a blood flow response, in contrast to those encoded. Furthermore, there appears to be material specificity for the types of items presented. Verbal items are more likely to activate dominant (left) hippocampal formation and parahippocampal areas. Items that are purely visuospatial rely on the right hippocampus. Tasks that require encoding of scenes or determining whether a scene is interior or exterior activate both hippocampal formations, presumably because both visuospatial and verbal strategies are used (Binder et al. 2008; Detre et al. 1998; Rabin et al. 2004). Such an explanation likely applies to mental navigation tasks (Roland hometown navigation) where a patient retraces steps through his or her home town (Block design) (Jokeit et al. 2001). There may be an anterior to posterior gradient based on novelty of items tested; novel items are processed in posterior hippocampus (Binder et al. 2005). Picture encoding tasks have been the most widely used. In normal populations there is equal activation in right and left hippocampal formation and parahippocampal gyrus. The activation is decreased in hippocampal formation/parahippocampal gyrus ipsilateral to the seizure focus. As a rule, volume averaging for hippocampal formation has not been performed as a complicating factor, but this may not be relevant for practical applications. Nonetheless, these paradigms have been proven useful.

Few studies have examined data on an individual basis. In general, fMRI memory tasks have less agreement with IAT on an individual basis than do language tasks (Detre et al. 1998). Unfortunately, there is poor correlation with general memory measures, but there is specific reliability for postoperative outcomes with the fMRI test (verbal, visuospatial) itself (Janszky et al. 2005; Powell et al. 2008; Rabin et al. 2004; Richardson et al. 2004). Thus, fMRI may be used to predict outcome performance, at least on a narrow range of measures. For memory paradigms to be clinically practical, it is likely that a panel of tasks that examines material specificity, encoding, and recall will need to be used (Golby et al. 2002; Powell et al. 2005, 2008).

Recent studies have stressed verbal encoding as a probe of verbal memory, which is of special interest in postoperative outcomes (Golby et al. 2001, 2002; Powell et al. 2005; Richardson et al. 2004). For these tasks, one expects greater activation in the left (or dominant) hippocampal formation and designed as a probe to predict postoperative verbal memory outcomes. There is increasing evidence that outcomes following hippocampal formation resection reflect activation in the resected hippocampus rather than activation in the nonresected hippocampal formation (Powell et al. 2008; Rabin et al. 2004; Richardson et al. 2004, 2006). Greater activation in the resected hippocampal formation for tasks is associated with greater postoperative deficit, regardless of contralateral activation. This supports the notion of hippocampal adequacy rather than hippocampal reserve. Finally,

it seems that verbal activation in hippocampal formation follows language dominance. The decreases in verbal memory attributed to memory paradigms may reflect the well-known reduction in verbal capacity when operating on the dominant temporal lobe, especially the mesial temporal lobe, for language (Binder et al. 2008). When dominance has not shifted there is little evidence for hippocampal compensation (Powell et al. 2007; Richardson et al. 2003).

Group studies suggest that there is less activation on the side ipsilateral to the seizure focus when scene encoding tasks are used (Bellgowan et al. 1998). These studies do not account for heterogeneity and individual results. Some investigators have suggested that hippocampus activation methods may be used to identify the side of seizure origin, but this is not the primary interest in memory studies (Jokeit et al. 2001). For tasks that yield bilateral hippocampus/parahippocampus activation, such as scene encoding, the side ipsilateral to the seizure focus usually exhibits less activation. Other studies of memory find that with diminished activation in hippocampus there is greater activation in dorsal lateral prefrontal cortex (Dupont et al. 2000), showing evidence of compensatory efforts that rely on alternative strategies to sustain memory function (e.g., working memory). Group studies do allow interrogation of data based on regression for performance and cognitive skills, but data for individuals are still lacking. Other data support impaired working memory systems that may have greater relevance for patient compensation and practical day-to-day living. Memory paradigms are only beginning to be designed for children and have not yet been applied to pediatric epilepsy populations.

EPILEPTOGENIC ZONE

Most imaging and neurophysiological techniques used to evaluate patients with localization-related epilepsy (e.g., structural MRI, PET, SPECT, video-EEG, MEG) are directed at identifying the epileptic zone to be targeted for resection. Unlike most methods, fMRI is primarily used to identify eloquent cortex to be spared during surgery. However, there are expanding efforts to use fMRI for seizure focus identification.

One such application uses fMRI to map homodynamic changes that occur in a seizure focus and in its propagation. In this regard, fMRI resembles ictal HMPAO/ECD SPECT (see Chapter 14), except that one can trace the temporal spread of the ictus and seizure propagation. However, such events are rare, as seizures must occur in the scanner and movement must be minimal. There are a few cases, mostly serendipitous, of ictal events occurring in the scanner (Detre et al. 1995; Jackson et al. 1994; Krings et al. 2000;

Schwartz et al. 1998). In such instances, the signal change associated with the seizures has generally been identified by clinical correlation (e.g., frequent simple partial seizures readily identifiable clinically) or by identification of a peculiar BOLD response. These studies show changes in CBF signal associated with the seizure and its propagation. More recently, efforts have been made to place patients in the MRI scanner for prolonged imaging with EEG recording after their medications have been discontinued for purposes of video-EEG seizure characterization and localization. In this manner, it is possible to capture seizures and examine their origin in some patients. More commonly, however, fMRI has been used for source localization of interictal spikes, comparable to the use of MEG (Gotman 2008). This approach presumes that the interictal source is the same as the ictal source and zone. To accomplish this goal, fMRI is used to identify the signal changes associated with an interictal spike to localize its source.

Obtaining EEG in the MRI scanner is not a simple matter, as the MRI environment is not conducive to EEG recording. Early and successful efforts monitored EEG in a quiet scanner; when a spike occurred, the scanner was engaged to image the brain. This strategy takes advantage of the observation that the peak hemodynamic response occurs approximately 5 seconds after the spike (Krakow et al. 1999; Symms et al. 1999). Current methods—using a series of filters, software processing, and nonmagnetic materials—allow for continuous scanning and continuous EEG acquisition. The data are then screened to identify time points when interictal spikes occurred (Al-Asmi et al. 2003; Lemieux 2004). Varying the hemodynamic response function can be used to model the optimal identification of signal change associated with spike activity (Bagshaw et al. 2004). These are the event-related methods described above. Data from these periods are compared to periods when the EEG is quiescent. In general, 5 to 30 events are needed for this analysis. Such data can be obtained in a substantial proportion of patients, but obviously depends on the interictal spike frequency and time possible to remain in the scanner.

Using this approach, interictal spikes can be readily mapped (Benar and Gotman 2002; Krakow et al. 2001). They have been mapped to mesial temporal structures in patients with mesial temporal sclerosis, to the margins of known structural lesions such as malformations of cortical development, and to neocortical foci in patients with normal MRI (Diehl et al. 2003; Kobayashi et al. 2005). However, there have not been many studies that have sought to compare such fMRI findings to localization from intracranial EEG monitoring (Benar et al. 2006; Lemieux et al. 2001).

Furthermore, fMRI can map signal changes associated with activity that is remote from the seizure origin and represents propagation from the primary site (Kobayashi et al. 2006). For example, temporal spikes may be associated with signal change in thalamus and contralateral temporal lobe. Such findings reinforce the important observation that local spikes may have widespread effects. In addition, one can discern areas of deactivation and may parse out differential effects of the spike and subsequent slow wave (Kobayashi et al. 2005). Examination of deactivation reveals maps that reflect the default network for interrupted cognition first described by Raichle at al. (2001) using ^{15}O-water PET. They have since been described using fMRI in the resting state, under anesthesia, and in absence epilepsy (Archer et al. 2003; Gotman et al. 2005; Laufs et al. 2006, 2007). Indeed, fMRI of spikes has been used to map not only primary generalized epilepsy of the absence type but also juvenile myoclonic epilepsy, as well as animal models of absence epilepsy (Aghakhani et al. 2004; Blumenfeld 2007; Nersesyan et al. 2004; Salek-Haddadi et al. 2003; Tenney et al. 2004). These studies have found heterogeneity of activation patterns, although most have confirmed the role of thalamus in spike propagation. Other brain regions are identified as being either active or deactivated. In general, these studies emphasize the observation that generalized epilepsy is restricted to a well-defined set of neural circuits.

Some fMRI studies have been used to identify signal change characteristics of the interictal and the preictal state. The former (Morgan et al. 2004) is based on the presumption that interictal activity will disrupt baseline CBF variance. The latter derives from studies that also presume differences in neuronal signature before seizures are organized into an ictal EEG pattern (Federico et al. 2005).

Finally, and briefly, the MRI technique of arterial spin labeling allows quantitative and absolute measures of blood flow. Arterial spin labeling studies have identified decreased CBF in the interictal state in temporal lobe epilepsy ipsilateral to the seizure focus (Lim et al. 2008; Wolf et al. 2001). These studies compare favorably with findings from ^{15}O-water PET. However, interictal CBF findings are not as reliable as ictal measures of CBF or resting interictal metabolic measurements using PET (Gaillard et al. 1995). Therefore, at present, arterial spin labeling MRI plays a limited role in seizure focus localization.

CONCLUSIONS

In summary, fMRI has entered standard clinical practice as a reliable and reproducible means of identifying motor, sensory, and language cortex in planning epilepsy surgery and has been validated by invasive means. There are, however, limitations and circumstances in which fMRI does not work. Overt disagreement with language fMRI is rare, but partial discordance occurs in 10% of patients. Patients with neocortical epilepsy and those with normal MRI are at greater risk for discordance. It is important to target brain regions selected for surgery with the proper task. When results are null, peculiar, and not reproducible, then invasive means should be used. Memory paradigms are beginning to be identified and will likely enter practice in the near future. As with language mapping, a panel of tasks will likely be necessary to delineate the several aspects of memory. Finally, spike-related fMRI may be useful in source localization of interictal spikes and their distributed network.

REFERENCES

Adcock, J. E., R. G. Wise, et al. 2003. Quantitative fMRI assessment of the differences in lateralization of language-related brain activation in patients with temporal lobe epilepsy. *Neuroimage* 18(2): 423–38.

Aghakhani, Y., A. P. Bagshaw, et al. 2004. fMRI activation during spike and wave discharges in idiopathic generalized epilepsy. *Brain* 127(Pt 5): 1127–44.

Ahmad, Z., L. M. Balsamo, et al. 2003. Auditory comprehension of language in young children: neural networks identified with fMRI. *Neurology* 60(10): 1598–605.

Al-Asmi, A., C. G. Benar, et al. 2003. fMRI activation in continuous and spike-triggered EEG-fMRI studies of epileptic spikes. *Epilepsia* 44(10): 1328–39.

Altman, N. R., and B. Bernal. 2001. Brain activation in sedated children: auditory and visual functional MR imaging. *Radiology* 221(1): 56–63.

Anderson, D. P., A. S. Harvey, et al. 2006. fMRI lateralization of expressive language in children with cerebral lesions. *Epilepsia* 47(6): 998–1008.

Archer, J. S., D. F. Abbott, et al. 2003. fMRI deactivation of the posterior cingulate during generalized spike and wave. *Neuroimage* 20(4): 1915–22.

Baciu, M. V., J. M. Watson, et al. 2003. Functional MRI reveals an interhemispheric dissociation of frontal and temporal language regions in a patient with focal epilepsy. *Epilepsy Behavior* 4(6): 776–80.

Bagshaw, A. P., Y. Aghakhani, et al. 2004. EEG-fMRI of focal epileptic spikes: analysis with multiple haemodynamic functions and comparison with gadolinium-enhanced MR angiograms. *Human Brain Mapping* 22(3): 179–92.

Bahn, M. M., W. Lin, et al. 1997. Localization of language cortices by functional MR imaging compared with intracarotid amobarbital hemispheric sedation. *AJR American Journal of Roentgenology* 169(2): 575–9.

Balsamo, L. M., B. Xu, et al. 2006. Language lateralization and the role of the fusiform gyrus in semantic processing in young children. *Neuroimage* 31(3): 1306–14.

Balsamo, L. M., B. Xu, et al. 2002. A functional magnetic resonance imaging study of left hemisphere language dominance in children. *Archives of Neurology* 59(7): 1168–74.

Bellgowan, P. S., J. R. Binder, et al. 1998. Side of seizure focus predicts left medial temporal lobe activation during verbal encoding. *Neurology* 51(2): 479–84.

Benar, C. G., and J. Gotman. 2002. Modeling of post-surgical brain and skull defects in the EEG inverse problem with the boundary element method. *Clinical Neurophysiology* 113(1): 48–56.

Benar, C. G., C. Grova, et al. 2006. EEG-fMRI of epileptic spikes: concordance with EEG source localization and intracranial EEG. *Neuroimage* 30(4): 1161–70.

Benke, T., B. Koylu, et al. 2006. Language lateralization in temporal lobe epilepsy: a comparison between fMRI and the Wada test. *Epilepsia* 47(8): 1308–19.

Berl, M. M., L. M. Balsamo, et al. 2005. Seizure focus affects regional language networks assessed by fMRI. *Neurology* 65(10): 1604–11.

Berl, M. M., C. J. Vaidya, et al. 2006. Functional imaging of developmental and adaptive changes in neurocognition. *Neuroimage* 30(3): 679–91.

Billingsley, R. L., M. P. McAndrews, et al. 2001. Functional MRI of phonological and semantic processing in temporal lobe epilepsy. *Brain* 124(Pt 6): 1218–27.

Binder, J. R., P. S. Bellgowan, et al. 2005. A comparison of two FMRI protocols for eliciting hippocampal activation. *Epilepsia* 46(7): 1061–70.

Binder, J. R., D. S. Sabsevitz, et al. 2008. Use of preoperative functional MRI to predict verbal memory decline after temporal lobe epilepsy surgery. *Epilepsia* 49(8): 1377–94.

Binder, J. R., S. J. Swanson, et al. 1996. Determination of language dominance using functional MRI: a comparison with the Wada test. *Neurology* 46(4): 978–84.

Blumenfeld, H. 2007. Functional MRI studies of animal models in epilepsy. *Epilepsia* 48 Suppl 4: 18–26.

Boatman, D., J. Freeman, et al. 1999. Language recovery after left hemispherectomy in children with late-onset seizures. *Annals of Neurology* 46(4): 579–86.

Bookheimer, S. Y., T. A. Zeffiro, et al. 1997. A direct comparison of PET activation and electrocortical stimulation mapping for language localization. *Neurology* 48(4): 1056–65.

Brazdil, M., P. Chlebus, et al. 2005. Reorganization of language-related neuronal networks in patients with left temporal lobe epilepsy: an fMRI study. *European Journal of Neurology* 12(4): 268–75.

Brewer, J. B., Z. Zhao, et al. 1998. Making memories: brain activity that predicts how well visual experience will be remembered. *Science* 281: 1185–87.

Briellmann, R. S., A. Labate, et al. 2006. Is language lateralization in temporal lobe epilepsy patients related to the nature of the epileptogenic lesion? *Epilepsia* 47(5): 916–20.

Briellmann, R. S., T. Little, et al. 2006. Pathologic and physiologic function in the subcortical band of double cortex. *Neurology* 67(6): 1090–3.

Brown, T. T., H. M. Lugar, et al. 2005. Developmental changes in human cerebral functional organization for word generation. *Cerebral Cortex* 15(3): 275–90.

Byars, A. W., S. K. Holland, et al. 2002. Practical aspects of conducting large-scale functional magnetic resonance imaging studies in children. *Journal of Child Neurology* 17(12): 885–90.

Carpentier, A., K. R. Pugh, et al. 2001. Functional MRI of language processing: dependence on input modality and temporal lobe epilepsy. *Epilepsia* 42(10): 1241–54.

Catani, M., M. P. Allin, et al. 2007. Symmetries in human brain language pathways correlate with verbal recall. *Proceedings of the National Academy of Sciences of the United States of America* 104(43): 163–8.

Catani, M., D. K. Jones, et al. 2005. Perisylvian language networks of the human brain. *Annals of Neurology* 57(1): 8–16.

Desmond, J. E., J. M. Sum, et al. 1995. Functional MRI measurement of language lateralization in Wada-tested patients. *Brain* 118: 1411–9.

Detre, J. A., L. Maccotta, et al. 1998. Functional MRI lateralization of memory in temporal lobe epilepsy. *Neurology* 50(4): 926–32.

Detre, J. A., J. I. Sirven, et al. 1995. Localization of subclinical ictal activity by functional magnetic resonance imaging: correlation with invasive monitoring. *Annals of Neurology* 38(4): 618–24.

Diehl, B., R. Prayson, et al. 2003. Hamartomas and epilepsy: clinical and imaging characteristics. *Seizure* 12(5): 307–11.

Dupont, S., P. F. Van de Moortele, et al. 2000. Episodic memory in left temporal lobe epilepsy: a functional MRI study. *Brain* 123 (Pt 8): 1722–32.

Federico, P., D. F. Abbott, et al. 2005. Functional MRI of the pre-ictal state. *Brain* 128(Pt 8): 1811–7.

Fernandez, G., A. de Greiff, et al. 2001. Language mapping in less than 15 minutes: real-time functional MRI during routine clinical investigation. *Neuroimage* 14(3): 585–94.

FitzGerald, D. B., G. R. Cosgrove, et al. 1997. Location of language in the cortex: a comparison between functional MR imaging and electrocortical stimulation. *AJNR American Journal of Neuroradiology* 18(8): 1529–39.

Fox, P. T., and M. E. Raichle. 1986. Focal physiological uncoupling of cerebral blood flow and oxidative metabolism during somatosensory stimulation of human subjects. *Proceedings of the National Academy of Sciences of the United States of America* 323: 806–809.

Frey, S., J. S. W. Campbell, et al. 2008. Dissociating the human language pathways with high angular resolution diffusion fiber tractography. *Journal of Neuroscience* 28(45): 11435.

Gaillard, W. D. 2004. Functional MR imaging of language, memory, and sensorimotor cortex. *Neuroimaging Clinics of North America* 14(3): 471–85.

Gaillard, W. D., L. Balsamo, et al. 2002. Language dominance in partial epilepsy patients identified with an fMRI reading task. *Neurology* 59(2): 256–65.

Gaillard, W. D., L. Balsamo, et al. 2004. fMRI language task panel improves determination of language dominance. *Neurology* 63(8): 1403–8.

Gaillard, W. D., L. M. Balsamo, et al. 2003. fMRI identifies regional specialization of neural networks for reading in young children. *Neurology* 60(1): 94–100.

Gaillard, W. D., M. M. Berl, et al. 2007. Atypical language in lesional and nonlesional complex partial epilepsy. *Neurology* 69(18): 1761–71.

Gaillard, W. D., S. Y. Bookheimer, et al. 2000. The use of fMRI in neocortical epilepsy. *Advances in Neurology* 84: 391–404.

Gaillard, W. D., S. Fazilat, et al. 1995. Interictal metabolism and blood flow are uncoupled in temporal lobe cortex of patients with complex partial epilepsy. *Neurology* 45(10): 1841–7.

Gaillard, W. D., L. Hertz-Pannier, L., et al. 2000. Functional anatomy of cognitve development: fMRI of verbal fluency in clhidren and adults. *Neurology* 54: 180–5.

Gaillard, W. D., M. Pugliese, et al. 2001. Cortical localization of reading in normal children: an fMRI language study. *Neurology* 57(1): 47–54.

Golby, A. J., R. A. Poldrack, et al. 2001. Material-specific lateralization in the medial temporal lobe and prefrontal cortex during memory encoding. *Brain* 124(Pt 9): 1841–54.

Golby, A. J., R. A. Poldrack, et al.2002. Memory lateralization in medial temporal lobe epilepsy assessed by functional MRI. *Epilepsia* 43(8): 855–63.

Gotman, J. 2008. Epileptic networks studied with EEG-fMRI. *Epilepsia* 49 Suppl 3: 42–51.

Gotman, J., C. Grova, et al. 2005. Generalized epileptic discharges show thalamocortical activation and suspension of the default state of the brain. *Proceedings of the National Academy of Sciences of the United States of America* 102(42): 15236–40.

Hadac, J., K. Brozová, et al. 2007. Language lateralization in children with pre- and postnatal epileptogenic lesions of the left hemisphere: an fMRI study. *Epileptic Disorders* 9(1): S19–27.

Hamberger, M. J. 2007. Cortical language mapping in epilepsy: a critical review. *Neuropsychology Review* 17(4): 477–89.

Hamberger, M. J., R. R. Goodman, et al. 2001. Anatomic dissociation of auditory and visual naming in the lateral temporal cortex. *Neurology* 56(1): 56–61.

Hamberger, M. J., W. T. Seidel, et al. 2007. Evidence for cortical reorganization of language in patients with hippocampal sclerosis. *Brain* 130(Pt 11): 2942–50.

Hammeke, T. A., F. Z. Yetkin, et al. 1994. Functional magnetic resonance imaging of somatosensory stimulation. *Neurosurgery* 35(4): 677–81.

Helmstaedter, C., N. E. Fritz, et al. 2006. Shift-back of right into left hemisphere language dominance after control of epileptic seizures: Evidence for epilepsy driven functional cerebral organization. *Epilepsy Research* 70(2–3): 257–62.

Hertz-Pannier, L., C. Chiron, et al. 2002. Late plasticity for language in a child's non-dominant hemisphere: a pre- and post-surgery fMRI study. *Brain* 125(Pt 2): 361–72.

Hertz-Pannier, L., W. D. Gaillard, et al. 1997. Noninvasive assessment of language dominance in children and adolescents with functional MRI: a preliminary study. *Neurology* 48(4): 1003–12.

Holland, S. K., E. Plante, et al. 2001. Normal fMRI brain activation patterns in children performing a verb generation task. *Neuroimage* 14(4): 837–43.

Holland, S. K., J. Vannest, et al. 2007. Functional MRI of language lateralization during development in children. *International Journal of Audiology* 46(9): 533–51.

Hunter, K. E., T. A. Blaxton, et al. 1999. (15)O water positron emission tomography in language localization: a study comparing positron emission tomography visual and computerized region of interest analysis with the Wada test. *Annals of Neurology* 45(5): 662–5.

Jack, C. R., R. M. Thompson, et al. 1994. Sensory motor cortex: correlation of presurgical mapping with functional MR imaging and invasive cortical mapping. *Radiology* 190: 85–92.

Jackson, G. D., A. Connelly, et al. 1994. Functional magnetic resonance imaging of focal seizures. *Neurology* 44(5): 850–6.

Jansen, J. F., A. P. Aldenkamp, et al. 2006. Functional MRI reveals declined prefrontal cortex activation in patients with epilepsy on topiramate therapy. *Epilepsy Behavior* 9(1): 181–5.

Janszky, J., H. Jokeit, et al. 2005. Functional MRI predicts memory performance after right mesiotemporal epilepsy surgery. *Epilepsia* 46(2): 244–50.

Janszky, J., M. Mertens, et al. 2006. Left-sided interictal epileptic activity induces shift of language lateralization in temporal lobe epilepsy: an fMRI study. *Epilepsia* 47(5): 921–7.

Jayakar, P., B. Bernal, et al. 2002. False lateralization of language cortex on functional MRI after a cluster of focal seizures. *Neurology* 58(3): 490–2.

Jokeit, H., M. Okujava, et al. 2001. Memory fMRI lateralizes temporal lobe epilepsy. *Neurology* 57(10): 1786–93.

Just, M. A., P. A. Carpenter, et al. 1996. Brain activation modulated by sentence comprehension. *Science* 274(5284): 114–6.

Kho, K. H., F. S. Leijten, et al. 2005. Discrepant findings for Wada test and functional magnetic resonance imaging with regard to language function: use of electrocortical stimulation mapping to confirm results. *Case report. Journal of Neurosurgery* 102(1): 169–73.

Kim, S. G., J. Ashe, et al. 1993. Functional imaging of human motor cortex at high magnetic field. *Journal of Neurophysiology* 69: 297–302.

Kobayashi, E., A. P. Bagshaw, et al. 2006. Temporal and extratemporal BOLD responses to temporal lobe interictal spikes. *Epilepsia* 47(2): 343–54.

Kobayashi, E., A. P. Bagshaw, et al. 2005. Intrinsic epileptogenicity in polymicrogyric cortex suggested by EEG-fMRI BOLD responses. *Neurology* 64(7): 1263–6.

Krakow, K., L. Lemieux, et al. 2001. Spatio-temporal imaging of focal interictal epileptiform activity using EEG-triggered functional MRI. *Epileptic Disorders* 3(2): 67–74.

Krakow, K., F. G. Woermann, et al. 1999. EEG-triggered functional MRI of interictal epileptiform activity in patients with partial seizures. *Brain* 122 (Pt 9): 1679–88.

Krings, T., R. Topper, et al. 2000. Hemodynamic changes in simple partial epilepsy: a functional MRI study. *Neurology* 54(2): 524–7.

Kwong, K. K., J. W. Belliveau, et al. 1992. Dynamic magnetic resonance imaging of human brain activity during primary sensory stimulation. *Proceedings of the National Academy of Sciences of the United States of America* 89(12): 5675–9.

Lanzenberger, R., G. Wiest, et al. 2005. FMRI reveals functional cortex in a case of inconclusive Wada testing. *Clinical Neurology & Neurosurgery* 107(2): 147–51.

Laufs, H., K. Hamandi, et al. 2007. Temporal lobe interictal epileptic discharges affect cerebral activity in default mode brain regions. *Human Brain Mapping* 28(10): 1023–32.

Laufs, H., U. Lengler, et al. 2006. Linking generalized spike-and-wave discharges and resting state brain activity by using EEG/fMRI in a patient with absence seizures. *Epilepsia* 47(2): 444–8.

Lee, D., S. J. Swanson, et al. 2008. Functional MRI and Wada studies in patients with interhemispheric dissociation of language functions. *Epilepsy & Behavior* 13(2): 350–6.

Lehericy, S., A. Biondi, et al. 2002. Arteriovenous brain malformations: is functional MR imaging reliable for studying language reorganization in patients? Initial observations. *Radiology* 223(3): 672–82.

Lehericy, S., L. Cohen, et al. 2000. Functional MR evaluation of temporal and frontal language dominance compared with the Wada test. *Neurology* 54(8): 1625–33.

Lehericy, S., H. Duffau, et al. 2000. Correspondence between functional magnetic resonance imaging somatotopy and individual brain anatomy of the central region: comparison with intraoperative stimulation in patients with brain tumors. *Journal of Neurosurgery* 92(4): 589–98.

Lemieux, L. 2004. Electroencephalography-correlated functional MR imaging studies of epileptic activity. *Neuroimaging Clinics of North America* 14(3): 487–506.

Lemieux, L., K. Krakow, et al. 2001. Comparison of spike-triggered functional MRI BOLD activation and EEG dipole model localization. *Neuroimage* 14(5): 1097–104.

Liegeois, F., A. Connelly, et al. 2008. Speaking with a single cerebral hemisphere: fMRI language organization after hemispherectomy in childhood. *Brain Language.* 106: 195–203.

Liegeois, F., A. Connelly, et al. 2004. Language reorganization in children with early-onset lesions of the left hemisphere: an fMRI study. *Brain* 127(Pt 6): 1229–36.

Liegeois, F., A. Connelly, et al. 2002. A direct test for lateralization of language activation using fMRI: comparison with invasive assessments in children with epilepsy. *Neuroimage* 17(4): 1861–7.

Lim, Y. M., Y. W. Cho, et al. 2008. Usefulness of pulsed arterial spin labeling MR imaging in mesial temporal lobe epilepsy. *Epilepsy Research* 82: 183–189.

Logothetis, N. K. 2003. The underpinnings of the BOLD functional magnetic resonance imaging signal. *Journal of Neuroscience* 23(10): 3963–71.

Malow, B. A., T. A. Blaxton, et al. 1996. Cortical stimulation elicits regionals distinctions in auditory and visual naming. *Epilepsia* 37(3): 245–252.

Mbwana, J., M. M. Berl, et al. 2009. Limitations to plasticity of language network reorganization in localization related epilepsy. *Brain* 132(2): 347–356.

Medina, L. S., B. Bernal, et al. 2005. Seizure disorders: functional MR imaging for diagnostic evaluation and surgical treatment—prospective study. *Radiology* 236(1): 247–53.

Medina, L. S., B. Bernal, et al. 2007. Role of functional MR in determining language dominance in epilepsy and nonepilepsy populations: a Bayesian analysis. *Radiology* 242(1): 94–100.

Moonen, C. T. W., and P. A. Bandettini. 2000. *Functional MRI.* Heidelberg: Springer.

Morgan, V. L., R. R. Price, et al. 2004. Resting functional MRI with temporal clustering analysis for localization of epileptic activity without EEG. *Neuroimage* 21(1): 473–81.

Nelson, L., S. Lapsiwala, et al. 2002. Preoperative mapping of the supplementary motor area in patients harboring tumors in the medial frontal lobe. *Journal of Neurosurgery* 97(5): 1108–14.

Nersesyan, H., F. Hyder, et al. 2004. Dynamic fMRI and EEG recordings during spike-wave seizures and generalized tonic-clonic seizures in WAG/Rij rats. *Journal of Cerebral Blood Flow Metabolism* 24(6): 589–99.

Pardo, J. V., and P. T. Fox. 1993. Preoperative assessment of the cerebral hemispheric dominance for language with CBF PET. *Human Brain Mapping* 1: 57–68.

Petersen, S. E., P. T. Fox, et al. 1988. Positron emission tomographic studies of the cortical anatomy of single word processing. *Nature* 331: 585–589.

Pouratian, N., S. Y. Bookheimer, et al. 2002. Utility of preoperative functional magnetic resonance imaging for identifying language cortices in patients with vascular malformations. *Journal of Neurosurgery* 97(1): 21–32.

Powell, H. W., M. J. Koepp, et al. 2004. The application of functional MRI of memory in temporal lobe epilepsy: a clinical review. *Epilepsia* 45(7): 855–63.

Powell, H. W., M. J. Koepp, et al. 2005. Material-specific lateralization of memory encoding in the medial temporal lobe: blocked versus event-related design. *Neuroimage* 27(1): 231–9.

Powell, H. W., G. J. Parker, et al. 2008. Imaging language pathways predicts postoperative naming deficits. *Journal of Neurology Neurosurgery & Psychiatry* 79(3): 327–330.

Powell, H. W., M. P. Richardson, et al. 2007. Reorganization of verbal and nonverbal memory in temporal lobe epilepsy due to unilateral hippocampal sclerosis. *Epilepsia* 48(8): 1512–25.

Powell, H. W., M. P. Richardson, et al. 2008. Preoperative fMRI predicts memory decline following anterior temporal lobe resection. *Journal of Neurology Neurosurgery & Psychiatry* 79(6): 686–693.

Pujol, J., J. Deus, et al. 1999. Cerebral lateralization of language in normal left-handed people studied by functional MRI. *Neurology* 52(5): 1038–43.

Pujol, J., L. Torres, et al. 1999. Functional magnetic resonance imaging study of frontal lobe activation during word generation in obsessive-compulsive disorder. *Biological Psychiatry* 45(7): 891–7.

Rabin, M. L., V. M. Narayan, et al. 2004. Functional MRI predicts post-surgical memory following temporal lobectomy. *Brain* 127(Pt 10): 2286–98.

Raichle, M. E., A. M. MacLeod, et al. 2001. A default mode of brain function. *Proceedings of the National Academy of Sciences U S A* 98(2): 676–82.

Ramsey, N. F., I. Sommer, et al. 2001. Combined analysis of language tasks in fMRI improves assessment of hemispheric dominance for language functions in individual subjects. *Neuroimage* 13: 719–733.

Rao, S. M., J. R. Binder, et al. 1993. Functional magnetic resonance imaging of complex human movements. *Neurology* 43: 2311–2318.

Richardson, M. P., B. A. Strange, et al. 2003. Preserved verbal memory function in left medial temporal pathology involves reorganisation of function to right medial temporal lobe. *Neuroimage* 20 Suppl 1: S112–9.

Richardson, M. P., B. A. Strange, et al. 2006. Memory fMRI in left hippocampal sclerosis: optimizing the approach to predicting postsurgical memory. *Neurology* 66(5): 699–705.

Richardson, M. P., B. A. Strange, et al. 2004. Pre-operative verbal memory fMRI predicts post-operative memory decline after left temporal lobe resection. *Brain* 127(Pt 11): 2419–26.

Ries, M. L., F. A. Boop, et al. 2004. Functional MRI and Wada determination of language lateralization: a case of crossed dominance. *Epilepsia* 45(1): 85–9.

Rosenberger, L. R., J. Zeck, et al. 2009. Interhemispheric and intrahemispheric language reorganization in complex partial epilepsy. *Neurology* 72(21): 1830–6.

Rother, J., R. Knab, et al. 2002. Negative dip in BOLD fMRI is caused by blood flow–oxygen consumption uncoupling in humans. *Neuroimage* 15(1): 98–102.

Roux, F. E., K. Boulanouar, et al. 2003. Language functional magnetic resonance imaging in preoperative assessment of language areas: correlation with direct cortical stimulation. *Neurosurgery* 52(6): 1335–47.

Roy, C. S., and C. S. Sherrington. 1890. On the regulation of blood flow to the brain. *Journal of Physiology* 11: 85–108.

Rutten, G. J., N. F. Ramsey, et al. 2002. FMRI-determined language lateralization in patients with unilateral or mixed language dominance according to the Wada test. *Neuroimage* 17(1): 447–60.

Rutten, G. J., N. F. Ramsey, et al. 2002. Development of a functional magnetic resonance imaging protocol for intraoperative localization of critical temporoparietal language areas. *Annals of Neurology* 51(3): 350–60.

Sabbah, P., F. Chassoux, et al. 2003. Functional MR imaging in assessment of language dominance in epileptic patients. *Neuroimage* 18(2): 460–7.

Sabsevitz, D. S., S. J. Swanson, et al. 2003. Use of preoperative functional neuroimaging to predict language deficits from epilepsy surgery. *Neurology* 60(11): 1788–92.

Salek-Haddadi, A., L. Lemieux, et al. 2003. Functional magnetic resonance imaging of human absence seizures. *Annals of Neurology* 53(5): 663–7.

Schlaggar, B. L., T. T. Brown, et al. 2002. Functional neuroanatomical differences between adults and school-age children in the processing of single words. *Science* 296(5572): 1476–9.

Schlosser, M. J., N. Aoyagi, et al. 1998. Functional MRI studies of auditory comprehension. *Human Brain Mapping* 6(1): 1–13.

Schwartz, T. H., S. R. Resor, Jr., et al. 1998. Functional magnetic resonance imaging localization of ictal onset to a dysplastic cleft with simultaneous sensorimotor mapping: intraoperative electrophysiological confirmation and postoperative follow-up: technical note. *Neurosurgery* 43(3): 639–45.

Smith, M. L., B. Bernal, et al. 2004. Severity of focal cortical dysplasia and functional organization of the brain. *Epilepsia* 45: 357.

Souweidane, M. M., K. H. Kim, et al. 1999. Brain mapping in sedated infants and young children with passive-functional magnetic resonance imaging. *Pediatric Neurosurgery* 30(2): 86–92.

Spreer, J., S. Arnold, et al. 2002. Determination of hemisphere dominance for language: comparison of frontal and temporal fMRI activation with intracarotid amytal testing. *Neuroradiology* 44(6): 467–74.

Springer, J. A., J. R. Binder, et al. 1999. Language dominance in neurologically normal and epilepsy subjects: a functional MRI study. *Brain* 122(Pt 11): 2033–46.

Staudt, M., W. Grodd, et al. 2001. Early left periventricular brain lesions induce right hemispheric organization of speech. *Neurology* 57(1): 122–5.

Staudt, M., K. Lidzba, et al. 2002. Right-hemispheric organization of language following early left-sided brain lesions: functional MRI topography. *Neuroimage* 16(4): 954–67.

Stern, C. E., S. Corkin, et al. 1996. The hippocampal formation participates in novel picture encoding: evidence from functional magnetic resonance imaging. *Proceedings of the National Academy of Sciences U S A* 93(16): 8660–5.

Symms, M. R., P. J. Allen, et al. 1999. Reproducible localization of interictal epileptiform discharges using EEG-triggered fMRI. *Physics in Medicine & Biology* 44(7): N161–8.

Szaflarski, J. P., J. R. Binder, et al. 2002. Language lateralization in left-handed and ambidextrous people: fMRI data. *Neurology* 59(2): 238–44.

Telfeian, A. E., C. Berqvist, et al. 2002. Recovery of language after left hemispherectomy in a sixteen-year-old girl with late-onset seizures. *Pediatric Neurosurgery* 37(1): 19–21.

Tenney, J. R., T. Q. Duong, et al. 2004. FMRI of brain activation in a genetic rat model of absence seizures. *Epilepsia* 45(6): 576–82.

Thiel, A., B. Schumacher, et al. 2006. Direct demonstration of transcallosal disinhibition in language networks. *Journal of Cerebral Blood Flow Metabolism* 26(9): 1122–7.

Thivard, L., J. Hombrouck, et al. 2005. Productive and perceptive language reorganization in temporal lobe epilepsy. *Neuroimage* 24(3): 841–51.

Vargha-Khadem, F., L. J. Carr, et al. 1997. Onset of speech after left hemispherectomy in a nine-year-old boy. *Brain* 120(Pt 1): 159–82.

Vargha-Khadem, F., E. B. Isaacs, et al. 1991. Development of language in six hemispherectomized patients. *Brain* 114(Pt 1B): 473–95.

Vitali, P., L. Minati, et al. 2008. Functional MRI in malformations of cortical development: activation of dysplastic tissue and functional reorganization. *Neuroimaging* 18(3): 296–305.

Voets, N. L., J. E. Adcock, et al. 2006. Distinct right frontal lobe activation in language processing following left hemisphere injury. *Brain* 129(Pt 3): 754–66.

Weber, B., J. Wellmer, et al. 2006. Left hippocampal pathology is associated with atypical language lateralization in patients with focal epilepsy. *Brain* 129(Pt 2): 346–51.

Wilke, M., S. K. Holland, et al. 2003. Language processing during natural sleep in a 6-year-old boy, as assessed with functional MR imaging. *AJNR American Journal of Neuroradiology* 24(1): 42–4.

Wise, R., F. Chollet, et al. 1991. Distribution of cortical neural networks involved in word comprehension and word retrieval. *Brain* 114: 1803–1817.

Woermann, F. G., H. Jokeit, et al. 2003. Language lateralization by Wada test and fMRI in 100 patients with epilepsy. *Neurology* 61(5): 699–701.

Wolf, R. L., D. C. Alsop, et al. 2001. Detection of mesial temporal lobe hypoperfusion in patients with temporal lobe epilepsy by use of arterial spin labeled perfusion MR imaging. *AJNR American Journal of Neuroradiology* 22(7): 1334–41.

Wood, A. G., A. S. Harvey, et al. 2004. Language cortex activation in normal children. *Neurology* 63(6): 1035–44.

Worthington, C., D. J. Vincent, et al. 1997. Comparison of functional magnetic resonance imaging for language localization and intracarotid speech amytal testing in presurgical evaluation for intractable epilepsy. *Preliminary results. Stereotactic & Functional Neurosurgery* 69(1–4 Pt 2): 197–201.

Yerys, B. E., K. F. Jankowski, et al. 2009. The fMRI success rate of children and adolescents: Typical development, epilepsy, attention deficit/hyperactivity disorder, and autism spectrum disorders. *Human Brain Mapping* 30:3426–35.

Yetkin, F. Z., S. Swanson, et al. 1998. Functional MR of frontal lobe activation: comparison with Wada language results. *AJNR American Journal of Neuroradiology* 19(6): 1095–8.

Yogarajah, M., H. W. Powell, et al. 2008. Tractography of the parahippocampal gyrus and material specific memory impairment in unilateral temporal lobe epilepsy. *Neuroimage* 40(4): 1755–64.

Yuan, W., J. P. Szaflarski, et al. 2006. fMRI shows atypical language lateralization in pediatric epilepsy patients. *Epilepsia* 47(3): 593–600.

Chapter 6

DIFFUSION MRI IN EPILEPSY

Rajkumar Munian Govindan and Harry T. Chugani

INTRODUCTION

Epilepsy is one of the most common disorders encountered in neurology practice. Seizures not only impair day-to-day activity and cognitive function, but also have a profound effect on brain development in the young (Helmstaedter 2002; Jokeit and Ebner 2002). This volume has provided an in-depth discussion of the many advances in neuroimaging that have been applied to the study of epileptic disorders. One of the most important of these is diffusion tensor magnetic resonance imaging (DT-MRI), briefly mentioned in Chapter 2. This technique allows, for the first time, an in vivo visualization and measurement of the properties of brain tracts, thus enabling the study of epileptic circuitry. In this chapter, we will briefly discuss the basic concepts of diffusion MRI, review findings from DT-MRI studies in epilepsy, and suggest future applications of diffusion MRI in epilepsy.

BROWNIAN MOTION

In water, the molecules of a solute disperse evenly in all directions by their random movements (Brown 1828). The rate at which the molecules diffuse depends upon the average speed of the randomly moving molecule as determined by the temperature and the concentration gradient of the molecule across various locations. This diffusion concept is simply explained by Fick's first law (equation 1: $J = -D.\Delta C$, where J is the diffusion vector, D is the diffusion coefficient, and ΔC is the concentration gradient of the molecule), whereas Einstein later explained it using a Gaussian displacement distribution model of diffusion for a specific timeframe and proposed the equation (equation 2: $x^2 = 6.D.t$, where x is the displacement, D is the diffusion coefficient, and t is the time). In both these equations, unlike the concentration gradient and the time, the diffusion coefficient D is an intrinsic property of a medium and depends upon the temperature, the size of the molecule, and other interactions this molecule might undergo during its random movement. In pure water, the diffusion coefficient $D = 3*10^{-3}$ mm^2/sec at 37 degrees Celsius. In biological tissues, water is the predominant medium but is not pure; its diffusion coefficient is determined by the interaction of the water molecule with other particles.

DIFFUSION MRI

In the past, measuring the diffusion coefficient values in a biological tissue was very difficult and cumbersome. Many studies were performed using dyes, electrolytes, or electrical gradient across regions to measure the diffusion coefficient of water (Sykova 2004). Most of these methods were invasive and could only be performed in vitro or on animals. In this regard, the invention of diffusion MRI is considered a giant technical leap to

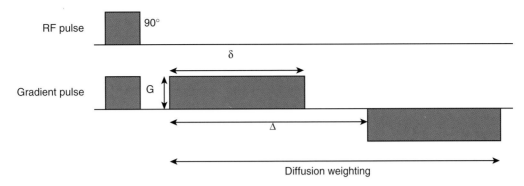

Figure 6.1 Stejskal and Tanner split pulse diffusion weighting gradient. The degree of diffusion weighting ('b') is measured using the expression "$b = (\delta \gamma G)^2.(\Delta - \delta/3)$", where γ is the gyromagnetic ratio, G is the amplitude of the magnetic field gradient pulses, δ is the duration of the gradient pulse, and Δ is the duration between the gradient pulses.

facilitate measurement of diffusion coefficients in biological tissue. Using this technique, it is now possible to measure diffusion coefficient values noninvasively in vivo with reasonably high spatial resolution.

The concept of diffusion MRI came about when Hahn (1950) recognized that the MR signal is sensitive to diffusion. He explained that the signal loss in a spin-echo (a 180-degree flipping pulse following the initial RF excitation) sequence was due to the molecular displacement by diffusion in an inhomogeneous magnetic field. Subsequently, Carr and Purcell (1954) proposed that if a controlled magnetic field gradient were to be applied during the spin-echo phase, the signal loss to the expected signal would be an indirect measure of the molecular displacement by diffusion. This concept was modified and refined by Stejskal and Tanner (1965) to include a split pulse gradient, which has more control over the signal acquired in a defined diffusion period (Fig. 6.1).

Initially, this technique was used to obtain the simple directionless scalar diffusion measurement (called diffusion weighted imaging [DWI]). Later, the methodology evolved to a more complex directional higher-order tensor model called diffusion tensor imaging (DTI) (Basser 1994). In this tensor model, the diffusion signals are measured in different diffusion gradients applied in various oriented planes in relation to the reference axis of the main magnetic field (B0).

DWI AND DTI

The first clinical application of DWI demonstrated that it is highly useful in the identification of acute decreases in diffusion during the early stages of brain ischemia, when other conventional imaging protocols (such as T1 and T2) typically show normal findings. On DWI, the regions with decreased diffusion appear as hyperintense areas (Moseley et al. 1990; Mukherjee

et al. 2008). To quantify the decrease in diffusivity using the apparent diffusion coefficient (ADC), a minimum of two MR signal measurements is needed—one without any diffusion weighting and other with a diffusion weighting gradient applied during the spin echo process (Le Bihan et al. 1986). The ratio of these two signals measures the signal attenuation by diffusion alone and eliminates the other components of the signal, such as T1- and T2-related decay signals, and gives an ADC image. When ADC values of different brain regions were visualized in the images, an interesting observation was noted (Moseley et al. 1990): the ADC values were different in specific regions with different orientations of the diffusion gradients (Fig. 6.2). This observation led to the important concept of diffusion anisotropy in MR imaging, although this concept was not new in the field of material science. If the ADC is the same in all applied gradients in different directions, the diffusion is considered isotropic, but if the ADC values are different, then the diffusion is considered anisotropic. In anisotropic diffusion, a higher-order tensor model is needed to represent the complex diffusion values. Conventionally, a tensor model with three component eigenvectors is used to represent a diffusion tensor, and it is mathematically expressed as a 3*3 matrix (Fig. 6.3). Using this tensor scheme, it is now possible to visualize the diffusion with its directional information using a color-coded image (Fig. 6.2).

Based on the tensor, many useful diffusion parameters can be calculated. The scalar values of the three eigenvectors denote the diffusivity in the corresponding directions. The average of these diffusion values gives the mean diffusivity (MD; different from the ADC mentioned earlier). An important and commonly used index of anisotropic diffusion called fractional anisotropy (FA) can also be calculated. FA is a measure of the variance of the three eigenvalues normalized to its mean diffusion values. In addition, other tensor-derived parameters such as linear, planar, and

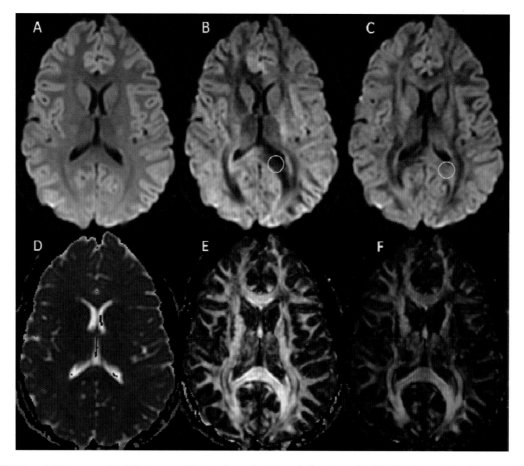

Figure 6.2 (A) Mean DWI image with diffusion sensitization from six different directions. (B, C) Diffusion-weighted images with diffusion-sensitizing gradients applied in two different directions. In these images, the diffusion values from the encircled regions interestingly depend upon the direction of the diffusion-sensitizing gradient and the orientation of the axonal fiber bundle. (D) Apparent diffusion coefficient (ADC) image. (E) Fractional anisotropy (FA) image. (F) Color-coded fractional anisotropy image (red: predominant fiber orientation in the left–right, transverse direction, green: predominant axonal bundle orientation in the anterior–posterior, transverse direction, blue: predominant orientation in the inferior–superior longitudinal direction).

spherical (triphasic) indices provide information about the diffusion shape, which is sensitive to diffusion change in a particular direction with respect to the orientation of the tensor ellipsoid (Fig. 6.3).

The valuable diffusion directional information thus collected can also be used to reconstruct the diffusion pathways. By linking diffusion directions across voxels, which are smoothly turning in direction, it is possible to approximately recreate white matter pathways. Using this principle, many tractographic methods are now available to isolate white matter tracts (Behrens et al. 2003; Mori et al. 1999). However, because only millimeter-size resolution is achievable in diffusion MRI, only a few major white matter tracts can be isolated using this technique.

DIFFUSION IN NEURAL TISSUE

In general, biological tissue is approximately 80% water, and the remaining 20% contains various other molecules of different sizes and shapes ranging from atomic-level solutes to macromolecules such as polypeptides and lipids. When these molecules combine and form larger cellular structures, thereby subdividing the medium into multiple intra-, extra-, and other cellular compartments, the free random movement of the water molecules is severely hindered. This restriction of free diffusion is expressed as a decrease in the measured diffusion coefficient. In neural tissue, gray matter and white matter have their own characteristic diffusion properties. In gray matter, tissue compartments are tightly packed, thus restricting water diffusion. However, they are oriented in random directions and hence restrict water movement equally in all directions (isotropic diffusion). In contrast, in the white matter, which mostly consists of axons and glial cells, the tissue compartments are longitudinally oriented parallel to the direction of the axon fibers. If sufficient numbers of axon fibers align parallel to each other, the diffusion of water is less restricted in the direction parallel to and more restricted in the direction perpendicular to the axons. This coherent arrangement of axons makes the diffusion in the white

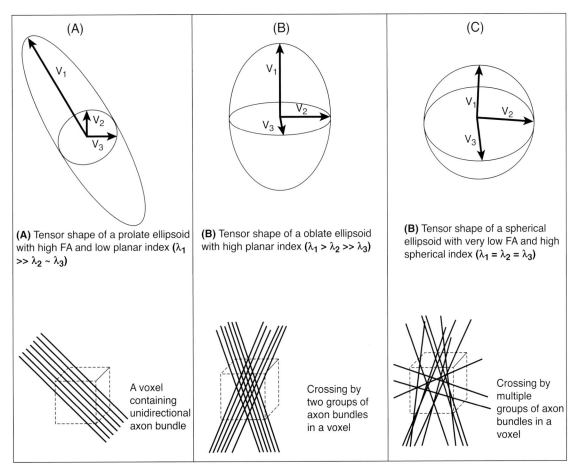

Figure 6.3 Graphic representation of the tensor ellipsoids where $V_{1, 2, 3}$ are the primary, secondary, and tertiary eigenvectors, respectively. Tensor shapes in voxel containing (A) single group of axon bundle, (B) two groups of crossing axon bundles, and (C) multiple groups of crossing axon bundles. In voxels with single group of axon bundle (e.g., median part of the corpus callosum), the primary eigenvector (V_1) represents diffusion parallel to the axon fibers and (V_2) and (V_3) represent diffusion perpendicular to the axon bundles. However, in voxels with crossing fibers (B, C) (e.g., most white matter regions of the cerebral cortex), the relation between the eigenvectors and the orientation of the axon bundle is not simple. In such voxels, measuring the parallel and perpendicular component of the diffusion separately is difficult, and other tensor-derived parameters such as triphasic indices may be helpful in providing this information (Govindan et al. 2008; Zhang et al. 2006).

matter anisotropic. However, it is unclear whether it is the cell membrane, intermembrane space, myelin sheath, microtubules, or neurofilaments that cause the diffusion anisotropy. Overall, the present consensus is that diffusion anisotropy in white matter mostly depends upon the three major microstructural characteristics of white matter tissue: the axonal density, coherent parallel arrangement of axons (Fig. 6.3), and myelin sheath thickness (Beaulieu 2002). This anisotropy combined with directional (parallel/perpendicular) diffusion measurements is, at present, the most sensitive index available to measure white matter structural integrity.

ICTAL AND POSTICTAL DIFFUSION CHANGES

Initial applications of diffusion MRI in epilepsy were in experimental studies on animal models of epilepsy.

These studies demonstrated the usefulness of diffusion MRI in the early detection of signal changes, which were not apparent on conventional MRI methods such as T1 or T2 images. Using DWI, this improved sensitivity for the early detection of an abnormal signal in acute events has also been demonstrated in other pathologic conditions, such as ischemic stroke, where the diffusion changes on DWI were the first to be detected. Indeed, this has led to widespread clinical application in stroke patients.

During an active seizure, the changes that occur in epileptic tissue can be subdivided chronologically into different phases based upon diffusion alterations (Yu and Tan 2008). In the initial phase, at the site of maximal neural activity, abnormally high electrical activity leads to a substantial increase in local cellular metabolism, which in turn leads to hyperperfusion (Bruehl et al. 1998; Szabo et al. 2005) without significant structural change or edema. During this phase, the diffusion changes are too subtle to be detected (i.e., there

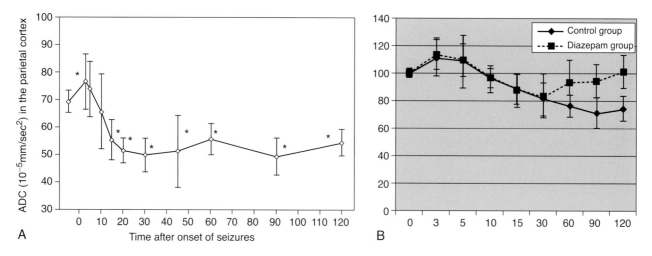

Figure 6.4 Acute changes (0–120 minutes) in the mean ADC values in rats following pilocarpine-induced seizures. The mean ADC values are increased in the initial 10 minutes following the onset of seizures (A, B). However, as the seizures continue, the mean ADC values decrease further below the baseline, but they subsequently recover and return to baseline following control of seizures (using diazepam)(B). Percentage ADC in the vertical axis indicates percentage increase in the ADC values compared to preictal values. Reprinted by permission from (A) Engelhorn, Hufnagel, et al. 2007, copyright by American Society of Neuroradiology and (B) Engelhorn, Weise, et al. 2007, copyright by Elsevier.

is no apparent change in the tissue microarchitecture detectable by diffusion MRI).

Following this short initial phase with persistent electrical activity, multiple tissue microstructural changes begin to appear. These changes are attributed to vasogenic extracellular edema with expansion of the vascular compartment and accumulation of water in the extracellular space. During this phase of predominantly vasogenic edema, an increase in ADC has been shown in animal studies (Engelhorn, Hufnagel, et al. 2007) (Fig. 6.4). In human studies, the findings have been less consistent in that increased ADC findings in the initial ictal period were reported in some studies (Hufnagel et al. 2003; Salmenpera, Simister, et al. 2006; Salmenpera, Symms, et al. 2006), but most studies have failed to demonstrate an increased ADC (Oh et al. 2004). In clinical settings, the likely reason for the difficulty in measuring the increased ADC is that this phase has a short duration (initial 10 to 15 minutes following seizure onset) (Fig. 6.4), and the clinical response time to acquire an MRI scan is often long.

With continued seizure activity, further changes appear in the neurons with high electrical activity and there is subsequent redistribution of ions (e.g., K$^+$) in the extracellular space and glial cells due to glial buffering (Prichard et al. 1995). During this third phase, the effect of cytotoxic edema predominates over vasogenic edema and the ADC decreases in the epileptic zone (Figs. 6.4 and 6.5). Most human and animal studies have shown decreased ADC in the epileptic zone during this phase (Auvin et al. 2007; Bhagat et al. 2001; Chu et al. 2001; Diehl et al. 2005; Ebisu et al.

1996; Hasegawa et al. 2003; Konermann et al. 2003; Oh et al. 2004; Parmar et al. 2006; Righini et al. 1994; Zhong et al. 1995). Thus, the *increased* ADC that is related to vasogenic edema is followed by *decreased* ADC due to cytotoxic edema, with significant overlap. Due to this overlap, the true pattern of ADC changes in these two phases is difficult to predict, and this might explain the inconsistent findings in both animal and human studies. Such difficulties have been noted even in a high-temporal-resolution experiment in an attempt to resolve these two phases (Zhong et al. 1997). Other potential reasons for the inconsistent findings could include differences in the mechanisms that cause seizures in humans and in animal models, as well as variations in the time period between the initiation of the seizure and the diffusion measurement. Therefore, in diffusion studies performed in the clinical setting, the time period between the onset of seizure and the MRI acquisition is critical for recording consistent diffusion abnormalities.

Phase four, the postictal phase, can either resolve or progress to an irreversible tissue injury. If the injury due to seizure activity progresses (Bhagat et al. 2005; Righini et al. 1994), a reversal of the ADC occurs and it becomes increased compared to the pre-ictal state and to the neighboring normal tissue. The reasons for the reversal of ADC to an increased level are due to neural cell death, acute inflammatory changes, and gliosis (Eidt et al. 2004; El-Koussy et al. 2002; Gong et al. 2008; Tokumitsu et al. 1997; Wall et al. 2000 (Fig. 6.6). During this process, the neural tissue loses its compartmental architecture, leading to increased ADC (Chu et al. 2001; Men et al. 2000; Nairismagi

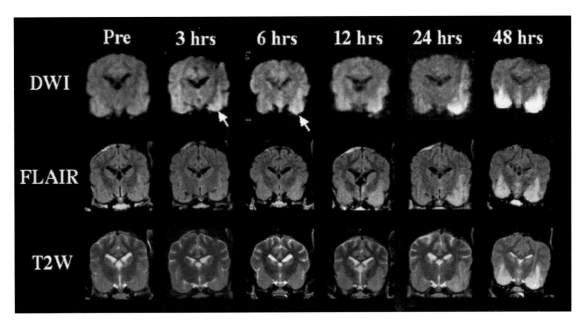

Figure 6.5 Sequence of DWI, FLAIR, and T2-weighted images of a dog with kainic acid-induced complex partial status epilepticus scanned between the preinduction and serially up to 48 hours following the induction of seizures. At 3 hours after the seizure onset, the DWI-weighted image showed hyperintensity with a decrease in ADC values and histopathology showed swelling of the nucleus of the neurons in the seizing zone (*arrow*). This figure also illustrates the sensitivity of DWI images in identifying early changes when other conventional images (FLAIR, T2W) appear normal. Reprinted by permission from Hasegawa et al. 2003, copyright by Elsevier.

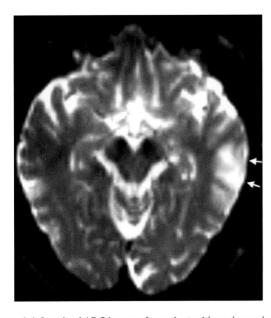

Figure 6.6 Post-ictal ADC image of a patient with prolonged new-onset partial seizures. Increased ADC values (hyperintense lesion in the left temporal cortex [*arrows*]) were noted in the seizure onset zone 7 days following the onset of the seizures. Histopathology of the resected tissue showed acute neuronal damage due to seizure activity.

et al. 2004; Parmar et al. 2006; Tokumitsu et al. 1997). On the other hand, if the ictal activity subsides without causing irreversible injury, a complete resolution with no residual diffusion change is noted (Buracchio et al.

2008; Calistri et al. 2003; Cohen-Gadol et al. 2004; Di Bonaventura et al. 2009; Flacke et al. 2000; Hasegawa et al. 2003; Kim et al. 2001; Lansberg et al. 1999; Li et al. 2003; Nakasu et al. 1995) (Fig. 6.7). Thus, in this phase, ADC increases in both scenarios (i.e., both with and without irreversible tissue injury), and a distinction between them is not clear, although irreversible injury also becomes apparent in the conventional MRI by this time. It has been suggested that in addition to the seizure-related destruction, concurrent repair or regenerative processes (Pitkanen and Lukasiuk 2009) might also contribute to the diffusion changes in the latter phase. However, not many experimental or clinical data are available to show the existence of diffusion changes related to repair or reorganization processes.

Interestingly, in both the animal and human studies, diffusion abnormalities were seen not only in the epileptic focus (Diehl et al. 1999) but also in regions distant from this focus. However, based on these studies, it is not clear whether the distant changes are secondary to propagation from the primary epileptic focus or they themselves are part of an epileptic network. The animal experiments show diffusion abnormalities in the amygdala, piriform cortex, and thalamus (Hasegawa et al. 2003; Nairismagi et al. 2004; Wall et al. 2000), whereas the human studies often demonstrate thalamic (Fig. 6.8) and hippocampal (Fig. 6.9) abnormalities (El-Koussy et al. 2002; Farina et al. 2004; Hufnagel et al. 2003; Katramados et al. 2009;

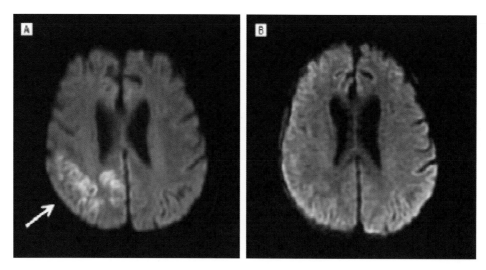

Figure 6.7 (A) DWI image during the post-ictal period following partial status epilepticus shows decreased ADC in the right parieto-occipital cortex (*arrow*). (B) Follow-up scan 4 weeks later shows complete resolution of the diffusion abnormality with control of seizures. Reprinted by permission from Buracchio et al. 2008, copyright by American Medical Association.

Konermann et al. 2003; Parmar et al. 2006; Szabo et al. 2005; Toledo et al. 2008; Wieshmann et al. 1999). In the clinical studies, such multifocal findings make diffusion MRI less useful in *localization* of the epileptic focus but occasionally useful in *lateralization* of the focus (Hakyemez et al. 2005; Hugg et al. 1999; Kantarci et al. 2002; Leonhardt et al. 2002; Londono et al. 2003; O'Brien et al. 2007; Wehner et al. 2007; Yoo et al. 2002) (Fig. 6.10).

During the ictal period, diffusion abnormalities are found mostly in the gray matter, although a few studies have shown abnormalities in the white matter. For example, increased ADC has been reported in the subcortical white matter regions underneath the epileptic cortex (Hisano et al. 2000; Lux et al. 1986; Wieshmann et al. 1997). Although anisotropy is a sensitive measure of diffusion, available data from a few studies showed no changes in anisotropy (Diehl et al. 2005). Hence, it appears that the diffusion parameter FA is less sensitive for demonstrating ictal changes. Studies examining ischemic cortical injuries, where the neurons are injured, have shown that the distal portions of axons exhibit progressive Wallerian degeneration with loss of anisotropy. Even though hyperperfusion occurs in the ictal zone, the tissue often suffers from relative ischemia due to the neural hyperactivity (Bruehl et al. 1998; Calistri et al. 2003; Szabo et al. 2005).

INTERICTAL DIFFUSION CHANGES

During the interictal period, diffusion abnormalities that have been identified are associated with primary lesions such as ischemic injury, tumor, tubers, and microcortical dysplasia (Eriksson et al. 2001; Gross et al. 2005; Jansen et al. 2003; Rugg-Gunn et al. 2001, 2002; Wieshmann et al. 1999). Diffusion abnormalities were also identified in regions at a distance from a variety of histopathologic cortical abnormalities (Dumas de la Roque et al. 2005; Focke et al. 2008; Thivard et al. 2006) (Fig. 6.11). Similar to diffusion abnormalities seen in the ictal and postictal periods, most interictal findings showed diffusion abnormalities associated with the epileptic focus and also remote from it (Gong et al. 2008; Kim et al. 2008). Unlike findings seen in the ictal and postictal periods, diffusion abnormalities seen in the interictal period were most often found in the white matter rather than gray matter regions. The reason for the absence of interictal findings in the gray matter is that the diffusion abnormalities associated with the ictal and postictal phases often resolve in the interictal period (see above). In the white matter, FA is always decreased, while ADC abnormalities are inconsistent (increased, decreased, or normal) (Arfanakis et al. 2002; Assaf et al. 2003; Concha et al. 2005; Eriksson et al. 2001; Focke et al. 2008; Govindan, Makki, et al. 2008; Kimiwada et al. 2006; Okumura et al. 2004; Thivard et al. 2005; Trivedi et al. 2006; Wehner et al. 2007). Several possible mechanisms might be responsible for such findings in the white matter.

First, as mentioned in the preceding section, it could be that proximal neural degeneration associated with chronic seizure activity may induce distal Wallerian degeneration of the axons, causing a decrease in FA. A decrease in FA with chronic seizures has been demonstrated in several studies (Rugg-Gunn et al. 2002). However, in addition to neuronal death, progressive degenerative changes such as axonal

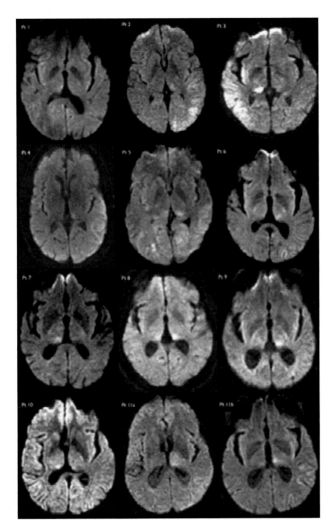

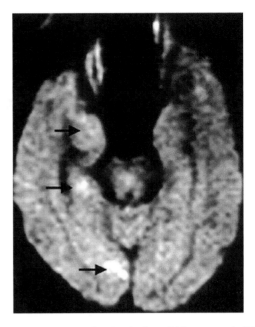

Figure 6.9 DWI image showing ipsilateral hippocampal diffusion abnormality (*arrows*) in a scan obtained 3 days after the onset of complex partial status epilepticus. Reprinted by permission from Kim et al. 2001, copyright by American Society of Neuroradiology.

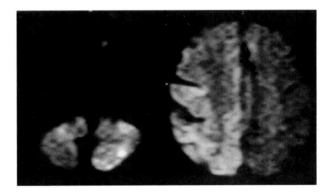

Figure 6.10 DWI image showing diffusion abnormalities in the entire right hemisphere, including the left cerebellar hemisphere (diaschisis effect), in a scan obtained 24 hours after the ictal onset. Reprinted by permission from Calistri et al. 2003, copyright by American Society of Neuroradiology.

Figure 6.8 DWI images of 11 patients showing ipsilateral thalamic diffusion abnormalities (hyperintense thalamic lesions with decrease in ADC values) in scans obtained within 5 days of seizure activity. Reprinted by permission from Katramados et al. 2009, copyright by John Wiley & Sons, Inc.

demyelination, formation of axonal spines, an increase in interstitial fluid volume due to edema, replacement of axons with glial cells, and astrocyte proliferation may all occur independently with chronic propagation of seizure activity (Sutula et al. 2003). In all these scenarios, the changes related to water diffusion are mostly in the direction of a loss of anisotropy. Multiple tissue structural components (see the section "Diffusion in Neural Tissue") might be involved in causing such diffusion changes, which are still poorly understood. Therefore, diffusion abnormalities in the white matter could be the result of progressive degenerative changes occurring in the epileptic cortex or independently in the underlying white matter with persistent seizure propagation, or both.

Another reason for the differential findings of decreased FA and inconsistent ADC findings in the

interictal state could be that the FA might be a more sensitive indicator in the white matter than the ADC in the gray matter for measuring subtle diffusion abnormalities during the interictal period (Focke et al. 2008). The possible presence of continuous subclinical seizure activity during the interictal period might result in these white matter findings with apparently normal-appearing gray matter regions.

Third, in many studies, decreases in FA values were noted not only in ipsilateral white matter regions/tracts but also in contralateral white matter regions/tracts (Arfanakis et al. 2002; Govindan, Makki, et al. 2008;

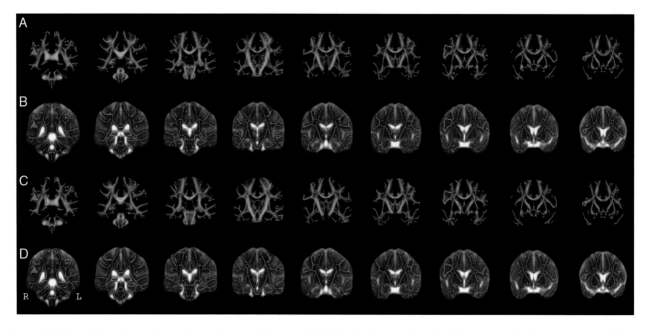

Figure 6.11 Voxel-based analysis showing widespread decrease in FA (A, C: left- and right-sided hippocampal sclerosis, respectively) and increase in ADC (B, D: left- and right-sided hippocampal sclerosis, respectively) values in unilateral mesial temporal lope epilepsy patients. Reprinted by permission from Focke et al. 2008, copyright by Elsevier. Red: voxels significantly different from healthy controls, green: skeleton voxels (TBSS; Smith et al. 2006).

Gross et al. 2006). In a few studies, such bilateral loss of anisotropy in epilepsy patients persisted even after the seizures were brought under control (Concha et al. 2007; Schoene-Bake et al. 2009). Not only were these findings seen in chronic epilepsy, but decreased FA was identified even in new-onset epilepsy patients who had experienced only a few seizures (Chugani et al. 2008). Based on these observations, it can be suggested that the overall anisotropy reduction in these patients may be a prevailing condition present even before the onset of clinical seizures. This state of reduced anisotropy could be related to the underlying primary pathology associated with a lowered seizure threshold. It may be the first hit of a two-hit hypothesis leading to the seizure onset (Lewis 2005). Alternatively, one could argue that the seizures themselves may result in a diffuse loss of anisotropy. Longitudinal DTI studies in epilepsy patients with proper control of other confounds, such as the potential effect of chronic medication (Wheless et al. 2009), may be useful in elucidating the mechanisms underlying decrease in anisotropy.

TRACTOGRAPHY AND FUTURE APPLICATIONS

Recent advances in tractographic techniques using diffusion MRI allows individual white matter tracts to be isolated and their diffusion properties measured. This technique is constantly improving and evolving at a rapid pace. Although several tractographic methods are available at present, the underlying concepts of these techniques are similar. The basic principle is to identify the directional diffusivity of water within a voxel and to use this directional information to connect to neighboring voxels with similar diffusion directionalities. However, these tractographic methods use very complex protocols that are time-consuming to execute even for a powerful personal computer.

Deterministic tractography is a commonly used fiber-tracking method due to its fast fiber-tracking protocol (Mori et al. 1999). Using this method, major white matter tracts (Fig. 6.12) can be isolated. However, this method has several limitations due to its inability to overcome crossing fibers within a voxel (Fig. 6.3). Under such circumstances, more robust multiple fiber-crossing tractographic methods are required to track white matter tracts more reliably (Behrens et al. 2003; Mori et al. 1999). In addition, since cortical white matter has complex networks of pathways, often the tract isolated is not homogeneous in its specificity to a particular white matter pathway because there are several regions in the isolated tract inclusive to other pathways. Although these are not of major concern in large pathways, such as corpus callosum or corticospinal tract, where axonal crossing is minimal, they are important when studying minor tracts, which are present exclusively in small regions. To overcome these problems and to improve the accuracy of identifying diffusion abnormalities in minor tracts, a method with

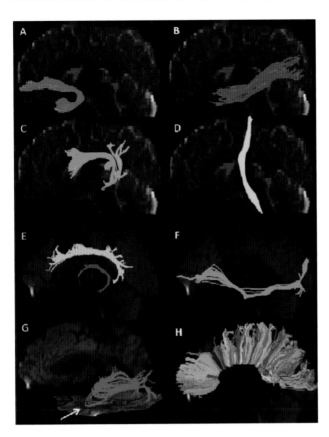

Figure 6.12 White matter tracts isolated using "DtiStudio" (Jiang et al. 2006). (A) Uncinate fasciculus. (B) Inferior longitudinal fasciculus. (C) Arcuate fasciculus; green: long segment, orange: posterior segment. (D) Corticospinal tract. (E) Gray: cingulum, blue: fornix. (F) Inferior fronto-occipital fasciculus. (G) Optic radiation, Meyer's loop: anterior portion of the optic radiation (*arrow*) extending into temporal lobe can be seen. (H) Corpus callosum.

high spatial resolution is needed. Voxel-based methods such as SPM or TBSS are more useful in studying minor tracts with subtle diffusion abnormalities. TBSS is a specialized technique for the study of cerebral white matter, making use of the intrinsic anisotropic properties of white matter to create a virtual tract skeleton that assists in tract comparisons across individuals (Smith et al. 2006).

Since diffusion MRI is sensitive enough to identify abnormalities in white matter regions during the ictal and interictal periods, diffusion imaging technique combined with tractographic and other voxel-based methods (such as TBSS) will help to reveal possible relationships between the diffusion changes related to tissue structure and the epilepsy.

In a study by Govindan, Makki et al (2008) on a group of children with left temporal lobe epilepsy, diffusion changes (FA and spherical index) in the left uncinate fasciculus showed the strongest correlation with the duration of epilepsy. This fasciculus, which is a component of the limbic system connecting the

temporal lobe with the inferior frontal lobe, probably plays a major role in the propagation of seizure activity to the frontal lobe (Chassoux et al. 2004; Lin et al. 2008; Rodrigo et al. 2007), and the persistence of abnormal electrical activity along this tract could account for the loss of anisotropy observed. In a further study (Chugani et al. 2008) using TBSS, abnormal white matter regions identified in children with new-onset epilepsy also showed a significant correlation between loss of anisotropy and duration of the epilepsy. Similarly, abnormal thalamocortical white matter regions identified in juvenile myoclonic epilepsy patients showed significant correlation between loss of anisotropy and frequency of generalized tonic-clonic seizures (Deppe et al. 2008). Therefore, these studies suggest a progressive loss of white matter integrity with epilepsy. Although many studies have shown abnormal findings in various tracts and regions, they did not show any correlation with duration of epilepsy (Deppe et al. 2008; Govindan, Makki, et al. 2008). These observations may suggest the possibility that different tracts are affected at different stages of the underlying pathologic process in epilepsy, and perhaps some tracts are more vulnerable than others.

The combination of highly sensitive indices (FA, ADC) of white matter structural integrity and the ability to isolate and study specific white matter tracts has allowed investigators to link epilepsy and the cognitive impairment so often seen in chronic epilepsy patients (Diehl et al. 2008; Govindan, Juhasz, et al. 2008; McDonald et al. 2008; Yogarajah et al. 2008). Although these studies have given only a glimpse of the crucial link between epilepsy, tissue damage, and cognitive impairment, this is an important area of investigation, and future studies will likely yield more answers to these important relationships.

Tractographic techniques can be used not only to study diffusion properties of a particular white matter tract or region, but also to provide morphologic information about white matter tracts. These morphologic analyses of white matter tracts in subjects with epilepsy have identified aberrant tracts in the brain (Eriksson et al. 2002). In neurosurgical practice, such morphologic information about white matter tracts can be useful for the accurate localization of cerebral cortical regions serving crucial neurologic functions. In some cases, the appearance of a larger tract on the contralateral hemisphere might give an indication that some functional reorganization to the contralateral hemisphere had already occurred (Govindan, Makki, et al. 2008; Rodrigo et al. 2008). For example, reorganization of the corticospinal tract or arcuate fasciculus contralateral to the side of surgery might indicate that their corresponding functions will less likely be affected after an ipsilateral surgical resection (Govindan, Chugani, et al. 2010) (Matsumoto et al. 2008; Powell et al. 2006;

Rodrigo et al. 2008). Similarly, tractography of Meyer's loop can locate the anterior extent of the optic radiation; this can be used as a guide to limit the extent and depth of temporal lobe resection and can avoid a postoperative contralateral superior quadrantanopsia (Chen et al. 2009; Kikuta et al. 2006; Powell et al. 2005; Taoka et al. 2008). Such neuronavigational uses of tractography can improve the precision and guide neurosurgical procedures in removing the epileptogenic cortex and avoid postsurgical complications (Nimsky et al. 2005; Romano et al. 2009). Moreover, tractography provides an advantage in this respect in that it can provide valuable functional localization noninvasively without active patient participation, an advantage particularly relevant in children. However, at present tractography alone is not reliable enough to suggest the presence or absence of a particular white matter tract and its associated functions, so it must be used in conjunction with other clinical data. This unreliability is because diffusion MRI is inherently low in spatial resolution, and validation of these tracts with robust tract-tracing methods is still ongoing. Therefore, for clinical use, the application of tractography must continue to be performed with some caution.

Another potential application, although preliminary, of diffusion MRI in epilepsy is in EEG source analysis (Haueisen et al. 2002). So far, epileptic source analysis has been performed using isotropic conductive head models. Since we now know that cerebral white matter is anisotropic, this added information combined with tractography can be used to estimate the anisotropic conductive head models. This additional information might be helpful in improving the accuracy of the epileptic source localization (Cook and Koles 2008; Rullmann et al. 2009).

CONCLUSIONS

In summary, diffusion MRI has provided us with a sensitive index to measure structural changes in neural tissue and, in addition, has provided tractography to isolate and study specific tracts and regions of the brain. Using this imaging tool, a number of abnormalities that were not previously apparent have been identified. In this chapter, we have discussed the common abnormalities identified and their implications in understanding the epileptic process, along with some clinical applications. In the future, diffusion MRI should be performed routinely in epilepsy patients in the clinical setting. Since diffusion changes are highly dynamic in the ictal and postictal periods, precise knowledge of the ictal and postictal duration from the onset of seizures should be recorded for a better understanding and calibration of diffusion changes. Most diffusion MRI studies are performed on a heterogeneous

group of patients with various etiologies; this heterogeneity often distorts the study results, where diffusion changes are very subtle. Therefore, future studies should consider better-controlled conditions (in homogeneous epileptic conditions and study populations). Since tractography techniques are still evolving, continued validation of tractographic tracts is needed to reliably use this method in clinical practice. Further improvement in these tractographic techniques and in the resolution of diffusion MRI could provide a giant step forward in the clinical and research applications of diffusion MRI.

REFERENCES

Arfanakis, K., B. P. Hermann, et al. 2002. Diffusion tensor MRI in temporal lobe epilepsy. *Magnetic Resonance Imaging* 20(7): 511–9.

Assaf, B. A., F. B. Mohamed, et al. 2003. Diffusion tensor imaging of the hippocampal formation in temporal lobe epilepsy. *AJNR American Journal of Neuroradiology* 24(9): 1857–62.

Auvin, S., L. Devisme, et al. 2007. Neuropathological and MRI findings in an acute presentation of hemiconvulsion-hemiplegia: a report with pathophysiological implications. *Seizure* 16(4): 371–6.

Beaulieu, C. 2002. The basis of anisotropic water diffusion in the nervous system: a technical review. *NMR Biomedicine* 15(7–8): 435–55.

Behrens, T. E., M. W. Woolrich, et al. 2003. Characterization and propagation of uncertainty in diffusion-weighted MR imaging. *Magnetic Resonance in Medicine* 50(5): 1077–88.

Bhagat, Y. A., A. Obenaus, et al. 2001. Magnetic resonance imaging predicts neuropathology from soman-mediated seizures in the rodent. *Neuroreport* 12(7): 1481–7.

Bhagat, Y. A., A. Obenaus, et al. 2005. Neuroprotection from soman-induced seizures in the rodent: evaluation with diffusion- and T2-weighted magnetic resonance imaging. *Neurotoxicology* 26(6): 1001–13.

Bruehl, C., G. Hagemann, et al. 1998. Uncoupling of blood flow and metabolism in focal epilepsy. *Epilepsia* 39(12): 1235–42.

Buracchio, T., S. L. Lewis, et al. 2008. Restricted diffusion on magnetic resonance imaging in partial status epilepticus. *Archives of Neurology* 65(2): 278–9.

Calistri, V., F. Caramia, et al. 2003. Visualization of evolving status epilepticus with diffusion and perfusion MR imaging. *AJNR American Journal of Neuroradiology* 24(4): 671–3.

Chassoux, F., F. Semah, et al. 2004. Metabolic changes and electro-clinical patterns in mesio-temporal lobe epilepsy: a correlative study. *Brain* 127(Pt 1): 164–74.

Chen, X., D. Weigel, et al. 2009. Prediction of visual field deficits by diffusion tensor imaging in temporal lobe epilepsy surgery. *Neuroimage* 45(2): 286–97.

Chu, K., D. W. Kang, et al. 2001. Diffusion-weighted magnetic resonance imaging in nonconvulsive status epilepticus. *Archives of Neurology* 58(6): 993–8.

Chugani, H. T., R. M. Govindan, et al. 2008. Tract-based analysis of cerebral white matter in children with recent-onset epilepsy. *Epilepsia* 49: 484.

Cohen-Gadol, A. A., J. W. Britton, et al. 2004. Transient cortical abnormalities on magnetic resonance imaging after status epilepticus: case report. *Surgical Neurology* 61(5): 479–82.

Concha, L., C. Beaulieu, et al. 2005. Bilateral limbic diffusion abnormalities in unilateral temporal lobe epilepsy. *Annals of Neurology* 57(2): 188–96.

Concha, L., C. Beaulieu, et al. 2007. Bilateral white matter diffusion changes persist after epilepsy surgery. *Epilepsia* 48(5): 931–40.

Cook, M. J., Z. J. Koles. 2008. The effect of tissue anisotropy on the EEG inverse problem. *Conference Proceedings IEEE Engineering Medicine Biological Soc 2008*: 4563–6.

Deppe, M., C. Kellinghaus, et al. 2008. Nerve fiber impairment of anterior thalamocortical circuitry in juvenile myoclonic epilepsy. *Neurology* 71(24): 1981–5.

Di Bonaventura, C., F. Bonini, et al. 2009. Diffusion-weighted magnetic resonance imaging in patients with partial status epilepticus. *Epilepsia* 50 Suppl 1: 45–52.

Diehl, B., R. M. Busch, et al. 2008. Abnormalities in diffusion tensor imaging of the uncinate fasciculus relate to reduced memory in temporal lobe epilepsy. *Epilepsia* 49(8): 1409–18.

Diehl, B., I. Najm, et al. 1999. Periictal diffusion-weighted imaging in a case of lesional epilepsy. *Epilepsia* 40(11): 1667–71.

Diehl, B., M. R. Symms, et al. 2005. Postictal diffusion tensor imaging. *Epilepsy Research* 65(3): 137–46.

Dumas de la Roque, A., C. Oppenheim, et al. 2005. Diffusion tensor imaging of partial intractable epilepsy. *European Radiology* 15(2): 279–85.

Ebisu, T., W. D. Rooney, et al. 1996. MR spectroscopic imaging and diffusion-weighted MRI for early detection of kainate-induced status epilepticus in the rat. *Magnetic Resonance in Medicine* 36(6): 821–8.

Eidt, S., E. J. Kendall, et al. 2004. Neuronal and glial cell populations in the piriform cortex distinguished by using an approximation of q-space imaging after status epilepticus. *AJNR American Journal of Neuroradiology* 25(7): 1225–33.

El-Koussy, M., J. Mathis, et al. 2002. Focal status epilepticus: follow-up by perfusion- and diffusion MRI. *European Radiology* 12(3): 568–74.

Engelhorn, T., A. Hufnagel, et al. 2007. Monitoring of acute generalized status epilepticus using multilocal diffusion MR imaging: early prediction of regional neuronal damage. *AJNR American Journal of Neuroradiology* 28(2): 321–7.

Engelhorn, T., J. Weise, et al. 2007. Early diffusion-weighted MRI predicts regional neuronal damage in generalized status epilepticus in rats treated with diazepam. *Neuroscience Letters* 417(3): 275–80.

Eriksson, S. H., F. J. Rugg-Gunn, et al. 2001. Diffusion tensor imaging in patients with epilepsy and malformations of cortical development. *Brain* 124(Pt 3): 617–26.

Eriksson, S. H., M. R. Symms, et al. 2002. Exploring white matter tracts in band heterotopia using diffusion tractography. *Annals of Neurology* 52(3): 327–34.

Farina, L., C. Bergqvist, et al. 2004. Acute diffusion abnormalities in the hippocampus of children with new-onset seizures: the development of mesial temporal sclerosis. *Neuroradiology* 46(4): 251–7.

Flacke, S., U. Wullner, et al. 2000. Reversible changes in echo planar perfusion- and diffusion-weighted MRI in status epilepticus. *Neuroradiology* 42(2): 92–5.

Focke, N. K., M. Yogarajah, et al. 2008. Voxel-based diffusion tensor imaging in patients with mesial temporal lobe epilepsy and hippocampal sclerosis. *Neuroimage* 40(2): 728–37.

Gong, G., L. Concha, et al. 2008. Thalamic diffusion and volumetry in temporal lobe epilepsy with and without mesial temporal sclerosis. *Epilepsy Research* 80(2–3): 184–93.

Gong, G., F. Shi, et al. 2008. Insights into the sequence of structural consequences of convulsive status epilepticus: a longitudinal MRI study. *Epilepsia* 49(11): 1941–5.

Govindan, R. M., C. Juhasz, et al. 2008. Abnormal diffusion of specific white matter regions in children with unilateral Sturge-Weber syndrome: correlation with epilepsy and cognitive functions. *Epilepsia* 49: 409–10.

Govindan, R. M., M. I. Makki, et al. 2008. Diffusion tensor analysis of temporal and extra-temporal lobe tracts in temporal lobe epilepsy. *Epilepsy Research* 80(1): 30–41.

Govindan, R.M., H.T. Chugani, et al. Presurgical prediction of motor functional loss using tractography. *Pediatric Neurology*, 43(1): 70–2.

Gross, D. W., A. Bastos, et al. 2005. Diffusion tensor imaging abnormalities in focal cortical dysplasia. *Canadian Journal of Neurologic Science* 32(4): 477–82.

Gross, D. W., L. Concha, et al. 2006. Extratemporal white matter abnormalities in mesial temporal lobe epilepsy demonstrated with diffusion tensor imaging. *Epilepsia* 47(8): 1360–3.

Hakyemez, B., C. Erdogan, et al. 2005. Apparent diffusion coefficient measurements in the hippocampus and amygdala of patients with temporal lobe seizures and in healthy volunteers. *Epilepsy Behavior* 6(2): 250–6.

Hasegawa, D., H. Orima, et al. 2003. Diffusion-weighted imaging in kainic acid-induced complex partial status epilepticus in dogs. *Brain Research* 983(1–2): 115–27.

Haueisen, J., D. S. Tuch, et al. 2002. The influence of brain tissue anisotropy on human EEG and MEG. *Neuroimage* 15(1): 159–66.

Helmstaedter, C. 2002. Effects of chronic epilepsy on declarative memory systems. *Progress in Brain Research* 135: 439–53.

Hisano, T., M. Ohno, et al. 2000. Changes in diffusion-weighted MRI after status epilepticus. *Pediatric Neurology* 22(4): 327–9.

Hufnagel, A., J. Weber, et al. 2003. Brain diffusion after single seizures. *Epilepsia* 44(1): 54–63.

Hugg, J. W., E. J. Butterworth, et al. 1999. Diffusion mapping applied to mesial temporal lobe epilepsy: preliminary observations. *Neurology* 53(1): 173–6.

Jansen, F. E., K. P. Braun, et al. 2003. Diffusion-weighted magnetic resonance imaging and identification of the epileptogenic tuber in patients with tuberous sclerosis. *Archives of Neurology* 60(11): 1580–4.

Jiang, H., P. C. van Zijl, et al. 2006. DtiStudio: resource program for diffusion tensor computation and fiber bundle tracking. *Computer Methods Programs Biomedicine* 81(2): 106–16.

Jokeit, H., A. Ebner. 2002. Effects of chronic epilepsy on intellectual functions. *Progress in Brain Research* 135: 455–63.

Kantarci, K., C. Shin, et al. 2002. Comparative diagnostic utility of 1H MRS and DWI in evaluation of temporal lobe epilepsy. *Neurology* 58(12): 1745–53.

Katramados, A. M., D. Burdette, et al. 2009. Periictal diffusion abnormalities of the thalamus in partial status epilepticus. *Epilepsia* 50(2): 265–75.

Kikuta, K., Y. Takagi, et al. 2006. Early experience with 3-T magnetic resonance tractography in the surgery of cerebral arteriovenous malformations in and around the visual pathway. *Neurosurgery* 58(2): 331–337.

Kim, H., Z. Piao, et al. 2008. Secondary white matter degeneration of the corpus callosum in patients with intractable temporal lobe epilepsy: a diffusion tensor imaging study. *Epilepsy Research* 81(2–3): 136–42.

Kim, J. A., J. I. Chung, et al. 2001. Transient MR signal changes in patients with generalized tonicoclonic seizure or status epilepticus: periictal diffusion-weighted imaging. *AJNR American Journal of Neuroradiology* 22(6): 1149–60.

Kimiwada, T., C. Juhasz, et al. 2006. Hippocampal and thalamic diffusion abnormalities in children with temporal lobe epilepsy. *Epilepsia* 47(1): 167–75.

Konermann, S., S. Marks, et al. 2003. Presurgical evaluation of epilepsy by brain diffusion: MR-detected effects of flumazenil on the epileptogenic focus. *Epilepsia* 44(3): 399–407.

Lansberg, M. G., M. W. O'Brien, et al. 1999. MRI abnormalities associated with partial status epilepticus. *Neurology* 52(5): 1021–7.

Le Bihan, D., E. Breton, et al. 1986. MR imaging of intravoxel incoherent motions: application to diffusion and perfusion in neurologic disorders. *Radiology* 161(2): 401–7.

Leonhardt, G., A. de Greiff, et al. 2002. Brain diffusion during hyperventilation: diffusion-weighted MR-monitoring in patients with temporal lobe epilepsy and in healthy volunteers. *Epilepsy Research* 51(3): 269–78.

Lewis, D. V. 2005. Losing neurons: selective vulnerability and mesial temporal sclerosis. *Epilepsia* 46 Suppl 7: 39–44.

Li, N., Z. Gong, et al. 2003. Water self-diffusion tensor changes in an avian genetic developmental model of epilepsy. *MAGMA* 16(3): 121–8.

Lin, J. J., J. D. Riley, et al. 2008. Vulnerability of the frontal-temporal connections in temporal lobe epilepsy. *Epilepsy Research* 82(2–3): 162–70.

Londono, A., M. Castillo, et al. 2003. Apparent diffusion coefficient measurements in the hippocampi in patients with temporal lobe seizures. *AJNR American Journal of Neuroradiology* 24(8): 1582–6.

Lux, H. D., U. Heinemann, et al. 1986. Ionic changes and alterations in the size of the extracellular space during epileptic activity. *Advances in Neurology* 44: 619–39.

Matsumoto, R., T. Okada, et al. 2008. Hemispheric asymmetry of the arcuate fasciculus: a preliminary diffusion tensor tractography study in patients with unilateral language dominance defined by Wada test. *Journal of Neurology* 255(11): 1703–11.

McDonald, C. R., M. E. Ahmadi, et al. 2008. Diffusion tensor imaging correlates of memory and language impairments in temporal lobe epilepsy. *Neurology* 71(23): 1869–76.

Men, S., D. H. Lee, et al. 2000. Selective neuronal necrosis associated with status epilepticus: MR findings. *AJNR American Journal of Neuroradiology* 21(10): 1837–40.

Mori, S., B. J. Crain, et al. 1999. Three-dimensional tracking of axonal projections in the brain by magnetic resonance imaging. *Annals of Neurology* 45(2): 265–9.

Moseley, M. E., Y. Cohen, et al. 1990. Diffusion-weighted MR imaging of anisotropic water diffusion in cat central nervous system. *Radiology* 176(2): 439–45.

Mukherjee, P., J. I. Berman, et al. 2008. Diffusion tensor MR imaging and fiber tractography: theoretic underpinnings. *AJNR American Journal of Neuroradiology* 29(4): 632–41.

Nairismagi, J., O. H. Grohn, et al. 2004. Progression of brain damage after status epilepticus and its association with epileptogenesis: a quantitative MRI study in a rat model of temporal lobe epilepsy. *Epilepsia* 45(9): 1024–34.

Nakasu, Y., S. Nakasu, et al. 1995. Diffusion-weighted MR in experimental sustained seizures elicited with kainic acid. *AJNR American Journal of Neuroradiology* 16(6): 1185–92.

Nimsky, C., O. Ganslandt, et al. 2005. Intraoperative diffusion-tensor MR imaging: shifting of white matter tracts during neurosurgical procedures—initial experience. *Radiology* 234(1): 218–25.

O'Brien, T. J., E. P. David, et al. 2007. Contrast-enhanced perfusion and diffusion MRI accurately lateralize temporal lobe epilepsy: a pilot study. *Journal of Clinical Neuroscience* 14(9): 841–9.

Oh, J. B., S. K. Lee, et al. 2004. Role of immediate postictal diffusion-weighted MRI in localizing epileptogenic foci of mesial temporal lobe epilepsy and non-lesional neocortical epilepsy. *Seizure* 13(7): 509–16.

Okumura, A., H. Fukatsu, et al. 2004. Diffusion tensor imaging in frontal lobe epilepsy. *Pediatric Neurology* 31(3): 203–6.

Parmar, H., S. H. Lim, et al. 2006. Acute symptomatic seizures and hippocampus damage: DWI and MRS findings. *Neurology* 66(11): 1732–5.

Pitkanen, A., K. Lukasiuk. 2009. Molecular and cellular basis of epileptogenesis in symptomatic epilepsy. *Epilepsy Behavior* 14 Suppl 1: 16–25.

Powell, H. W., G. J. Parker, et al. 2005. MR tractography predicts visual field defects following temporal lobe resection. *Neurology* 65(4): 596–9.

Powell, H. W., G. J. Parker, et al. 2006. Hemispheric asymmetries in language-related pathways: a combined functional MRI and tractography study. *Neuroimage* 32(1): 388–99.

Prichard, J. W., J. Zhong, et al. 1995. Diffusion-weighted NMR imaging changes caused by electrical activation of the brain. *NMR Biomedicine* 8(7–8): 359–64.

Righini, A., C. Pierpaoli, et al. 1994. Brain parenchyma apparent diffusion coefficient alterations associated with experimental complex partial status epilepticus. *Magnetic Resonance Imaging* 12(6): 865–71.

Rodrigo, S., C. Oppenheim, et al. 2007. Uncinate fasciculus fiber tracking in mesial temporal lobe epilepsy. Initial findings. *European Radiology* 17(7): 1663–8.

Rodrigo, S., C. Oppenheim, et al. 2008. Language lateralization in temporal lobe epilepsy using functional MRI and probabilistic tractography. *Epilepsia* 49(8): 1367–76.

Romano, A., G. D'Andrea, et al. 2009. Pre-surgical planning and MR-tractography utility in brain tumour resection. *European Radiology* [e-pub June 16].

Rugg-Gunn, F. J., S. H. Eriksson, et al. 2001. Diffusion tensor imaging of cryptogenic and acquired partial epilepsies. *Brain* 124(Pt 3): 627–36.

Rugg-Gunn, F. J., S. H. Eriksson, et al. 2002. Diffusion tensor imaging in refractory epilepsy. *Lancet* 359(9319): 1748–1751.

Rullmann, M., A. Anwander, et al. 2009. EEG source analysis of epileptiform activity using a 1 mm anisotropic hexahedra finite element head model. *Neuroimage* 44(2): 399–410.

Salmenpera, T. M., R. J. Simister, et al. 2006. High-resolution diffusion tensor imaging of the hippocampus in temporal lobe epilepsy. *Epilepsy Research* 71(2–3): 102–6.

Salmenpera, T. M., M. R. Symms, et al. 2006. Postictal diffusion weighted imaging. *Epilepsy Research* 70(2–3): 133–43.

Schoene-Bake, J. C., J. Faber, et al. 2009. Widespread affections of large fiber tracts in postoperative temporal lobe epilepsy. *Neuroimage* 46: 569–76.

Smith, S. M., M. Jenkinson, et al. 2006. Tract-based spatial statistics: voxelwise analysis of multi-subject diffusion data. *Neuroimage* 31(4): 1487–505.

Sutula, T. P., J. Hagen, et al. 2003. Do epileptic seizures damage the brain? *Current Opinion Neurology* 16(2): 189–95.

Sykova, E. 2004. Diffusion properties of the brain in health and disease. *Neurochemistry International* 45(4): 453–66.

Szabo, K., A. Poepel, et al. 2005. Diffusion-weighted and perfusion MRI demonstrates parenchymal changes in complex partial status epilepticus. *Brain* 128(Pt 6): 1369–76.

Taoka, T., M. Sakamoto, et al. 2008. Diffusion tensor tractography of the Meyer loop in cases of temporal lobe resection for temporal lobe epilepsy: correlation between postsurgical visual field defect and anterior limit of Meyer loop on tractography. *AJNR American Journal of Neuroradiology* 29(7): 1329–34.

Thivard, L., C. Adam, et al. 2006. Interictal diffusion MRI in partial epilepsies explored with intracerebral electrodes. *Brain* 129(Pt 2): 375–85.

Thivard, L., S. Lehericy, et al. 2005. Diffusion tensor imaging in medial temporal lobe epilepsy with hippocampal sclerosis. *Neuroimage* 28(3): 682–90.

Tokumitsu, T., A. Mancuso, et al. 1997. Metabolic and pathological effects of temporal lobe epilepsy in rat brain detected by proton spectroscopy and imaging. *Brain Research* 744(1): 57–67.

Toledo, M., J. Munuera, et al. 2008. MRI findings in aphasic status epilepticus. *Epilepsia* 49(8): 1465–9.

Trivedi, R., R. K. Gupta, et al. 2006. Diffusion tensor imaging in polymicrogyria: a report of three cases. *Neuroradiology* 48(6): 422–7.

Wall, C. J., E. J. Kendall, et al. 2000. Rapid alterations in diffusion-weighted images with anatomic correlates in a rodent model of status epilepticus. *AJNR American Journal of Neuroradiology* 21(10): 1841–52.

Wehner, T., E. Lapresto, et al. 2007. The value of interictal diffusion-weighted imaging in lateralizing temporal lobe epilepsy. *Neurology* 68(2): 122–7.

Wheless, J. W., L. Carmant, et al. 2009. Magnetic resonance imaging abnormalities associated with vigabatrin in patients with epilepsy. *Epilepsia* 50(2): 195–205.

Wieshmann, U. C., C. A. Clark, et al. 1999. Water diffusion in the human hippocampus in epilepsy. *Magnetic Resonance Imaging* 17(1): 29–36.

Wieshmann, U. C., C. A. Clark, et al. 1999. Reduced anisotropy of water diffusion in structural cerebral abnormalities demonstrated with diffusion tensor imaging. *Magnetic Resonance Imaging* 17(9): 1269–74.

Wieshmann, U. C., M. R. Symms, et al. 1997. Diffusion changes in status epilepticus. *Lancet* 350(9076): 493–4.

Yogarajah, M., H. W. Powell, et al. 2008. Tractography of the parahippocampal gyrus and material specific memory impairment in unilateral temporal lobe epilepsy. *Neuroimage* 40(4): 1755–64.

Yoo, S. Y., K. H. Chang, et al. 2002. Apparent diffusion coefficient value of the hippocampus in patients with hippocampal sclerosis and in healthy volunteers. *AJNR American Journal of Neuroradiology* 23(5): 809–12.

Yu, J. T., L. Tan. 2008. Diffusion-weighted magnetic resonance imaging demonstrates parenchymal pathophysiological changes in epilepsy. *Brain Research Review* 59(1): 34–41.

Zhang, J., P. C. van Zijl, et al. 2006. Image contrast using the secondary and tertiary eigenvectors in diffusion tensor imaging. *Magnetic Resonance in Medicine* 55(2): 439–49.

Zhong, J., O. A. Petroff, et al. 1997. Reversible, reproducible reduction of brain water apparent diffusion coefficient by cortical electroshocks. *Magnetic Resonance in Medicine* 37(1): 1–6.

Zhong, J., O. A. Petroff, et al. 1995. Barbiturate-reversible reduction of water diffusion coefficient in flurothyl-induced status epilepticus in rats. *Magnetic Resonance in Medicine* 33(2): 253–6.

Chapter 7

MAGNETOENCEPHALOGRAPHY-BASED SOURCE IMAGING FOR EPILEPSY AND LANGUAGE LOCALIZATION

Robert C. Knowlton and Lawrence W. Ver Hoef

INTRODUCTION

Magnetoencephalography (MEG) is a remarkable technology used to record spontaneous and evoked magnetic fields generated by brain neuronal activity. Recordings are performed in a superconducting environment with induction coils submerged in liquid helium at near absolute zero temperature. Modern systems use whole-head detector arrays to record in vivo the exceedingly small magnetic fields (10^{-12} T) generated by intraneuronal currents of the human brain. Although analogous to the electroencephalogram (EEG) in that both measure and record signal reflecting neuronal activity, fundamental differences exist (Cuffin and Cohen 1979). Today's MEG systems allow almost instantaneous high-resolution (100 to 300 channels) recordings of cortical function and dysfunction that are neither attenuated nor distorted by the skull and other variable intervening tissue layers between the scalp and brain. Historically, these technical attributes have created the tendency to use MEG for source localization more than EEG. High-resolution

EEG recording combined with advanced modeling techniques may overcome some of the source localization challenges of EEG, but the use of such methods has been studied little to date for clinical application (Ahnlide et al. 2007; Brodbeck et al. 2009; Plummer et al. 2008). In contrast, MEG has been studied and used extensively toward clinical application since the inception of multidetector array systems in the early 1990s. In fact, in the United States, MEG-based source localization—called magnetic source imaging (MSI) when combined with structural imaging—received FDA approval for clinical use in 1997 and was given Current Procedural Terminology (CPT) codes for epilepsy localization and presurgical brain mapping in 2003.

Source analysis is the critical component of MEG that converts the standard of inferring location from two-dimensional scalp-recorded waveforms (as has been done with EEG in epilepsy since the 1930s) to three-dimensional brain location that can be visualized on structural or functional anatomical imaging. To determine the location of a source generator(s) in the brain from scalp MEG or EEG, advanced signal processing is necessary to solve what is called the *inverse problem*. Detailed examination of the inverse problem and solutions is far beyond the scope of this chapter. An excellent review is provided by Plummer et al. (2008). In summary, the basic computation compares the measured field pattern at the scalp to a computer-simulated field pattern derived from equations for source estimates placed in different locations inside the brain and with varying orientation at each region. Usually, a least squares difference is measured between the observed and computed field patterns (forward solution), and is minimized iteratively until an optimal fit is obtained. The forward solution with the best fit may be chosen to represent the inverse solution.

Different models for source localization begin with the set of conditions used for the forward problem in order to arrive at a computed solution. The set of conditions represents the volume conductor—a head model created by definitions of compartments, surfaces, and conductivities. Computation of the projected field (lead field) from a source generator to the scalp surface where recordings are made must use some form of a head model. The choice of model for the forward problem can range from a simple sphere based on the scalp surface to complex multilayered realistic head models derived from segmented structural imaging (typically MRI) that includes separate conductivities for brain, cerebrospinal fluid, skull, and scalp.

Differential sensitivity to forward models is one aspect of source localization that can separate MEG and EEG. Theoretically and empirically, MEG is less dependent on a requirement for complex real-head models. As mentioned earlier, the relative ease and computational efficiency of spherical head modeling has allowed MEG to be much more readily used than EEG for source localization in the clinical environment. With improvement in computer processing speed, network access to digital imaging, and software ease of use, this difference may be diminished to the point that EEG source localization can be more readily employed for clinical application.

What remains the greatest challenge for both EEG and MEG source localization is the inverse problem. In contrast to the forward problem, no unique solution exists. Constraints on possible solutions need to be used. Some constraints such as limiting the source space to that of the cortical mantle are obvious and very likely to be valid. Others, such as limitation to specific brain regions, must be assumed on prior knowledge and may not be valid. It is the differences in constraint conditions that distinguish inverse models.

The two fundamental types of inverse approaches are dipole and distributed source modeling. Dipole modeling requires an assumption on the number of sources generating the observed signal at a given instance or time frame. Dipole(s) representing the source (conceptually) can be allowed to move over time—different location at each successive time point over the duration of an event of interest with temporal resolution dictated by sampling frequency. Conversely, dipoles can be fixed in position with rotation and other parameters free to change over the time interval. Figure 7.1 shows an example of an epileptic spike (detected on MEG and not EEG) that is amenable to single equivalent current dipole modeling fixed in location with freedom for rotation. More complex dipole models attempt to account for multiple overlapping sources in space and time, a context that may apply to some interictal epileptiform disturbances (e.g., secondary bilateral synchrony). For the majority of spikes and sharp waves a single source may be safely assumed and the main issue is propagation—avoiding the risk of localizing the destination versus the source of the spike.

Before discussing dipole modeling further, some explanation of what dipoles actually are is necessary. In source localization the dipole is an artificial representation of the putative source's maximal current (MEG)/potential (EEG). In contrast to EEG, where the source is created by summated extracellular membrane depolarization current, MEG source signal is generated by intracellular (mainly dendritic) current. For both MEG and EEG the dipole model can represent only an estimate of the source by a location, direction, and strength. Arguably, the location parameter is the least accurate since a point in space cannot represent a source(s) generated by an extended area of cortex. A point source dipole will be only a mathematical estimate that may be located within or near the actual tissue generating the measured signal. Empirically, the estimates can be remarkably accurate (Fig. 7.1), particularly with the uncomplicated focal spikes seen in many epilepsy patients.

Yet despite nearly two decades of MEG clinical investigation, controversy and questions remain as to what contribution MEG adds to EEG and the role that it plays among other established epilepsy imaging tests and intracranial EEG (icEEG). This chapter will focus mainly on MEG epilepsy localization and language mapping. MEG presurgical brain mapping is well established for primary sensory (visual, somatosensory, and auditory) and motor modalities. These are fairly straightforward tests similar to evoked potentials but with the added value of 3D localization. The work that has been done with language lateralization and mapping will be included in this chapter because this is one of the most challenging brain mapping clinical applications. A substantial number of studies have been performed with MEG and clinical validation of language mapping. Language mapping is probably

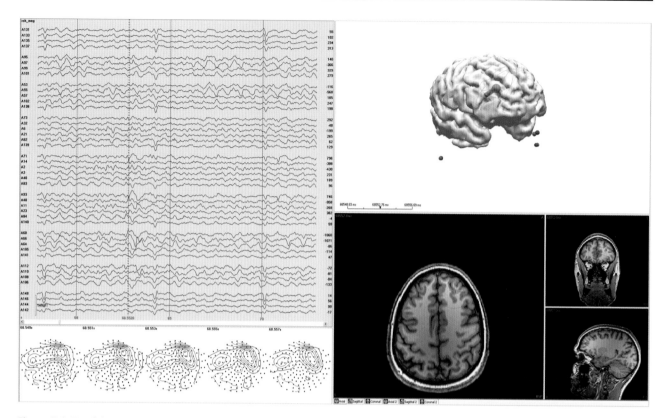

Figure 7.1 Top left: MEG signal versus time tracing showing a subset of the total 148 channels of the recording system in a longitudinal montage (anterior to posterior) starting from left (higher channels) to central (middle channels) to right (bottom channels). MEG spike peak in right frontal channels is centered at 68.552 sec as delineated by the vertical time bar. Bottom left: Magnetic flux contours at four successive latencies (2-msec interval) surrounding the spike peak. Isofield contours show a unifocal dipole maxima and minima over the right frontal polar region with a mostly horizontal orientation. Top right: 3D rendering of segmented brain surface from MRI with dipole source localization estimate shown as a small red sphere with a vector orientation tail. The surrounding ellipsoids reflect the 95% confidence volume for the source estimate. Bottom right: Orthogonal MRI slices through dipole source location.

best served by MEG or its combination with functional MRI (fMRI) such that high spatial and temporal resolution is provided to resolve networked areas of brain processing that are likely to overlap. The application of fMRI in language mapping is discussed in detail in Chapter 5.

SPIKE SOURCE LOCALIZATION

Before discussing MEG source localization for epilepsy, the first question that should be asked is whether accurate localization of interictal epileptiform discharges (spikes and sharp waves) is of value. This question is made obvious because localization for epilepsy surgery is conceptually based on determining where seizures, not spikes, arise. Although seizures can be captured, recorded, and even localized by MEG (Assaf et al. 2003; Eliashiv et al. 2002; Tilz et al. 2002), it is a rare exception that an ictal event occurs during the scan; it is not expected in the routine study. Thus, it has to be understood that the information provided by MEG spike source localization, even if technically

accurate, may not reflect the actual localization of the patient's epilepsy, the onset region of his or her habitually recurrent spontaneous seizures. In most clinical scenarios, however, completely false localizing spikes should be recognizable. The history and seizure semiology alone should be helpful in discerning which spikes are most related to the patient's habitual seizures. Also, as will be discussed later, spikes seen at the scalp by either EEG or MEG should be not be confused with those recorded at the cortex, where terms or concepts such as "irritative zones" are used. Spikes recordable at the scalp are a strongly selected subset of robust, large-amplitude discharges that contrast with other scattered spikes that are exclusive to the electrocorticogram (Ray et al. 2007; Tao et al. 2005). In neocortical epilepsies (lateral temporal and extratemporal), where MEG is probably of greatest value (see below), frequent unifocal spikes that tightly cluster on source localization appear to have a strong correlation with seizure onsets recorded with icEEG (Knowlton et al. 2006, 2008; Minassian, et al. 1999; Oishi et al. 2006). Still, ultimately, the potential value of spike localization has to be determined on a case-by-case basis.

SENSITIVITY

If the value of spike localization can be accepted, at least in some proportion of cases, then the next most important question is that of sensitivity for detecting spikes of interest in an MEG examination. This question also brings up the first issue of clinically significant potential difference between MEG and EEG: is either MEG or EEG more sensitive for the detection of spikes? Multiple, some interrelated, variables are involved in the criteria that have to be met for a spike to be recordable at the scalp: extent of depolarized cortex (simultaneous or sufficiently overlapping by cortico-cortical propagation), depth from surface, amplitude, dipolar orientation, and conductivity of intervening tissues all are important. To what degree, and which of these variables, has a differential effect on EEG versus MEG may result in a detection sensitivity difference. Depth is a heavily weighted variable, and in this case EEG might have a slight advantage because MEG detectors are not as close to the scalp as EEG electrodes. This might be more than offset, however, by the attenuation from conductivity differences caused by the skull that are not applicable to MEG.

The extent of involved cortex required to detect a spike signal at the scalp is a most interesting variable that has been increasingly studied and may indeed be different for MEG than EEG. From temporal lobe studies of simultaneous icEEG, it has been estimated that at least 6 to 8 cm^2 of basal lateral cortex is necessary for MEG detection of spikes (Baumgartner et al. 2000; Mikuni et al. 1997; Oishi et al. 2002). In one recent study, spikes seen only in the most distal (mesial) contacts of a depth electrode were detected with MEG, but the extent of involvement of adjacent mesial basal cortex was not sampled (Santiuste et al. 2008). For spikes in the lateral convexity (longitudinal frontal sulcus), only 3 to 4 cm^2 was necessary with MEG recording (Oishi et al. 2002). For EEG the number of 6 cm^2 has been used widely for decades, since the 1965 study by Cooper et al. (1965). This estimate was based on an in vitro experiment that did not include background noise. A more recent in vivo study with subdural grids over the anterior lateral temporal cortex found that very few spikes involving less than 10 cm^2 were recognizable on the scalp EEG, and that most typical anterior temporal lobe spikes reflected 20 to 30 cm of cortical source area (Tao et al. 2005). Together, these findings suggest that MEG may have a better sensitivity than EEG. Unfortunately, no simultaneous scalp EEG, MEG, and icEEG studies that would allow direct comparison have been reported.

Several studies have compared detection of spikes in routine examinations with scalp EEG and MEG. Most are series of temporal lobe epilepsy patients and there is only one with high-density EEG recording (Iwasaki et al. 2005; Leijten et al. 2003; Lin et al. 2003; Zijlmans et al. 2002). From these, no clear differences are seen; most spikes are detected by both modalities, and only small percentages are detected by only one. One exception is posterior lateral temporal sources, where MEG had higher yields (Lin et al. 2003). This increase in sensitivity may also herald the same for extratemporal convexity regions, especially if sources involve sulcal banks producing more tangentially oriented dipoles (e.g., the longitudinal frontal sulci, the intraparietal sulcus, and both banks of the sylvian fissure). It is valuable to remember that over two thirds of the cortical mantle is located in sulcal walls and depths.

The orientation of the source dipole is also an important factor, a limitation that will apply more to MEG, which cannot record purely radial sources (e.g., those confined to the crown of gyrus, which is a highly unlikely physiologic circumstance). In one sense, this putative limitation of MEG can be an attribute for localization by giving rise to a more geometrically simple and more spatially limited source to model. EEG has an increase in contribution from volume currents that are further spatially and temporally blurred by the skull.

Whether MEG is more sensitive than EEG is still not clear, but the likelihood that it is for many neocortical sources has provoked much of the enthusiasm for its use as a tool in epilepsy evaluation. If MEG does detect more spikes than EEG in neocortical epilepsy, a new challenge arises: how to reliably identify true epileptiform discharges on MEG alone. Confounding sharp transients of no epileptiform significance have not been well defined as they have been in EEG. Also, MEG spikes coincident with EEG discharges have different morphologic characteristics (de Jongh et al. 2005; Fernandes et al. 2005). Most of the differences consist of spatial and temporal blunting (duration and sharpness) of the EEG, presumed to reflect volume current propagation through surrounding tissues of varying conductivity. This has an amplified effect in disturbed brain and skull regions such as cystic lesions and prior craniotomies, not uncommon scenarios in epilepsy surgery. This difference has a more important role in regard to dipole modeling accuracy than sensitivity, but it is another factor that adds to the problem of more widespread use of MEG. Clearly, more training in MEG interpretation in clinical neurophysiology is needed.

ACCURACY

Regardless of whether MEG is more sensitive than EEG, another potential advantage remains for MEG: specifically, source localization accuracy. It is this area that has been assumed to be a forte of MEG. The key features of MEG that lend to an advantage are (1) absence of magnetic field distortion and attenuation by highly variable conductivities between brain and sensor that apply to EEG and (2) the ease of very-high-density sampling. Yet for both MEG and EEG, solving the inverse problem remains challenging, and numerous assumptions have to be taken into account. If sources of interest are unifocal (not overlapping either spatially or temporally with other sources) and limited in extent, then the single equivalent current dipole (ECD) model is likely to be appropriate. Indeed, with MEG mapping of focal evoked fields (e.g., somatosensory or auditory), a high degree of accuracy on the order of millimeters has been demonstrated in

normal and abnormal brains, including in patients with tumors and other destructive lesions (Gallen et al. 1993; Sobel et al. 1993; Sutherling 2001). However, epilepsy spikes can be much more complicated and, as discussed above, and involve a relatively large amount of cortex, even if they are considered single and "focal." Extended source models based on current distribution of a fixed set of dipoles using minimum norm estimation are theoretically better than ECD modeling of most extended spike sources (Fuchs et al. 1999). Figure 7.2 shows the distributed source modeling of the same spike localized with single ECD modeling. Moreover, many spike discharges as visualized at the scalp are complex and likely comprise overlapping sources. For these cases, the single ECD model should

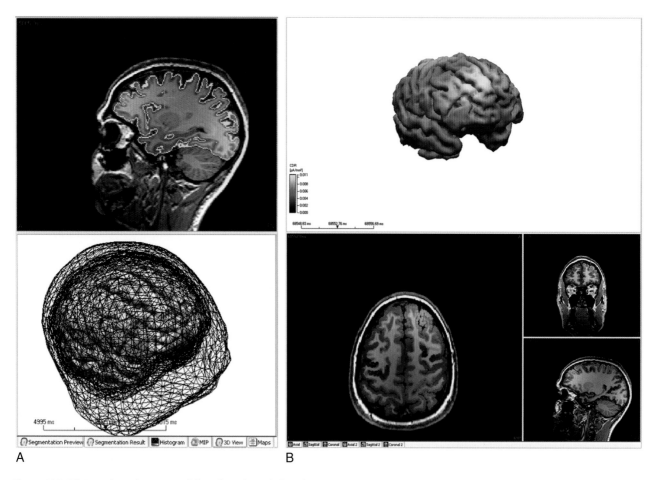

A   B

Figure 7.2 (A) Boundary element modeling (based on skull and tissue segmentation of the MRI) was used for the forward calculations to determine the source localization with either dipole or distributed source modeling. No appreciable difference was seen with equivalent current dipole localization between the single sphere and boundary element forward models. (B) 3D rendering of the segmented brain surface from MRI with minimum norm computed distributed source localization of the same spike shown in Figure 7.1. The boundary element model shown in (A) was used as the forward model, including the confinement of source contribution to the cortical mantle. Note that the cerebellum is excluded from the brain volume for modeling, reflecting the assumption that cerebellar cortex does not contribute to spike sources.

not be expected to provide a satisfactory answer; multidipole spatiotemporal modeling should be considered for such discharges (Stephen et al. 2003). Ideally, for this problem, an a priori knowledge of plausible physiologic sources should be available for the model. One example of where this might be possible is secondary bilateral synchrony of overlapping mesial frontal lobe sources. It is still important to emphasize that although limited by strict assumptions about the source, only the ECD model to date has been investigated to any extent by clinical validation.

VALIDATION

Numerous direct and indirect approaches have been aimed at determining the accuracy of MEG source localization of epilepsy. The direct methods use either implanted dipoles or simultaneous icEEG–MEG recordings. Indirect methods include measures of co-localization with epileptogenic tissue either visualized on imaging or delineated with icEEG, and then ideally confirmed by surgical resection and histopathology.

Recordings with implanted dipoles (created by a pair of special electrodes included at icEEG electrode implantation) with precise knowledge of location provide the rigor of validation similar to phantom studies but with in vivo characterization of effects from intervening tissue and skull of the human head. Estimates of error include means that range from a few millimeters (Rose et al. 1991) to nearly 2 cm (Balish et al. 1991). Error was shown to be greatly dependent on both signal-to-noise and depth. Although of value, it is noted that all such studies were performed with only single- or seven-channel instruments that required several instrument repositionings to fully sample the observed field patterns. Also, radiographs were used to determine the locations of the implanted dipoles. Both of these aspects of earlier recordings contribute to error measures.

Simultaneous icEEG and large-array MEG studies offer the best opportunity to validate source localization of spontaneous epileptiform discharges. The few studies that have been done have all confirmed that MEG spike source localization was *roughly* concordant with the electrocortigraphic mapping of spikes (Baumgartner et al. 1997; Oishi et al. 2002). Only one study included an extratemporal lobe spike source (Oishi et al. 2006). None included quantitative error estimates. Some caution regarding precision has to be considered in these types of studies because complete characterization of sources is not always possible with the limited placement of intracranial electrodes required for clinical use. Also, surgical dressings and electrode connectors increase the distance between brain and detectors and further decrease signal-to-noise.

The bulk of proof-of-principal clinical validation attempts involved correlation of spike dipole source localization with ultimate surgical localization. In lesional cases, studies have consistently shown MEG to be concordant with icEEG findings, including various tumors and intrinsically epileptogenic developmental lesions (Bast et al. 2004; Knowlton et al. 1997; Morioka et al. 1999). Figure 7.3 provides an example of icEEG validation of the spike sources seen in Figures 7.1 and 7.2. Although the recordings were not acquired simultaneously with MEG, the consistency of the largest-amplitude spikes (the only discharges likely to be detected by scalp EEG/MEG) allows for inference that the spikes reflect what has been localized with MEG. In addition to validation, such cases demonstrate the ability of MEG spike localization to delineate the topographic relation of epileptogenic tissue to the lesion as visualized on imaging (Hader et al. 2004). Even co-localization with cryptogenic lesions (not seen on MRI) has provided clinical validity (Knowlton et al. 1997).

In contrast to mostly proof-of-principle and technical validation is the challenge of generalizable clinical validation. An obvious initial approach has been to study MEG prediction of invasive gold standards for epilepsy localization. The first standard may be considered icEEG localization of seizures, an ultimate arbiter in surgical decision making that is not influenced by the many uncontrolled variables in surgical outcome. If MEG spike localization correlated with icEEG seizure localization, then a foundation from which an MEG impact on the surgical evaluation could begin to be established. The potential roles of a relatively high-sensitivity, noninvasive test would be numerous, stretching from a screening tool with high specificity for surgical candidates deemed most appropriate for further evaluation, to adding localizing information not available from other established tests, to improving icEEG placement, to replacing other more expensive tests (ictal single photon emission computed tomography), even possibly icEEG in a subset of cases. Studies specifically addressing prediction of icEEG demonstrate that highly localized MEG studies are concordant with seizure onsets recorded with subdural grid recordings (Knowlton et al. 2008; Mamelak et al. 2002; Minassian et al. 1999; Oishi et al. 2006).

Other studies with relatively large series of broadly selected surgical candidates have attempted to address additional issues of clinical value. However, it first needs to be mentioned that studies investigating the impact of a test in the context of epilepsy surgery are fraught with difficulties unlike studies of standard diagnostic tests. Protocols for surgery evaluations are highly nonstandardized across centers and are tailored

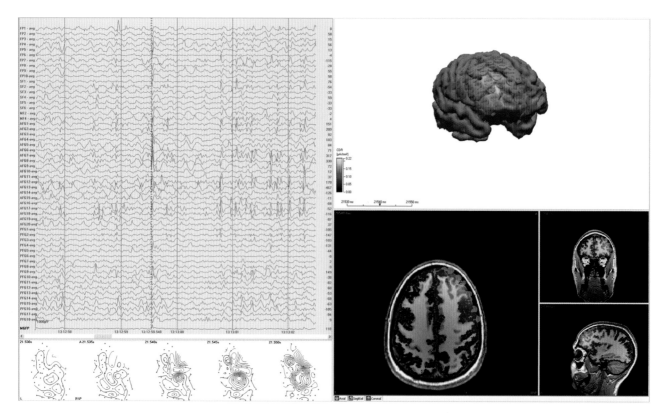

Figure 7.3 Top left: Intracranial EEG with grid and strip subdural electrodes placed over the right dorsal lateral and frontal polar regions show multiple spikes. A spike with large amplitude and extent centered at 21.540 msec was selected for analysis because it is representative of what would likely be recorded at the scalp. Bottom left: Isopotential field contours for the selected spike. Top right: 3D rendering of the segmented brain surface from MRI, including subdural electrodes localized from co-registered post-implantation CT scan, shows the spike source localization from the minimum norm computed distributed source localization. Bottom right: Orthogonal MRI slices through the distributed source localization of the electrocortigraphy-recorded spike. The findings are concordant with the MEG dipole and distributed sources seen in Figures 7.1 and 7.2.

frequently on a case-by-case basis even within centers. Also, sensitivity and specificity can often not be reliably obtained: decisions to proceed with further evaluation are often subjective; icEEG may yield an incorrect answer leading to no surgery or the wrong surgery, and not infrequently surgical outcomes are affected by other factors independent of test localization accuracy (e.g., limited resection).

Despite these major issues, investigators have diligently tried to deal with them in design and analysis. Stefan et al. (2003) examined MEG performed in a broadly collected group of 455 patients with intractable epilepsy, 50% of whom were considered treatable with surgery. To address many of the above issues, they measured MEG agreement with an ultimate suspected localization of the patient's epilepsy based on all tests available and by consensus from multiple investigators. In addition, contribution to the localization answer was measured using a five-point rating scale taking into account disagreement, no contribution, agreement, additional information, and novel influence on surgery decision.

Two large studies from the University of Texas at Houston Laboratory examined the relative accuracy and contribution of MEG to the most established non-invasive tests of localization: ictal and interictal scalp EEG with video (VEEG) and MRI (Pataraia et al. 2004; Wheless et al. 1999). Concordance measures were based on degree of resection overlap with and without analysis including surgical outcome. Unique in this work was that MEG was considered experimental and therefore not used in decision making to define the region of resection.

These and other studies have consistently shown an overall sensitivity between 70% and 80% for a positive MEG study—spikes captured and satisfactory ECD source localization achieved. No significant difference stands out between temporal and extratemporal lobe epilepsy, although some disparity is noted, including that which may be related to varying whole-head instrument coverage of the inferior temporal region (Leijten et al. 2003). The various measures of diagnostic localization accuracy were greater for MEG than for VEEG. This is not surprising, especially in extratemporal lobe epilepsy, where ictal scalp EEG recordings are frequently nonlocalizing due to artifact and rapid propagation. This should not be interpreted to mean that VEEG is unnecessary; rather, it should strongly suggest that MEG could be contributory. Indeed, a common conclusion from each of the studies was that MEG added value in approximately 35% to 40% of cases with inconclusively localizing VEEG. Moreover, many cases with normal or nonlocalizing MRI can also be added to this group.

CLINICAL UTILITY OF MSI IN EPILEPSY SURGERY

As with most imaging tests in epilepsy surgery, the level of evidence supporting the clinical role of MSI is limited. No randomized studies to determine the clinical utility of any epilepsy imaging tests exist. This may be partly explained by the many issues complicating such studies. First, what evidence of technical and clinical validity that does exist raises an ethical issue of withholding test results in one group of patients, and it is not clear that equipoise would exist. Second, matching patient groups would be challenging, if not impossible, given the great heterogeneity of neocortical and nonlesional epilepsy patients (arguably every patient represents a unique epilepsy). Third, a wide range of practice variation is present across epilepsy surgery centers in both evaluation approaches and final surgical decision-making preferences. An added complication is that tests like MSI in epilepsy surgery are not simply diagnostic—aiding in the determination of who should and should not be treated with surgery—as a *test sort* role. MSI also may affect overall outcome measures, most importantly the probability of seizure-free outcome, or cure rate. The studies that do offer some evidence of clinical validity—diagnostic value in regard to prediction of seizure-free outcome—are compromised by inherent selection and ascertainment bias. Also, nearly all studies that show an association between MSI results and other imaging tests as well as icEEG do not allow conclusions as to whether the health outcomes were improved by the additional test data. This assessment is drawn from a Blue Cross/Blue Shield policy review based on published literature up to mid 2008 (BCBS 2009). Cited as representative studies in the assessment are two papers from a prospective observational study performed at our center that detail the diagnostic characteristics of MSI in a nonlesional epilepsy surgery cohort. Predictive values based on the sensitivities and specificities measured relative to either icEEG or surgical outcomes were comparable and nonredundant to positron emission tomography of glucose metabolism (FDG PET) and ictal SPECT, but values of 70% to 75% are not sufficient to be used

as a sorting tool alone. What is not mentioned in the assessment is that MSI is not interpreted and used in isolation. Indeed, MSI combined with concordant PET or ictal SPECT had specificities near 90%, values that may be acceptable when taken into account with other supporting clinical data warranting a move to proceed with surgery.

The greatest problem of MSI as a patient selection tool is the problem of false-negative results. Negative results that are due to the absence of capturing epileptiform disturbance during a recording session should be interpreted only as nondiagnostic. To be distinguished are results in which source localization attempts fail and the MSI is interpreted as "nonlocalized." Whether the result is a false or true negative is very important. True negatives could be used to influence a case away from further surgical evaluation or even a failed surgery.

At this point, with the common clinical use of the single ECD model, the false-negative rate (around 50%) is too high. Thus, techniques, both in acquisition (sensitivity) and source localization analysis (specificity), need improvement if MSI is to play more potent patient selection role. Attempts to increase sensitivity include detection and localization of slow wave and high-frequency oscillations. For complex epileptiform disturbances that cannot be localized by single ECD modeling, spatial-temporal dipole and distributed source models offer the possibility of increasing both sensitivity and specificity; however, studies to technically and clinically validate localization results remain to be done.

Regardless of the present limitations in MSI sensitivity, the positive predictive value of a conclusively localized study should not be ignored. False-positive localization can be a risk, but the possibility can be mitigated by interpretation in the context of other electroclinicoanatomical data available in surgery evaluations. When MSI spike source estimates are highly localized (tightly clustered, consistent in dipole orientation, and temporally stable) and concordant with clinical impression, the association with accurate localization of the epileptogenic zone is strong. In this setting MSI may affect not only the evaluation strategy but also the outcome—a most important contribution to test utility.

The test effect on "cure rate" does not need to be large to create a scenario in which evaluation strategies that include use of the test become preferred. Two recent studies reveal some support for a test effect on outcome by demonstrating modification of icEEG plans before and after blinded MSI results were provided (Knowlton et al. 2009; Sutherling et al. 2008). In both studies it can be inferred that some patients would likely have failed surgery due to false localization from incorrect or insufficient icEEG coverage of the seizure onset zone. In other cases false-negative icEEG localization would have led to no surgery in patients who became seizure-free with appropriate localization that resulted from MSI-modified icEEG coverage. Even though the studies are strengthened by use of blinding, allowing some determination of MSI effect on decision making and outcome, conclusions have to be limited to suggestions rather than firm changes in clinical practice. Neither study was designed or powered to provide this level of evidence. Further, the wide practice variation in surgical evaluation strategies in nonlesional, mostly neocortical epilepsy surgery limits the generalizability of the findings. Nonetheless, demonstrating the possibility of a likely test effect on cure rate should evoke enthusiasm for determining the actual impact of MEG-based spike source localization.

MEG LANGUAGE MAPPING

The main utility of MEG in the management of epilepsy patients is in source localization of epileptiform spikes, but it also may be useful in presurgical planning to map eloquent cortex noninvasively. Aphasia or dysphasia associated with injury to language-specific cortex is potentially the most devastating disabling complication of resective epilepsy surgery. Because the ability to communicate is an essential cognitive function, severe impairments in this domain, particularly if receptive language is impaired, can affect quality of life even more severely than hemiplegia. Therefore, a noninvasive tool to localize language-specific cortex accurately or even just lateralize the dominant hemisphere would be very helpful for surgical planning and estimation of surgical risk.

Language mapping with MEG poses definite challenges over mapping of primary sensory (somatosensory, visual, auditory) cortex. Primary sensory stimulation robustly activates a discrete cortical patch for a relatively brief duration that is tightly time-locked to stimulus onset. By contrast, receptive language activity occurs over a wider cortical network with a more complex pattern of synaptic firing occurring over a longer duration that is variable in latency. These factors make it less amenable to dipole modeling, which assumes a point source of coherent current flow. Numerous experimental language activation paradigms have been tried, but the method with the most clinical validation is the verbal recognition memory paradigm developed by the MEG/MSI lab at the University of Texas Houston Health Sciences Center (Breier et al. 1998; Zouridakis et al. 1998). The Houston group and several other laboratories, including ours, have employed this method or slight variations on it in clinical practice for several years.

To briefly describe the method, the patient is first exposed visually or aurally to a list of approximately 30 abstract nouns (e.g., truth, victory). Then three blocks of 40 words, including the original 30 words and 10 new words (also abstract nouns), are presented serially to the patient while neuromagnetic data are acquired. Data are collected in 1200-ms epochs starting 200 ms before stimulus presentation and continuing until 1000 ms after the stimulus presentation onset. The patient is instructed to pay careful attention to each word and decide if it is one of the words from the initial list or a new word and to lift his or her index finger if it is recognized from the initial list. The patient's response is not recorded, nor are the data segregated for analysis by familiar versus novel words; rather, the purpose of asking the patient to indicate recognition is to keep the patient attentive to the stimuli as they are presented. No significant difference in the degree or location of receptive language cortex activation between familiar versus novel words has been seen with this method. A second run of three blocks of 40 words each is then repeated. The epochs of each run are averaged, yielding an averaged event-related waveform for each sensor, as shown in Figure 7.4, for each run. ECD analysis is performed for each sample over the interval from 200 to 800 ms post-stimulus onset. For each time sample, an automated algorithm selects the best group of channels for each hemisphere from which to derive the source localization. Dipole localizations are calculated at each time sample, and only those dipoles that meet a certain threshold of goodness of fit and confidence volume are retained. A statistical algorithm then compares the location and latency of each dipole derived from each of the two runs and generates a rank-ordered list of the dipoles that are most reproducible in space and latency within and between both runs. The best 60% of the dipole locations from that list are retained. Most often some degree of activity is seen in both the right and left hemispheres, but the test is felt to be lateralizing for hemispheric dominance if there is more than a 10% difference between the number of dipoles that localize to one hemisphere over the other. An example of a cluster of language source localizations in a patient with brain tumor is shown in Figure 7.5.

As a verbal recognition stimulation paradigm, this method shows the most robust activity in the posterior superior temporal gyrus (Breier et al. 1998), in the region of Wernicke's area. As with most cognitive functional imaging techniques, other areas are activated as well, but less so with this technique than others, especially fMRI (discussed in Chapter 5). The language-specific activation is similar whether the stimulus is presented visually or audibly (Papanicolaou et al. 1999). The results of this method have been shown to be stable and reproducible across serial examinations

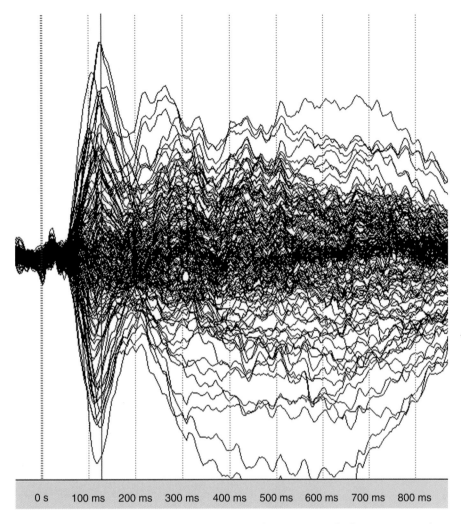

0 s 100 ms 200 ms 300 ms 400 ms 500 ms 600 ms 700 ms 800 ms

Figure 7.4 MEG receptive language event-related waveforms: the 148 overlaid tracings in the figure represent the neuromagnetic activity from the whole-head magnetometer array. Each line represents the event-related magnetic field magnitude measured from one of the 148 sensors. The data shown are averaged from all epochs (n = 120) from before stimulus onset (0 ms) to approximately 900 ms after stimulus onset. The narrow deflection around 100 ms represents primary auditory processing of the presented words, and the broad deflection from approximately 200 ms to 800 ms represents the late language components that are analyzed for source localization.

in the same patients (Simos et al. 2005) as well as demonstrating good interrater reliability (Lee et al. 2006).

Papanicolaou et al. (2004) compared the lateralization of the dominant hemisphere as predicted by MEG with the intracarotid amobarbital test/Wada test (Loring et al. 1990; Wada and Rasmussen 1960) as a gold standard in 85 patients undergoing evaluation for epilepsy surgery. For each test, dominance was categorized as left, right, or bilateral. There was 87% complete agreement between the tests. Of the 11 patients with discordant results, all occurred in the situation where one test predicted bilateral dominance while the other predicted unilateral dominance—that is, there were no cases where MEG predicted dominance exclusively on one side while the Wada test indicated dominance exclusively on the contralateral side. In most of these cases (7 of 11), it was a matter of MEG overestimating the degree of right hemisphere activity

and predicting bilateral dominance when Wada showed left dominance. It bears mentioning that in the context of a presurgical epilepsy evaluation, the significant question is usually not whether the patient is left, right, or bilaterally dominant, but rather whether the hemisphere under evaluation for surgery contributes to language processing. As such, an argument was made that MEG results compared to Wada should be considered in each hemisphere independently. From this perspective, they showed that MEG had 98% sensitivity for detecting the presence of language-specific activity and 83% specificity. However, their population included only three (4%) right-dominant patients, one of whom was classified as bilaterally dominant by MEG. With so few right-dominant cases, it is very difficult to prove with confidence that this paradigm can or cannot determine language laterality with a high degree of accuracy. Also, 21% of their

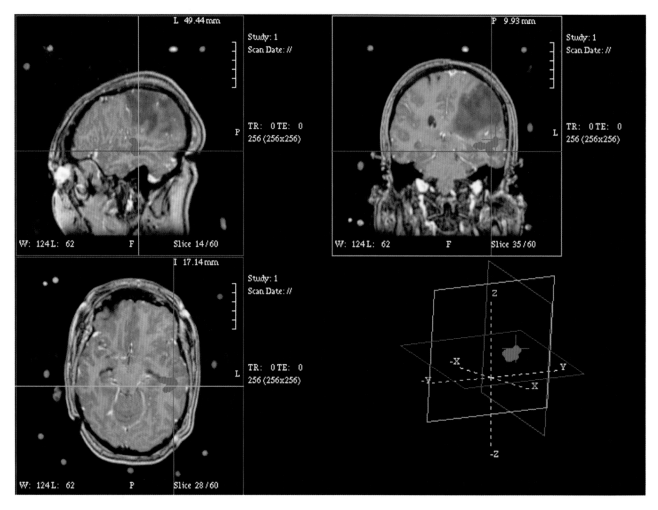

Figure 7.5 MEG language mapping source localizations overlain on MRI. The red circles represent the most temporally and spatially consistent dipole sources acquired during the language task. The cluster of dipoles is centered in the left superior temporal gyrus, which is displaced slightly inferiorly by the large frontoparietal tumor.

population was found to be bilaterally dominant by Wada testing, which is surprisingly high.

Two other laboratories have published similar results using an identical or nearly identical paradigm. Doss et al. (2009) used the same technique in a series of 35 consecutive patients undergoing evaluation for epilepsy or tumor resective surgery and compared MEG results to Wada test findings. They found 69% of cases had complete agreement between MEG and Wada as being left, right, or bilaterally dominant. Of the 11 cases where discordant results were found, 10 were the result of one test showing bilaterality and the other showing unilaterality. One case in their series had completely discordant results in which MEG showed right dominance and Wada showed left dominance. When examining only the hemisphere under consideration for treatment, these investigators found that they correctly detected dominance for language with 80% sensitivity and the absence of dominance with 100% specificity. Much like the Papanicolaou

series, there was an unexpectedly high rate of bilateral dominance (29%) shown by the Wada test. Maestu et al. (2002) reported a series of 21 patients studied with a Spanish version of this language task. Only eight of these patients also had a Wada test performed. Seven of these were left-handed and found to be left language dominant by both MEG and Wada, and the eighth patient was found to be bilaterally dominant by Wada and right dominant by MEG.

Of 108 cases performed in our laboratory using the technique described above, only a small minority of whom had Wada tests performed, we have had two cases of false lateralization where MEG clearly showed right hemisphere dominance in patients who subsequently were found to be left hemisphere dominant by Wada testing. In both cases, the patients were being evaluated for epilepsy surgery involving the left hemisphere, and relying upon MEG alone to determine hemispheric dominance could have been potentially disastrous. To date, no centers that we are aware of consider MEG to be a confident substitute for the Wada test to the point of ceasing to do Wada tests when clearly indicated.

Bowyer et al. (2004) have used MEG data for language mapping using a different analysis model. Instead of applying the single dipole ECD model that the other laboratories mentioned had used, they applied a distributed source current density model known as MR-FOCUSS that allows the source to be localized to multiple distributed points instead of just a single point source at a given point in time. This is attractive because the magnetic fields associated with language activity are often quite complex and not well modeled as a single point source, thus requiring a loosening of acceptability criteria (e.g., confidence volume, goodness of fit, correlation) that would not be considered acceptable for epileptic spike localization. They have studied two separate tasks, one designed to activate receptive language cortex and the other to activate expressive language cortex. In an initial study of 18 right-handed healthy controls and 24 right-handed patients with epilepsy, they found activity in the superior temporal gyrus, supramarginal gyrus, and angular gyrus in each subject with the receptive language task and the inferior frontal gyrus with the expressive language task. They then compared this method with the Wada test in patients undergoing evaluation for epilepsy surgery (Bowyer et al. 2005). Of 27 patients studied, 24 had clearly lateralizing Wada test results, and in all but one of these cases (96% agreement) the degree of activity in the inferior frontal gyrus (Broca's area) predicted the side of Wada language lateralization. In the three cases that were not well lateralized with the Wada test, definitive lateralization was determined with direct cortical stimulation, which showed that MEG had correctly predicted the language dominant hemisphere in one of those three, yielding an overall 89% success rate. However, their methodology requires that only the MEG activity in Broca's area during the expected latency interval (396 to 460 ms) of expressive language activity be used to calculate the laterality index. Using Wernicke's area activity from the receptive language task or the total activity from the entire language processing, they examined the interval for each of the two tasks and found that neither performed particularly well. As with the other studies, very few right-hemisphere-dominant subjects were included, only 2 out of 27 in this series.

These studies represent significant and important progress toward the goal of accurate and reliable noninvasive language mapping. They show that MEG can measure cognitive evoked fields in a clinically meaningful way. Each study shows a good degree of correlation with the reference test. However, the consistent weakness of these studies is that they have relatively

few right-hemisphere-dominant subjects. With no more than three right-dominant subjects in any single study, it is very difficult to prove with a high degree of precision how accurate the test is at detecting and discriminating right-dominant subjects. Merely having low numbers does not prove that the methodologies above are not potentially useful, and if more right-dominant subjects can be studied in the future the confidence in the study will improve significantly. Also, all of these studies had a correlation with the Wada test of less than 90%. To replace or even significantly supplant the Wada test in clinical practice on the level of individuals, an extremely high correlation with the Wada test or some other gold standard will be necessary.

Aside from lateralization, the other utility of noninvasive mapping is to localize receptive language cortex to a focal cortical region within the dominant hemisphere. This information could be used preoperatively to evaluate the likelihood of inflicting a deficit for a given resection area thought to be in the neighborhood of receptive language cortex and could help decide if further intracranial investigation is worth undertaking. If intracranial electrodes are placed, noninvasive language mapping could potentially guide placement of the electrode grid for direct cortical mapping with electrical stimulation. In subjects with brain tumor, this information could also help surgeons decide whether an awake craniotomy is necessary and guide where to begin cortical stimulation, thereby reducing time spent in the operating room.

The Houston group also reported a series of 13 consecutive patients with both preoperative MEG language mapping and mapping with direct cortical stimulation (Simos et al. 1999). These subjects were a mixture of epilepsy and tumor patients. They found that in all of the cases the locations where electrical stimulation was found to interrupt language function were within the bounds of the area predicted by the MEG technique, although the area predicted by MEG was more extensive and often extended deep into sulci or the sylvian fissure, areas not easily accessed by electrical stimulation. The exact location of effective stimulation varied from case to case, including the posterior and anterior aspects of the superior temporal gyrus, or middle temporal gyrus, and in two cases there were two separate and discrete areas in the superior temporal gyrus that interrupted language function on stimulation and correlating with separate and distinct areas predicted by MEG.

These data are very encouraging and suggest that MEG may be independently useful for localizing language eloquent cortex within a given hemisphere. However, at this point, MEG language mapping should only be used to help guide intraoperative cortical stimulation or placement of an electrode grid; it should not replace direct stimulation until larger studies prove accuracy. Since resection of a tumor or an epileptogenic region nearly always occurs in the context of a single hemisphere in question, the issue of lateralization accuracy compared to the Wada test is not quite as great because MEG language mapping commonly produces some degree of bilateral activity even if the laterality index predicts a clearly unilateral dominance of activity. In other words, even when MEG language mapping falsely shows bilateral language activity, the localization within the truly dominant hemisphere may be correct.

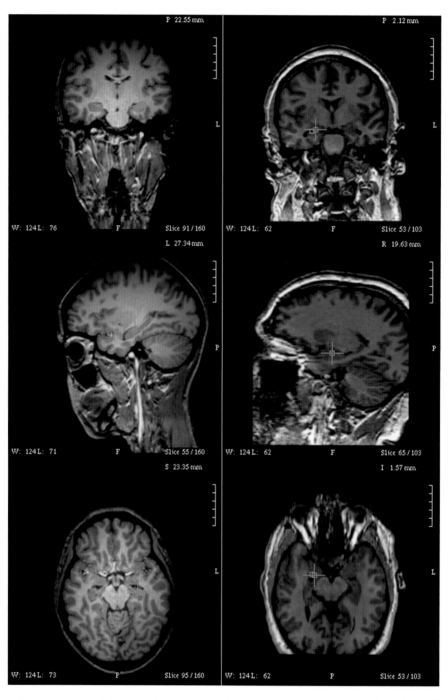

Figure 7.6 Hippocampal dipoles detected during verbal recognition language task. The images on the right are from a healthy control subject and show MEG dipole sources localizing to the left hippocampus during the verbal recognition task used for receptive language mapping. Images on the left show an epilepsy patient who has left mesial temporal sclerosis (MTS) who showed activity in the right hippocampus during the verbal recognition task but not on the left, suggesting left MTS patients may recruit the right mesial temporal structures during recognition memory tasks. The lateral temporal dipoles were deleted from these images for clarity.

MEG MEMORY MAPPING

The Wada test provides not only information on hemispheric language dominance but also memory support. Poor recall of objects presented during the post-injection period suggests that the mesial temporal structures of the injected hemisphere are contributing minimally to memory performance and resection of these structures is unlikely to cause significant memory decline. The language task described above involves not only a receptive language activity but also a verbal recognition memory component and has been shown to elicit a small amount of mesial temporal activity as well as lateral temporal activity (Breier et al. 1998), thought to represent accessing of hippocampal memory networks. Papanicolaou et al. (2002) studied normal individuals using the language paradigm described above as well as a similar visual pictorial recognition paradigm in which kaleidoscope images were presented for learning and recognition instead of abstract nouns. They found that word stimuli preferentially activated the left mesial temporal area, while the kaleidoscope images preferentially activated the right mesial temporal lobe.

Our laboratory reported the results of MEG language mapping in normal controls and a series of patients with intractable epilepsy and evidence of left mesial temporal sclerosis (MTS). We found that all six (100%) of the left MTS patients but only two (28%) normal control subjects had right mesial temporal activity ($p < 0.02$). Two (33%) left MTS patients and six (86%) normal control subjects had left mesial temporal activity ($p = 0.27$) (Ver Hoef et al. 2008). Figure 7.6 shows MEG dipoles that localize to the left hippocampus in a normal control subject and the right hippocampus of a left MTS patient. These findings are consistent with the hypothesis that patients with left MTS are more likely to use right mesial temporal structures when accessing verbal memory than normal individuals. The small sample size of this study precludes its clinical applicability, but if this method or another similar technique could be shown to predict post-temporal lobectomy memory outcome, it would be an important adjunct to the presurgical epilepsy evaluation, particularly since the Wada test does not perfectly predict postoperative memory impairment, and a true gold standard exists (i.e., postoperative memory performance).

CONCLUSIONS

MEG-EEG comparison studies independently recognize that the modalities are complementary, whether in the context of better characterization of sources for optimal modeling (Fuchs et al. 1998) or in the clinical role of combining rapidly acquired accurate spike source localization with ictal neurophysiology from long-term EEG recording and implicit localization from neuroimaging. The historical limitation of MEG availability for clinical application is rapidly diminishing. It should soon be feasible to answer more difficult questions about the role of MEG, particularly those with the largest impact on both efficacy and cost of epilepsy surgery: (1) improved early patient selection, (2) increasing the accuracy of icEEG sampling, (3) reducing the proportion of patients who require invasive studies, and most importantly (4) improving the total number of patients rendered seizure-free. Once combined with validated noninvasive brain mapping, especially language and memory (with or without fMRI techniques), MEG may not only offer an improved method of surgical evaluation, but also increase the opportunity for more epilepsy surgery candidates to actually have this potent treatment of a lifelong disabling disorder.

REFERENCES

Ahnlide, J. A., I. Rosen, P. Linden-Mickelsson Tech, et al. 2007. Does SISCOM contribute to favorable seizure outcome after epilepsy surgery? *Epilepsia* 48: 579–88.

Assaf, B. A., K. M. Karkar, K. D. Laxer, et al. 2003. Ictal magnetoencephalography in temporal and extratemporal lobe epilepsy. *Epilepsia* 44: 1320–7.

Balish, M., S. Sato, P. Connaughton, et al. 1991. Localization of implanted dipoles by magnetoencephalography. *Neurology* 41: 1072–6.

Bast, T., O. Oezkan, S. Rona, et al. 2004. EEG and MEG source analysis of single and averaged interictal spikes reveals intrinsic epileptogenicity in focal cortical dysplasia. *Epilepsia* 45: 621–31.

Baumgartner, C., E. Pataraia, G. Lindinger, et al. 2000. Neuromagnetic recordings in temporal lobe epilepsy. *Journal of Clinical Neurophysiology* 17: 177–89.

Blue Cross/Blue Shield. 2009. *Special Report: MEG and MSI for the Purpose of Presurgical Localization of Epileptic Lesions—A Challenge for Technology Evaluation.* Chicago.

Bowyer, S. M., J. E. Moran, K. M. Mason, et al. 2004. MEG localization of language-specific cortex utilizing MR-FOCUSS. *Neurology* 62: 2247–55.

Breier, J. I., P. G. Simos, G. Zouridakis, et al. 1998. Relative timing of neuronal activity in distinct temporal lobe areas during a recognition memory task for words. *Journal of Clinical & Experimental Neuropsychology* 20: 782–90.

Brodbeck, V., A. M. Lascano, L. Spinelli, et al. 2009. Accuracy of EEG source imaging of epileptic spikes in patients with large brain lesions. *Clinical Neurophysiology* 120: 679–85.

Cooper, R., A. L. Winter, H. J. Crow, et al. 1965. Comparison of subcortical, cortical and scalp activity using chronically indwelling electrodes in man. *Electroencephalography Clinical Neurophysiology* 18: 217–28.

Cuffin, B. N., & D. Cohen. 1979. Comparison of the magnetoencephalogram and electroencephalogram. *Electroencephalography Clinical Neurophysiology* 47: 132–46.

de Jongh, A., J. C. de Munck, S. I. Goncalves, et al. 2005. Differences in MEG/EEG epileptic spike yields explained by regional differences in signal-to-noise ratios. *Journal of Clinical Neurophysiology* 22: 153–8.

Eliashiv, D. S., S. M. Elsas, K. Squires, et al. 2002. Ictal magnetic source imaging as a localizing tool in partial epilepsy. *Neurology* 59: 1600–10.

Fernandes, J. M., A. M. da Silva, G. Huiskamp, et al. 2005. What does an epileptiform spike look like in MEG? Comparison between coincident EEG and MEG spikes. *Journal of Clinical Neurophysiology* 22: 68–73.

Fuchs, M., M. Wagner, T. Kohler, et al. 1999. Linear and nonlinear current density reconstructions. *Journal of Clinical Neurophysiology* 16: 267–95.

Fuchs, M., M. Wagner, H. A. Wischmann, et al. 1998. Improving source reconstructions by combining bioelectric and biomagnetic data. *Electroencephalography Clinical Neurophysiology* 107: 93–111.

Gallen, C., D. Sobel, J. Lewine, et al. 1993. Neuromagnetic mapping of brain function. *Radiology* 187: 863–7.

Hader, W. J., M. Mackay, H. Otsubo, et al. 2004. Cortical dysplastic lesions in children with intractable epilepsy: role of complete resection. *Journal of Neurosurgery* 100: 110–7.

Iwasaki, M., E. Pestana, R. C. Burgess, et al. 2005. Detection of epileptiform activity by human interpreters: blinded comparison between electroencephalography and magnetoencephalography. *Epilepsia* 46: 59–68.

Knowlton, R. C., R. Elgavish, J. Howell, et al. 2006. Magnetic source imaging versus intracranial electroencephalogram in epilepsy surgery: a prospective study. *Annals of Neurology* 59: 835–42.

Knowlton, R. C., R. A. Elgavish, N. Limdi, et al. 2008. Functional imaging: I. Relative predictive value of intracranial electroencephalography. *Annals of Neurology* 64: 25–34.

Knowlton, R. C., K. D. Laxer, M. J. Aminoff, et al. 1997. Magnetoencephalography in partial epilepsy: clinical yield and localization accuracy. *Annals of Neurology* 42: 622–31.

Knowlton, R. C., S. N. Razdan, N. Limdi, et al. 2009. Effect of epilepsy magnetic source imaging on intracranial electrode placement. *Annals of Neurology* 65: 716–23.

Lee, D., S. M. Sawrie, P. G. Simos, et al. 2006. Reliability of language mapping with magnetic source imaging in epilepsy surgery candidates. *Epilepsy Behavior* 8: 742–9.

Leijten, F. S., G. J. Huiskamp, I. Hilgersom, et al. 2003. High-resolution source imaging in mesiotemporal lobe epilepsy: a comparison between MEG and simultaneous EEG. *Journal of Clinical Neurophysiology* 20: 227–38.

Lin, Y. Y., Y. H. Shih, J. C. Hsieh, et al. 2003. Magnetoencephalographic yield of interictal spikes in temporal lobe epilepsy. Comparison with scalp EEG recordings. *Neuroimage* 19: 1115–26.

Loring, D. W., K. J. Meador, G. P. Lee, et al. 1990. Cerebral language lateralization: evidence from intracarotid amobarbital testing. *Neuropsychologia* 28: 831–8.

Maestu, F., T. Ortiz, A. Fernandez, et al. 2002. Spanish language mapping using MEG: a validation study. *Neuroimage* 17: 1579–86.

Mamelak, A. N., N. Lopez, M. Akhtari, et al. 2002. Magnetoencephalography-directed surgery in patients with neocortical epilepsy. *Journal of Neurosurgery* 97: 865–73.

Mikuni, N., T. Nagamine, A. Ikeda, et al. 1997. Simultaneous recording of epileptiform discharges by MEG and subdural electrodes in temporal lobe epilepsy. *Neuroimage* 5: 298–306.

Minassian, B. A., H. Otsubo, S. Weiss, et al. 1999. Magnetoencephalographic localization in pediatric epilepsy surgery: comparison with invasive intracranial electroencephalography. *Annals of Neurology* 46: 627–33.

Morioka, T., S. Nishio, H. Ishibashi, et al. 1999. Intrinsic epileptogenicity of focal cortical dysplasia as revealed by magnetoencephalography and electrocorticography. *Epilepsy Research* 33: 177–87.

Oishi, M., S. Kameyama, H. Masuda, et al. 2006. Single and multiple clusters of magnetoencephalographic dipoles in neocortical epilepsy: significance in characterizing the epileptogenic zone. *Epilepsia* 47: 355–64.

Oishi, M., H. Otsubo, S. Kameyama, et al. 2002. Epileptic spikes: magnetoencephalography versus simultaneous electrocorticography. *Epilepsia* 43: 1390–5.

Papanicolaou, A. C., P. G. Simos, J. I. Breier, et al. 1999. Magnetoencephalographic mapping of the language-specific cortex. *Journal of Neurosurgery* 90: 85–93.

Papanicolaou, A. C., P. G. Simos, E. M. Castillo, et al. 2002. The hippocampus and memory of verbal and pictorial material. *Learning Memory* 9: 99–104.

Papanicolaou, A. C., P. G. Simos, E. M. Castillo, et al. 2004. Magnetocephalography: a noninvasive alternative to the Wada procedure. *Journal of Neurosurgery* 100: 867–76.

Pataraia, E., P. G. Simos, E. M. Castillo, et al. 2004. Does magnetoencephalography add to scalp video-EEG as a diagnostic tool in epilepsy surgery? *Neurology* 62: 943–8.

Plummer, C., A. S. Harvey, M. Cook. 2008. EEG source localization in focal epilepsy: where are we now? *Epilepsia* 49: 201–18.

Ray, A., J. X. Tao, S. M. Hawes-Ebersole, et al. 2007. Localizing value of scalp EEG spikes: a simultaneous scalp and intracranial study. *Clinical Neurophysiology* 118: 69–79.

Rose, D. F., S. Sato, E. Ducla-Soares, et al. 1991. Magnetoencephalographic localization of subdural dipoles in a patient with temporal lobe epilepsy. *Epilepsia* 32: 635–41.

Santiuste, M., R. Nowak, A. Russi, et al. 2008. Simultaneous magnetoencephalography and intracranial EEG registration: technical and clinical aspects. *Journal of Clinical Neurophysiology* 25: 331–9.

Simos, P. G., A. C. Papanicolaou, J. I. Breier, et al. 1999. Localization of language-specific cortex by using magnetic source imaging and electrical stimulation mapping. *Journal of Neurosurgery* 91: 787–96.

Simos, P. G., S. Sarkari, E. M. Castillo, et al. 2005. Reproducibility of measures of neurophysiological activity in Wernicke's area: a magnetic source imaging study. *Clinical Neurophysiology* 116: 2381–91.

Sobel, D., C. Gallen, et al. 1993. Locating the central sulcus: comparison of MR anatomic and magnetoencephalographic functional methods. *AJNR American Journal of Neuroradiology* 14: 915–26.

Stefan, H., C. Hummel, G. Scheler, et al. 2003. Magnetic brain source imaging of focal epileptic activity: a synopsis of 455 cases. *Brain* 126: 2396–405.

Stephen, J. M., C. J. Aine, D. Ranken, et al. 2003. Multidipole analysis of simulated epileptic spikes with real background activity. *Journal of Clinical Neurophysiology* 20: 1–16.

Sutherling, W. 2001. Localization precision of whole cortex neuromagnetometer system for human epilepsy studies. *Epilepsia* 42 (supp 7).

Sutherling, W. W., P. H. Crandall, L. D. Cahan, et al. 1988. The magnetic field of epileptic spikes agrees with intracranial localizations in complex partial epilepsy. *Neurology* 38: 778–86.

Sutherling, W. W., A. N. Mamelak, D. Thyerlei, et al. 2008. Influence of magnetic source imaging for planning intracranial EEG in epilepsy. *Neurology* 71: 990–6.

Tao, J. X., A. Ray, S. Hawes-Ebersole, et al. 2005. Intracranial EEG substrates of scalp EEG interictal spikes. *Epilepsia* 46: 669–76.

Tilz, C., C. Hummel, B. Kettenmann, et al. 2002. Ictal onset localization of epileptic seizures by magnetoencephalography. *Acta Neurologica Scandinavica* 106: 190–5.

Ver Hoef, L. W., S. Sawrie, J. Killen, et al. 2008. Left mesial temporal sclerosis and verbal memory: a magnetoencephalography study. *Journal of Clinical Neurophysiology* 25: 1–6.

Wada, J., and T. Rasmussen. 1960. Intracarotid injection of sodium amytal for the lateralization of cerebral speech dominance. Experimental and clinical observations. *Journal of Neurosurgery* 17: 266–82.

Wheless, J. W., L. J. Willmore, J. I. Breier, et al. 1999. A comparison of magnetoencephalography, MRI, and V-EEG in patients evaluated for epilepsy surgery. *Epilepsia* 40: 931–41.

Zijlmans, M., G. M. Huiskamp, F. S. Leijten, et al. 2002. Modality-specific spike identification in simultaneous magnetoencephalography/electroencephalography: a methodological approach. *Journal of Clinical Neurophysiology* 19: 183–91.

Zouridakis, G., P. G. Simos, J. I. Breier, et al. 1998. Functional hemispheric asymmetry assessment in a visual language task using MEG. *Brain Topography* 11: 57–65.

Chapter 8

POSITRON EMISSION TOMOGRAPHY: GLUCOSE METABOLISM STUDIES IN TEMPORAL LOBE EPILEPSY

Thomas R. Henry

Physiologic brain imaging with positron emission tomography (PET) can map numerous physiochemical brain processes. Mapping of neuronal energy metabolism by measurement of glucose consumption is the principal clinical application of PET in epilepsy evaluation. Mapping of neurotransmitter systems is performed with positron-emitter-labeled ligands and precursors of neurotransmitters. These are discussed in Chapters 11, 12, and 13. Since this is the first of six chapters describing applications of PET in epilepsy, we begin with a brief narrative on PET methodology.

METHODS OF POSITRON EMISSION IMAGING IN THE EPILEPSIES

Clinical and research studies with PET require the sophisticated physics (for generation of positron-emitting radionuclides), neurochemistry (for radiopharmaceutical preparation), and computing (for image reconstruction and analysis) widely available in nuclear medicine facilities. Clinical cyclotrons can produce positron-emitting isotopes of fluorine (^{18}F, half-life of 110 minutes), carbon (^{11}C, half-life of 20 minutes), nitrogen (^{13}N, half-life of 10 minutes), and oxygen (^{15}O, half-life of 2 minutes). Radiochemists have perfected reaction sequences to rapidly incorporate these radionuclides into a wide variety of labeled organic molecules, which can be administered intravenously in high purity to image many neurochemical sites and brain processes of interest to epileptologists. The accuracy of PET measurement and anatomical display is determined by the biochemical and physical properties of the selected radiopharmaceutical tracer (Table 8.1) and its mathematical model, performance characteristics of the tomographic instrument, scanning procedure, and other factors. The spatial resolution of PET imaging has increased over years of development, based on improvements in detector function and geometry, and in image reconstruction (Tai et al. 2008; Turkheimer et al. 2008; Wahl 2009). In recent years the fusion of PET with X-ray computed tomographs has greatly benefited whole-body imaging for oncology

Table 8.1 Positron-emitting radiopharmaceuticals used in PET studies of epilepsy

Functions	Radiopharmaceuticals
Glucose metabolism	2-deoxy-2-[^{18}F]fluoro-D-glucose (FDG)
Oxygen metabolism and extraction ratio	[^{15}O]O$_2$
Cerebral blood flow	[^{15}O]O$_2$, [^{15}O]H$_2$O, [^{15}O]CO$_2$, [^{13}N]NH$_3$
Central benzodiazepine receptor distribution	[^{11}C]flumazenil (formerly [^{11}C] RO15-1788) [^{18}F]fluoroethylflumazenil
N-methyl-D-aspartate receptor distribution	(S)-[N-methyl-^{11}C]ketamine
Serotonin synthesis	[^{11}C]Alpha-methyl-tryptophan
Serotonin-1A receptor distribution	[^{11}C]WAY100635, [^{18}F] FCWAY, [^{18}F] MPPF*
Dopamine synthesis (dopa uptake)	[^{18}F]Fluoro-l-DOPA
Dopamine-2/3 receptor distribution	[^{18}F]Fallypride
Muscarinic cholinergic receptor distribution	[^{11}C]N-methyl piperidyl benzilate
Opiate receptor distribution	[^{11}C]Carfentanil (mu-receptors) [^{18}F]Cyclofoxy (mu-/kappa-receptors) [^{11}C]Diprenorphine (mu-/kappa-/delta-receptors)
Drug distribution	[^{11}C]Phenytoin [^{11}C]Valproate
Monoamine oxidase B distribution (glial density)	[^{11}C]Deuterium-deprenyl
Peripheral benzodiazepine receptor distribution (microglial density)	[^{11}C]PK-11195

*[11C]WAY 100 635 is [O-methyl-11C]-N-(2-(4-(2-methoxyphenyl)-1-piperazinyl)ethyl)-N-(2-pyridinyl) cyclohexanecarboxamide trihydrochloride. [18F]FCWAY is [18F]trans-4-fluoro-N-2-[4-(2-methoxyphenyl)piperazin-1-yl] ethyl]-N-(2-pyridyl)cyclohexanecarboxamide (FCWAY). [18F] MPPF is 2'-methoxyphenyl-(N-2'-pyridinyl)-p-18F-fluoro-benzamidoethylpiperazine.

applications (Blodgett et al. 2007). While PET-CT does not appear to offer similar benefit for brain imaging in the epilepsies, CT artifacts do not degrade 2-deoxy-2-[^{18}F]fluoro-D-glucose (FDG) images of the brain (Fig. 8.1). In the near future, PET-MRI instruments likely will confer the ability to simultaneously acquire complementary physiologic data, such as FDG uptake and fMRI, and thus offer unique opportunities to study a disorder with rapid shifts in functional state such as epilepsy (Schlemmer et al. 2008). Several reviews have covered general and epilepsy-related aspects of PET methodology in detail (Frey 1999, 2000; Henry et al. 1993a; Votaw 1995, 2000). Recently these PET methods have been applied in experimental epilepsy models (Dedeurwaerdere et al. 2007; Mirrione et al. 2006),

permitting serial metabolic and ligand studies of ictogenesis and epileptogenesis.

The performance of each PET tracer and PET scanning system must be considered in four dimensions of physiologic imaging: process, temporal, contrast, and spatial resolutions. *Process* resolution is the accuracy of a tracer kinetic method in measuring the intended biochemical process. *Temporal* resolution is the duration of brain function represented in any PET data set. *Contrast* resolution ("signal-to-noise ratio") is determined by the ability of a PET system to accurately measure the activity of positron-emitting tracer within the object scanned. *Spatial* resolution is determined by the ability of an imaging system to detect subdivisions of the object scanned to support image reconstruction that renders the subdivisions in accurate position and shape. Each dimension of a volume of tissue must be at least twice the linear resolution of the imaging system, if the volume is to be accurately resolved in space and functional intensity on the image (Mazziotta et al. 1981). Structures smaller than this will have their functional activity averaged with those of adjacent structures (the partial volume effect). The higher spatial resolution of current PET tomographs, compared with those reported in earlier FDG imaging research, has been shown to generate more sensitive and accurate detection of hypometabolism, with greater ability to correlate FDG image coordinates with brain MRI locations (Henry et al. 1993b). Epileptologists who use MRI in research are accustomed to spatial resolution and signal-to-noise ratio in determining which reported findings are supported by the imaging techniques. Results of PET-based epilepsy research must be critically analyzed with respect to all four dimensions of resolution in physiologic imaging.

Interictal FDG PET is readily available in clinical PET centers, while research centers typically provide FDG and multiple other PET radiotracers. Clinical PET centers are financially supported mainly by whole-body FDG PET, used to screen for metastases of solid tumors. The relatively long half-life of ^{18}F (about 2 hours), the common use of highly standardized protocols for synthesizing FDG, and the availability of high-resolution tomographic cameras all serve to make FDG imaging practical and affordable in an advanced oncology center. Epileptologists can easily arrange for brain FDG imaging in a clinical PET center, which provides the multidisciplinary expertise required for safe and accurate PET imaging. However, clinical epileptologists will need to understand essentials of PET methodology and FDG physiology in order to apply FDG images in presurgical epilepsy evaluations. Following intravenous injection of radiolabeled FDG, patients are observed for 30 to 45 minutes, and then scanning is performed. During the observation period after FDG injection, the labeled FDG circulates

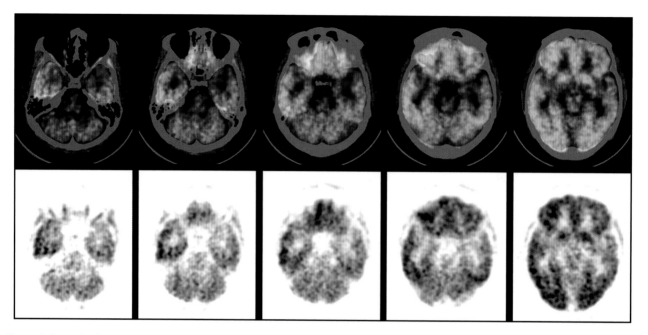

Figure 8.1 Interictal FDG PET-CT images of a limbic TLE patient. The upper row shows FDG activity in color and X-ray CT in gray. The CT has higher spatial resolution than the PET images, and on each image plane the skull (CT) partly covers the cerebral metabolism (PET); this is particularly evident over the inferior frontal lobe in the second and third planes from the left. As shown in the lower rows, the FDG images should be viewed without the CT in order to analyze the metabolic anatomy accurately. In this case the CT component of the images appears to offer little diagnostic advantage in recognizing the interictal hypometabolism of the left temporal and inferior frontal cortex (on the image at right), but the acquisition of the FDG images with a PET-CT instrument also should cause no particular difficulties.

through cerebral arterioles and capillaries, with diffusion into brain tissue; FDG is taken up by neurons and other cells, and phosphorylated as is glucose; unlike glucose, however, FDG does not enter the rest of the Krebs cycle and remains in place as ^{18}F decays and emits positrons (Phelps et al. 1979). The tomograph detects oppositely directed, high-energy photons produced in positron decay. Image data usually are reconstructed into a set of axial FDG activity images, which are viewed and interpreted by a nuclear medicine physician.

Evaluation of FDG images is complex with respect to temporal resolution, but otherwise fairly straightforward. The FDG kinetics generate a nonlinear temporal resolution, in that glucose metabolism is averaged over about 40 minutes, with earlier periods during scanning weighted more heavily in this average. The tracer kinetic model of FDG requires steady-state conditions for absolute measurements of glucose metabolic rate, so only relative comparison of metabolism within different regions of the image set can be made if a single seizure occurs during FDG imaging (Phelps et al. 1979). Ictal FDG PET studies cannot be quantified because glucose metabolism is not at steady state (Phelps et al. 1979). Dynamic $[^{15}\text{O}]\text{H}_2\text{O}$ PET imaging of cerebral blood flow (CBF) is in theory superior for ictal scanning of single seizures compared to either FDG PET or single photon emission

computed tomography (SPECT) techniques, owing to its superior temporal resolution and the possibility of fully quantifying CBF (without the requirement of correction for nonlinear activity–CBF relationships, as occur with SPECT agents). In practice the short half-life of ^{15}O and the usually unpredictable timing of seizure onsets render ictal $[^{15}\text{O}]\text{H}_2\text{O}$ PET impossible, except for the study of reflex seizures. Relative increases and decreases in ictal regional metabolism have been observed with FDG PET (Meltzer et al. 2000). Ictal FDG studies are most useful when the duration of continuous seizure activity approximates the duration of FDG uptake and phosphorylation following bolus FDG injection (i.e., when seizures last 10 minutes or longer). Epilepsia partialis continua is required for "purely" ictal FDG scanning (Hajek et al. 1991; Palmini et al. 2005). Occurrence of a brief complex partial seizure shortly after FDG injection may actually be associated with false normalization of apparent FDG activity, presumably due to averaging of interictal hypometabolism and ictal hypermetabolism in the same region (Henry et al. 1993a).

Many centers perform continuous scalp EEG monitoring immediately prior to and following FDG administration, including for outpatient PET. Continuous EEG is useful in determining wake–sleep state, frequency of interictal epileptiform discharges, and occurrence of electrographic seizures. Scalp electrodes do not significantly attenuate or scatter the high-energy (511 keV) photons that are produced by positron annihilation. Some centers do not routinely perform EEG monitoring because this slightly increases the cost of FDG scanning, and because some believe that subclinical or unreported seizures rarely occur in the imaging suite and that single seizures do not alter FDG images (Barrington et al. 1998). The latter point has been disproved (see, e.g., the case presented in Henry et al. 1993a). Nonetheless, the cost–benefit ratio of continuous EEG during clinical FDG studies has not been established. Continuous EEG monitoring is standard in PET research protocols, not only for FDG but also for other radiopharmaceuticals; focal seizures cause marked focal increases in CBF and therefore cause marked increases in delivery of any PET ligand to areas of maximal seizure involvement, resulting in altered physiologic images.

Structural imaging data should guide anatomical analysis of PET images. An individual's MRI and PET images can be co-registered and then viewed side-by-side, or with superimposition of the functional and structural images (Fig. 8.2). Accurate PET–MRI co-registration permits comparison of anatomically specific metabolic measurements of the individual with normal subjects' means and variances of regional metabolism (Drzezga et al. 1999). In addition to providing an anatomical framework in which to evaluate PET images qualitatively or statistically, a PET subject's MRI data might be used to reduce partial volume effects in the PET reconstruction (Baete et al. 2004a, 2004b).

Statistical parametric imaging detects some abnormalities that cannot be appreciated with qualitative interpretation. For example, unilateral temporal lobe epilepsy (TLE) often causes bilateral temporal hypometabolism with marked asymmetry of temporal metabolism (with lower FDG activity on the epileptogenic side). Bilateral but asymmetric temporal lobe hypometabolism can be detected readily with statistical parametric imaging techniques, but usually appears only as unilateral temporal hypometabolism on visual interpretation. Quantitative analyses that determine an asymmetry index also will fail to detect bilateral temporal hypometabolism, although the temporal lobe with relatively greater metabolic decrease will be accurately noted as the more hypometabolic. Issues regarding the construction of regions of interest, for regional sampling of FDG activity, have been previously discussed (Henry et al. 1993a). Despite the advantages of statistical parametric imaging techniques, visual interpretation and quantification of asymmetry remain useful in current clinical applications, as unilateral TLE often has asymmetric, bilateral temporal hypometabolism interictally.

Effects of antiepileptic drugs on cerebral glucose metabolism have not generally been considered to affect clinical applications of FDG PET. Barbiturates and benzodiazepines appear to reduce glucose utilization diffusely over the brain (Theodore et al. 1986b; Volkow et al. 1995). Other antiepileptic drugs likely reduce FDG uptake less severely but also diffusely over the brain, although many newer antiepileptic drugs have not been fully studied (Gaillard et al. 1996; Joo et al 2006; Theodore 1988; Theodore et al. 1986a, 1989). Other PET ligands may have specific interactions with antiepileptic drugs and other clinically used agents, many of which will be obvious based on the biochemical model of the PET ligand.

Epilepsy research has used a variety of positron-emitter-labeled ligands and precursors of neurotransmitters (Table 8.1). Imaging of neurotransmitter systems often reveals abnormalities that are not simple maps of the ablative effects of epilepsy-associated cerebral lesions, and similarly are not generated by interictal cerebral hypoperfusion (Bouilleret et al. 2008; Bouvard et al. 2005; Chugani et al. 1998; Didelot et al. 2008; Frost et al. 1988; Hammers et al. 2002; Henry et al. 1993; Juhasz et al. 1999; Juhasz et al. 2003; Koepp et al. 1997, 1998; Kumlien et al. 1999; Liew et al. 2009; Leveque et al. 2003; Mayberg et al. 1991; Merlet et al. 2004; Pennell et al. 1999; Richardson et al. 1996; Ryvlin et al. 1999; Savic et al. 1988, 2004; Szelies et al. 1996; Theodore et al. 1992a, 2006; Toczek et al. 2003; Werhahn et al. 2006). These studies are reviewed in the following chapters. Rarely, the distributions of glial cell types in epilepsy and the cerebral kinetics of antiepileptic drug have been studied with PET (Banati et al. 1999l Baron et al. 1983; Kumar et al. 2008; Kumlien et al. 1995; Ramsay 1983).

STUDIES OF TLE WITH GLUCOSE METABOLIC IMAGING

Mesial (Limbic) TLE

Hypometabolism of one temporal lobe (Figs. 8.2, 8.3, and 8.4, and 8.5), or asymmetric bitemporal hypometabolism (i.e., bilateral temporal lobe hypometabolism with more severe hypometabolism of one temporal lobe) (Fig. 8.6), is usually found on interictal FDG PET in adults and children with refractory mesial TLE (Abou-Khalil et al. 1987; Arnold et al. 1996; Blum et al. 1998; Bouilleret et al. 2002a; Engel et al. 1982a, 1982c, 1982d, 1990; Hajek et al. 1993, 1994; Henry et al. 1990, 1993a, 1993b, 1993d, 1994; Knowlton et al. 1997; Koutroumanidis et al. 2000; Kuhl et al. 1980; Lee et al. 2009; Leiderman et al. 1992; Nickel et al. 2003; Radtke et al. 1993; Ryvlin et al. 1991, 1995; Sackellares et al. 1990; Sadzot et al. 1992; Sperling et al.1990; Stefan

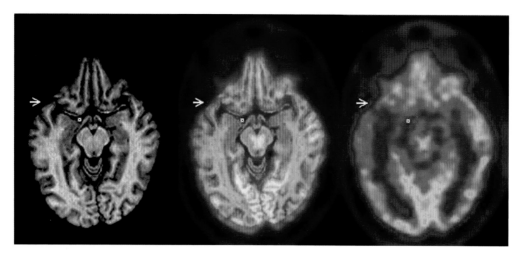

Figure 8.2 Co-registered axial image plane of MRI and interictal FDG PET images of a mesial TLE patient. The gray-scale MR image (on the left) and the color PET image (on the right) are co-registered in the center image. The MRI and PET data were re-oriented parallel to a line through the anterior and posterior commissures. A widespread area of reduced FDG activity is evident on the left side of the PET image; inspection of the PET image alone does not clarify whether the reduction extends from mesial structures (at the dot internal to the brain FDG image) of the temporal lobe into the basal frontal lobe, nor whether the lateral temporal hypometabolism (at the arrow) extends above the sylvian fissure. The dot and arrowhead appear at the same coordinates in the MRI and the co-registered MRI-PET images as in the PET image, clarifying that all sites with severe hypometabolism are confined to the temporal lobe.

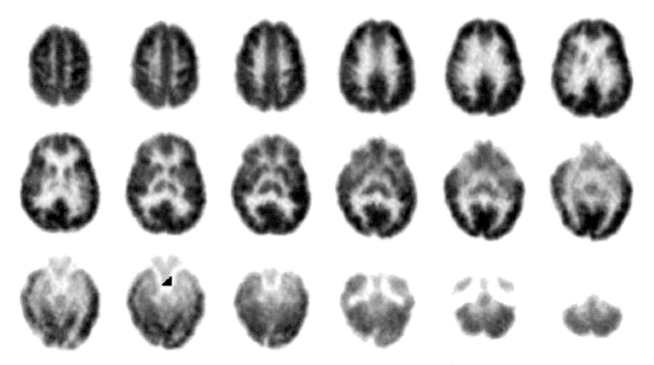

Figure 8.3 Interictal FDG PET images of a mesial TLE patient. These transaxially oriented images show left anterior hippocampal hypometabolism (*arrowhead*), which is more severe than the reduction in FDG activity in the adjacent inferior-lateral temporal regions. No extratemporal abnormalities are evident. The patient's brain MRI was normal. Mild hippocampal sclerosis was present in tissue resected on the side of hypometabolism and of extracranially recorded EEG ictal onsets. Seizures ceased after resection.

et al. 1987; Swartz et al. 1992; Theodore 1988; Theodore et al. 1986, 1990, 1983, 1992b; Valk et al. 1993). Qualitative visual analysis of FDG scans, obtained with high-performance tomographs, currently detects unilateral (or bilateral, but asymmetric) temporal lobe hypometabolism in over 70% of refractory TLE patients. Higher-resolution tomographic systems support a higher detection rate for hypometabolism, and support greater concordance among readers, in qualitative interpretation of FDG imaging

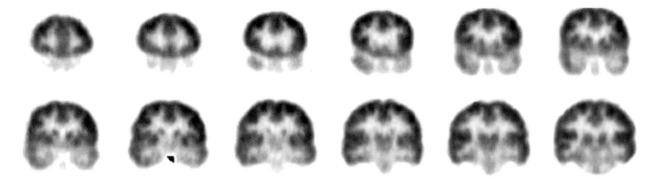

Figure 8.4 Interictal FDG PET images of a mesial TLE patient. These coronally oriented images were reconstructed from the same FDG data as shown in **Figure 8.3**. The mesial > lateral temporal hypometabolism is evident (at *arrowhead* and on adjacent planes). On each row the coronal images are arranged with the most anterior plane to the left and 4-mm spacing. Subject left is displayed on image right.

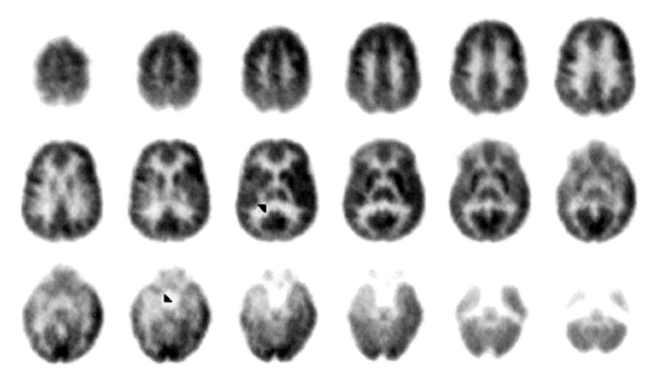

Figure 8.5 Interictal FDG PET images of a mesial TLE patient. These images show severe hypometabolism of the right anterior hippocampus (*lower arrowhead*) and moderate hypometabolism of the ipsilateral temporal neocortex and thalamus (*upper arrowhead*). Mild hypometabolism is also seen diffusely over the dorsolateral frontal and parietal cortex ipsilaterally. The patient's brain MRI showed mild bilateral hippocampal atrophy. Moderate hippocampal sclerosis was present in tissue resected on the side of hypometabolism and of intracranially recorded EEG ictal onsets. Seizures ceased after resection.

in localization-related epilepsies (Henry et al. 1993b). With quantitative analysis, detection of significant temporal lobe hypometabolism may exceed 90% in this group (Kang et al. 2001; Knowlton et al. 1997; Van Bogaert et al. 2000).

Temporal lobe hypometabolism usually extends over mesial and lateral portions of an interictally dysfunctional temporal lobe, on FDG scans in mesial temporal lobe epilepsy (Henry et al. 1990, 1993d; Sackellares et al. 1990; Valk et al. 1993). Regional hypometabolism in mesial TLE typically is diffuse, with graded demarcations from adjacent areas of normal metabolism, and with a relatively large area of hypometabolism. Even in the presence of a temporal lobe foreign-tissue lesion, patients with refractory mesial temporal seizures usually have widespread temporal lobe hypometabolism, rather than focal hypometabolism restricted to the site of the lesion. The lateral temporal hypometabolism often appears more severe than the mesial temporal hypometabolism of an

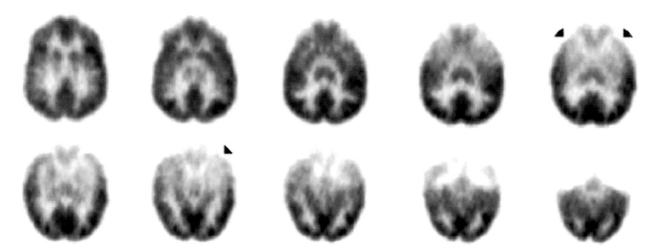

Figure 8.6 Interictal FDG PET images of a mesial TLE patient. These images show bilateral mesial temporal hypometabolism (*arrowheads* on image at upper right), which is more severe on the left (*arrowhead* on image on lower row). The patient's brain MRI showed mild left hippocampal atrophy. Moderate hippocampal sclerosis was present in tissue resected on the side of the more severe hypometabolism and of intracranially recorded EEG ictal onsets. Seizures ceased after resection.

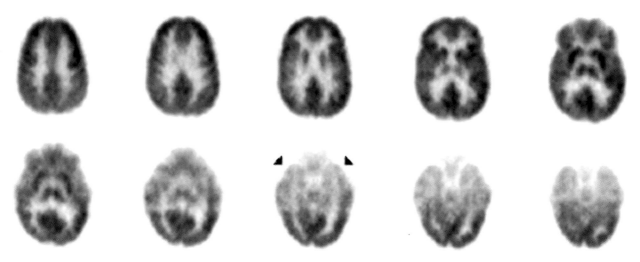

Figure 8.7 Interictal FDG PET images of a mesial TLE patient. These images show bilateral mesial temporal hypometabolism (*arrowheads* on image at middle of lower row), which is symmetric. The patient's brain MRI was normal. Extracranially recorded EEG ictal onsets were artifactually obscured, in some instances with prolonged right temporal ictal discharges seen in later periods during complex partial seizures. Intracranially recorded EEG ictal onsets occurred independently over each hippocampus, in approximately equal numbers. Resective surgery was not performed.

affected temporal lobe, on qualitative scan interpretation and even with quantification, when using older tomographs with lower spatial resolution (Henry et al. 1993d; Sackellares et al. 1990). However, using an ultra-high-resolution tomograph, one study of mesial TLE found that small volumes of anterior mesial temporal structures were more severely hypometabolic than were any other temporal or extratemporal areas in many mesial TLE patients (Valk et al. 1993). As shown in Figure 8.3, current tomographs more often provide FDG scans that show mesial temporal > lateral temporal hypometabolism of the affected temporal lobe. This suggests that partial-volume averaging of severe hypometabolism in the epileptogenic amygdala-hippocampus together with less depressed metabolism of adjacent basal temporal areas may cause the mesial temporal areas to appear less severely hypometabolic than they actually are, using older clinical PET systems. In contrast to lateralized temporal lobe predominance of metabolic dysfunction most often observed in refractory TLE, some patients have symmetric hypometabolism of both temporal lobes

(Fig. 8.7) (Blum et al. 1998; Kim et al. 2006). Normal interictal metabolism also occurs in refractory mesial TLE, but normal FDG scans are more common in nonrefractory than in refractory patients (Gaillard et al. 2002; Matheja et al. 2001).

Many TLE patients have unilateral frontal, parietal, thalamic, or basal ganglial hypometabolism ipsilateral to temporal hypometabolism, but occipital hypometabolism is rare in mesial TLE (Arnold et al. 1996; Bouilleret et al. 2002a; Henry et al. 1990, 1993d; Lee et al. 2009; Nelissen et al. 2006; Rusu et al. 2005; Sadzot et al. 1992; Sperling et al. 1990a). The temporal hypometabolism is nearly always more severe than is any extratemporal hypometabolism. The thalamus ipsilateral to the affected temporal lobe is the extratemporal site most likely to demonstrate hypometabolism in mesial TLE (Henry et al. 1990, 1993d). Thalamic asymmetries in FDG activity are mainly dorsal (Fig. 8.5), and in some cases are associated with dorsal thalamic atrophy on structural MRI (Juhasz et al. 1999). The ipsilateral putamen is significantly more likely to be interictally hypometabolic in patients whose complex partial seizures involve dystonic posturing than in those without ictal hemidystonia (Rusu et al. 2005). Interestingly, TLE patients with normal basal ganglial structure on MRI and normal striatal FDG activity may nonetheless have reduced striatal [^{18}F]fluoro-l-DOPA activity bilaterally on PET (Bouilleret et al. 2008). The cortical hypometabolic area typically is contiguous across its entire temporal and extratemporal extent (Fig. 8.4). In particular, the insular and inferior frontal regions are most often the portions of the ipsilateral frontal lobe that are hypometabolic in association with temporal lobe hypometabolism (Arnold et al. 1996; Bouilleret et al. 2002a; Henry et al. 1993d; Nickel et al. 2003). Bilateral cerebellar hypometabolism is also common (Theodore et al. 1987a). Thus, interictal FDG PET in refractory mesial TLE patients usually reveals unilateral diffuse regional hypometabolism of one mesial-lateral temporal area, with or without ipsilateral extratemporal cortical hypometabolism or contralateral temporal hypometabolism; ipsilateral extratemporal hypometabolism almost always appears to be less severe than does the temporal lobe hypometabolism.

The pathophysiologic basis of regional hypometabolism, imaged with FDG interictally in TLE, currently is unclear. Ablative structural lesions must contribute to localized decreases in glucose metabolism. Nonetheless, it has been recognized for some time that the volume of hypometabolism is greater than the volume of associated structural lesions, in localization-related epilepsies (Engel et al. 1982a). Acute-subacute cerebral infarction is associated with hypometabolism at the site of neuronal loss, and additional extra-infarctional sites of hypometabolism are

considered to represent "diaschisis," as passive and usually impersistent effects of a focal injury on remote brain regions that receive projections from the damaged area (Meyer et al. 1987). Neuronal loss and diaschisis were considered the causes of the anatomically distributed interictal hypometabolism in TLE patients with hippocampal sclerosis. This hypothesis was refuted, however, by a study of quantified preoperative FDG PET in patients whose resected temporal tissue underwent quantitative neuronal volumetric densitometry (Henry et al. 1994). Subsequent studies, using various methodologies, confirmed this observation (Carne et al. 2004; Dlugos et al. 1999; Foldvary et al. 1999; Lamusuo et al. 2001). Similarly, several studies of MRI volumetry and interictal FDG PET found that hippocampal atrophy and temporal lobe hypometabolism are not highly correlated in mesial TLE (Gaillard et al. 1995; Knowlton et al. 2001; O'Brien et al. 1997; Theodore et al. 2001). Further, MR spectroscopic determination of the neuron-specific peaks of N-acetyl aspartate (NAA) also found limited association of mesial temporal glucose hypometabolism and NAA decreases (Achten et al. 1998; Knowlton et al. 2002). While neuronal loss and diaschisis probably cause some of the disseminated glucose metabolic depression in mesial TLE, other factors must also influence regional metabolism interictally. Indeed, surgical ablation of epileptogenic temporal lobe tissue might be expected to increase diaschisis effects on extratemporal glucose metabolism. Instead, comparisons of preoperative and postoperative FDG scans have shown postoperative increases in FDG activity of the contralateral temporal lobe and of ipsilateral thalamus and frontal sites (Dupont et al. 2001; Hajek et al. 1994; Spanaki et al. 2000). Somewhat different findings were generated with group averaging and statistical parametric mapping of preoperative and post-temporal resection FDG data, in that a combination of focally increased and focally decreased FDG activity was observed ipsilateral to resection, with little change contralaterally (Joo et al. 2005).

Several pathophysiologic explanations of interictally reduced regional FDG activity have been proposed, in addition to diaschisis resulting from focal sites of neuronal loss. These include reduced transmembrane glucose transport rates and reduced mitochondrial glucose oxidation of viable neurons in sites of ictal onset and habitual propagation (Reutens et al. 1998; Vielhaber et al. 2003). On comparing the anatomical distributions of ictal hyperperfusion (using SPECT) and interictal glucose hypometabolism (using FDG PET) within individual TLE patients, it is evident that many such patients have an identical or highly similar distribution of ictal hyperperfusion–interictal hypometabolism that predominates in the temporal lobe and thalamus ipsilateral to the epileptogenic site (including but extending beyond the electrographic ictal onset zone), often with less severe involvement of ipsilateral frontoparietal and basal ganglial sites and of contralateral temporal cortex (Henry et al. 2005); one exception is the occipital hyperperfusion often observed in the absence of occipital hypometabolism in TLE. Possibly long-duration postictal dysfunctions may underlie some of the reduction in FDG activity, as suggested by differential associations of specific distributions of extrahippocampal hypometabolism with specific patterns of electrographic seizure propagation in groups with unilateral hippocampal sclerosis (e.g., patients with bitemporal hypometabolism having earlier spread of ictal discharges from one hippocampus to the other) (Chassoux et al. 2004; Lee et al. 2009; Savic et al. 1997). The presence and severity of focal polymorphic delta slowing often increase on scalp EEG postictally, and several studies have reported the association of interictal temporal lobe hypometabolism with ipsilateral temporal delta slowing on EEG (Erbayat et al. 2005; Koutroumanidis et al. 1998). However, not all investigators have observed this association (Engel et al. 1982d). Further, focal polymorphic delta activity occurs in the absence of postictal states, and it must be considered pathophysiologically nonspecific.

Altered energy use in neurotransmitter metabolism might mediate such spatial relationships between ictal dysfunctions and postictal dysfunctions, as suggested by a study using MR spectroscopic determination of the glutamate–glutamine peaks in which localized interictal decreases and ictal increases of FDG activity and glutamate–glutamine peaks were coupled (Pfund et al. 2000). Dual pathology undetectable with MRI, specifically microscopic cortical dysplasia accompanying some but not all cases of hippocampal sclerosis, might generate some of the heterogeneity of FDG topography in TLE (Diehl et al. 2003). At present the diagnostically robust patterns of interictal glucose hypometabolism in TLE are not fully explained by macrostructural, microstructural, and biochemical alterations.

Peri-ictal [^{18}F]FDG PET studies have shown a complex time course of regional cerebral metabolic rates for glucose (CMR_{Glc}) alterations following seizures. In a group of patients with complex partial seizures who had PET at different intervals following the most recent seizure, quantified regional metabolic alterations evolved for more than 48 hours after a single complex partial seizure (Leiderman et al. 1994). The most severe regional hypometabolism occurred more than 48 hours after the seizure, the least severe hypometabolism occurred at 24 to 48 hours postictally, and metabolism was intermediate in the first 24 hours pos-

tictally. In a study in which [^{18}F]FDG studies were performed on average less than 60 hours after the most recent seizure, the type of seizures that preceded the scan had a strong influence on the regional distribution of hypometabolism (Savic et al. 1997). In general, the most localized ictal discharges preceded scans with the smallest volumes of hypometabolism, and secondarily generalized seizures preceded scans with the most widespread patterns of unilateral hypometabolism. In both lesional and non-lesional partial epilepsies, the volume of hypometabolism expands with increasing numbers of seizures over the course of the epilepsy, even with non-progressive lesions (Benedek et al., 2006; Matheja et al. 2001), and in mesial TLE the severity of mesial temporal hypometabolism increases with increasing duration of epilepsy (Theodore et al. 2004).

Focal mesial temporal *hyper*metabolism sometimes occurs interictally in children with mesial TLE, but it rarely occurs in adults with localization-related epilepsies (Chugani et al. 1993a; Engel et al. 1982c; Theodore et al. 1983). Continuous or repetitive focal mesial temporal seizures, which are subclinical and not detectable with scalp electrodes, may cause "interictal" deep temporal hypermetabolism (Sperling et al. 1995). Alternatively, there may be interictal epileptogenic processes that may be peculiar to childhood, and that may generate greater glucose metabolism interictally. The latter speculation is encouraged by the presence of interictal regional hypermetabolism in some young children with the Sturge-Weber syndrome or with infantile spasms, which does not occur in older children with the Sturge-Weber syndrome or with the Lennox-Gastaut syndrome (a frequent "endpoint" for patients with infantile spasms earlier in life), the older children having exclusively hypometabolism or normal metabolism interictally.

Ictal or peri-ictal (representing mixed ictal–postictal–interictal states during the FDG uptake period) FDG scans are difficult to obtain and to interpret. True ictal imaging with FDG is restricted to status epilepticus due to the relatively poor temporal resolution of the FDG method. Occurrence of a single complex partial seizure during the FDG uptake period may be associated with the usual interictal findings of unilateral temporal hypometabolism. In one reported case, a partial seizure occurred about 2 minutes after FDG injection and the scan appeared normal; the same patient later had marked hypometabolism of the epileptogenic temporal lobe on an interictal FDG scan (Henry et al. 1993a). Presumably ictal hypermetabolism was averaged with interictal–postictal hypometabolism over the temporal lobe to cause "normalization" of FDG activity on the peri-ictal scan. In another case, a TLE patient had repeated complex partial seizures following FDG injection, and the scan showed hypermetabolism over the epileptogenic temporal lobe, with ipsilateral frontal and thalamic metabolic increases (Engel et al. 1983). Alterations on ictal and peri-ictal FDG images likely reflect ictal dysfunction at the site of ictal onset, but also disturbances in areas of ictal propagation, and interictal and postictal dysfunction in these areas. It is difficult or impossible to sort out the relative contributions of these various factors to a single set of FDG images.

Cerebral glucose metabolism and CBF normally are coupled (increasing and decreasing in parallel with changes in synaptic activity within each region of cortex), but interictal PET measurements show uncoupling of CBF and FDG activity in TLE (Gaillard et al. 1995; Lee DS et al. 2001). Interictal CBF imaging with PET often shows "diffuse" regional hypoperfusion, consisting of a relatively large area of hypoperfusion with indistinct boundaries from adjacent areas of normal CBF, and with inhomogeneous severity of hypoperfusion (Bernardi et al. 1983; Franck et al. 1985; Kuhl et al. 1980; Leiderman et al. 1992). Interictal regional CBF decreases often occur predominantly contralateral to the ictal onset zone in mesial TLE (Leiderman et al. 1992; Theodore et al. 1994). Ictal CBF imaging of complex partial seizures with [^{15}O] H$_2$O is nearly impossible to obtain, given the 2-minute half-life of oxygen-15, except with seizure induction by proconvulsant drugs or during complex partial status epilepticus (Theodore et al. 1996). For these reasons, ictal imaging and resting interictal imaging with [^{15}O] H$_2$O have no clinical role in presurgical evaluation. It has been suggested, however, that detection of regional glucose metabolic-CBF uncoupling might be more

sensitive in detecting epileptogenic tissue than is FDG mapping alone (Zubal et al. 2000).

Basal and Lateral (Neocortical) TLE

Interictal FDG PET often demonstrates a region of pathologic hypometabolism in adults and children with refractory partial seizures of neocortical (extralimbic) temporal origin (Hajek et al. 1993, 1994; Henry et al. 1991, 1993a; Radtke et al. 1994; Sperling et al. 1990; Swartz et al. 1989; Theodore et al. 1986). In patients with a single neocortical site of ictal onset, interictal FDG PET usually demonstrates a single region of hypometabolism (Fig. 8.8), but normal metabolism also is frequently observed. Compared with non-lesional mesial TLE, non-lesional neocortical epilepsies are more likely to have normal interictal FDG PET studies (Henry et al. 1991; Radtke et al. 1994). Interictal focal neocortical areas of *hyper*metabolism may occur in early childhood epilepsies (Chugani et al. 1993a) but have not been reported in adults. In many lesional neocortical epilepsies, the hypometabolic region is small, sharply circumscribed, and co-localized with a focal structural lesion detected with MRI; a similar relationship of "matching" focal PET hypometabolism and focal MRI lesion rarely is observed in mesial TLE (Henry et al. 1991). Many individuals with lesional or non-lesional neocortical localization-related epilepsies have a more widespread hypometabolic zone, which has graded transitions from areas of severe hypometabolism to areas of normal metabolism, similar to patterns of hypometabolism in mesial TLE. When associated with a lesion, a

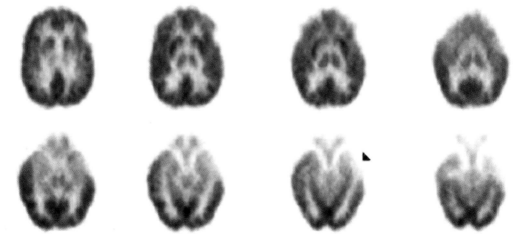

Figure 8.8 Interictal FDG PET images of a neocortical TLE patient. These images show severe hypometabolism of the lateral and inferior temporal neocortex (*arrowhead*) and moderate hypometabolism of the ipsilateral mesial temporal structures. The patient's brain MRI was normal. Focal cortical dysplasia was present in tissue resected at the site of severe hypometabolism and of intracranially recorded EEG ictal onsets. Seizures were reduced by greater than 90% after resection.

diffuse hypometabolic area of neocortex often is much larger than any associated structural imaging abnormality and than any histopathologic lesion (Fig. 8.8), as also is observed in mesial TLE. In the absence of a structural lesion on MRI, the volume of diffuse regional hypometabolism sometimes is fairly small in neocortical epilepsies. Larger areas of hypometabolism often include mesial temporal, thalamic, and basal ganglial hypometabolism ipsilateral to the neocortical site of hypometabolism. Hypometabolism over an entire hemisphere is rare, as is symmetric bilateral hypometabolism, in unilateral neocortical epilepsies. The degree of hypometabolism usually varies across a region of diffuse hypometabolism. The zone of most severe hypometabolism, excluding the site of a foreign-tissue lesion, usually contains the electrophysiologically defined ictal onset zone (Henry et al. 1993a).

PRESURGICAL EVALUATION

Planning Surgery of Localization-Related Epilepsies

Single regions of interictal hypometabolism on FDG PET are highly associated with the region that can be resected to control seizures in localization-related epilepsies. In the syndrome of medically refractory mesial TLE, strong support for anterior temporal resection *without* prior intracranial EEG monitoring is provided by the presence of most severe dysfunction in one temporal lobe, on interictal FDG PET, if other noninvasively acquired data support this localization. Specifically, unilaterally predominant hypometabolism supports temporal resection, in the absence of intracranial EEG recordings, when (1) extracranial EEG recordings show temporal ictal onsets exclusively on the side of functional imaging abnormality; (2) MRI is normal, or nonspecifically abnormal, as in the case of puncta of subcortical white matter abnormalities, or MRI shows hippocampal atrophy, malformation of cortical development, foreign-tissue lesion, or encephalomalacia in the same temporal lobe; and (3) other noninvasively acquired data are not discordant with this localization) (Engel et al. 1990). When brain MRI is normal in the syndrome of refractory mesial TLE, interictal FDG PET can detect temporal lobe hypometabolism (Carne et al. 2004, 2007; Henry et al. 1993b; Knowlton et al. 1997; Uijl et al. 2007; Willmann et al. 2007). In the syndrome of mesial TLE, when interictal FDG PET shows most severe abnormality in one temporal lobe, this does not alone establish that all seizures are arising from that temporal lobe (as discussed further below). Thus, intracranial EEG will be necessary when FDG or ictal CBF abnormalities are not supported by ictal extracranial EEG localization, and

when FDG or ictal CBF abnormalities contradict other localizing abnormalities. In some cases of refractory localization-related epilepsy that have normal brain MRI and non-localizing ictal scalp EEG, the finding of unilateral temporal lobe (or of asymmetric bitemporal) hypometabolism may strongly support intracranial EEG monitoring (Uijl et al. 2007; Willmann et al. 2007).

In extratemporal lobe epilepsies and in localization-related epilepsies that cannot be fully characterized by electroclinical manifestations, ictal CBF and interictal FDG abnormalities cannot be used to determine the margin of cortical resection, but can be used with other data to determine sites that should be monitored with intracranial electrodes (Henry et al 1991; So et al. 2000). Current evidence demonstrates that PET and SPECT data are not redundant with electrophysiologic data nor with structural imaging data. These functional imaging modalities sometimes provide evidence of falsely localized extracranial ictal EEG data, or evidence that EEG and MRI falsely suggested unifocal ictal onsets in patients who actually have two independent ictal onset zones (Henry et al. 1999a). The cost-effectiveness of performing one of these functional imaging modalities in all patients before resective epilepsy therapy is unknown. Based on currently available information, however, it is reasonable to perform either interictal FDG PET or ictal/interictal SPECT in all patients with localization-related epilepsies before resective surgery, in addition to ictal recordings with extracranial EEG, MRI, and neuropsychometric studies.

Unilateral temporal lobe hypometabolism is "falsely lateralized" (located contralateral to the intracranially recorded site of ictal onset, in patients with single ictal onset zone) in approximately 1% to 2% of patients, in series in which potential sources of imaging artifact and unreliable forms of quantitative analysis were excluded. Prior intracranial surgery, including depth electrode placement, can produce temporal lobe hypometabolism that is falsely lateralized with respect to intracranially recorded temporal lobe ictal onsets and to the side of subsequent, efficacious resection (Engel et al. 1990). Imaging artifacts also can be produced by unrecognized errors in cranial positioning, errors of improperly aligned images in attenuation correction, and other aspects of imaging; visual image analysis should be used to exclude these artifacts before any automated quantitative image analysis. Volume-of-interest–based quantitative analysis should sample regions whose volumes are in the range of the usual volume of the interictally hypometabolic area of TLE, and techniques that do not use predefined volumes of interest, such as statistical parametric mapping, should use a volume threshold to avoid detection of potentially misleading, tiny foci of statistically significant hypometabolism, at least for application in presurgical evaluation. Continuous EEG monitoring can be performed during FDG scanning and sometimes can exclude unintentional ictal scanning that could lead to misinterpretation of FDG images (Henry et al. 1993a). There is a case report of a patient who did not have subjective or objective clinical changes or scalp EEG changes during "interictal" FDG scanning, which appeared to show falsely lateralized temporal lobe hypometabolism (Sperling et al. 1995). In fact, the scan probably showed correctly lateralized ictal hypermetabolism. Subsequent intracerebral recordings showed frequently recurrent seizures confined to one hippocampus (without subjective or objective behavioral change and without scalp EEG change). Visual interpretation relies on detecting asymmetry, so hypermetabolism on one side may appear to give the impression of hypometabolism on the other side. The investigators suggested that relative quantification of temporal and occipital lobe metabolism may support distinction of temporal lobe hypermetabolism on one side from temporal lobe hypometabolism on the other side (Sperling et al. 1995). As is true of all noninvasive means of localizing the epileptogenic zone, presurgical application of interictal FDG PET in partial epilepsies should be limited to correlation with other studies used to regionalize the ictal onset zone.

Cerebral MRI is essential in detection of hippocampal sclerosis, neoplasia, vascular malformations, other foreign-tissue lesions, ablative lesions, and malformations of cortical development (Duncan et al. 1997; Kuzniecky et al. 2005). Cerebral structural abnormalities are highly but not completely correlated with the epileptogenic zone. In some cases, a small foreign-tissue lesion may be located distant from the ictal onset zone, although most cerebral lesions are located near ictal onset zones and this topographic relationship is especially strong in the case of cavernomas. In cases of a large area of encephalomalacia, porencephaly, or cerebral maldevelopment, the ictal onset zone may be much smaller than the lesion; even when extracranial EEG recordings suggest that the ictal onset zone is near the lesion, it often is not desirable or necessary to resect the entire lesion when the exact location of the ictal onset zone is unclear; sometimes such lesions are distant from the region of ictal onset. In groups of patients with tuberous sclerosis and other conditions with longstanding multifocal lesions, individual patients can have a single ictal onset zone, or multiple independent ictal onset zones, or even generalized-onset seizures. Optimal choice of intracranial electrode placements is necessary for successful localization of the electrophysiologic ictal onset zone, when noninvasive data do not suffice. Interictal metabolic and ictal perfusion information may be combined with other data to direct intracranial electrode placement to sites of possible ictal onset (Muzik et al. 2000). Regional hypometabolism or ictal hyperperfusion can suggest otherwise unsuspected possible sites

of ictal onset, in order to avoid intracranial monitoring procedures that record ictal propagation patterns but fail to record earliest ictal onset patterns (evidenced by absence of ictal discharges recorded during earliest behavioral manifestations). The absence of any hypometabolism obviously does not rule out localization-related epilepsy. Similarly, regional hypometabolism strongly suggests that seizures may begin somewhere near or within the region of hypometabolism, but does not rule out multiple areas of ictal onset both within and beyond the hypometabolic cortex. At the current time many epilepsy surgery programs offer temporal lobe resection to a patient who has refractory complex partial seizures with semiology characteristic of mesial TLE, without prior physiologic imaging or intracranial EEG monitoring, if the patient has unilateral temporal lobe spikes interictally and ictal onsets on extracranial EEG, and has hippocampal atrophy or specific mesial temporal lesions ipsilaterally on MRI, in the absence of contradictory information on neuropsychometric or other standard studies. In some programs confirmatory information would be sought with interictal FDG PET or ictal SPECT in such a patient, although no detailed cost–benefit analysis of this additional physiologic imaging has been reported.

Unilateral temporal lobe hypometabolism has been reported in patients who have bilateral independent hippocampal ictal onsets recorded with intracranial electrodes during habitual complex partial seizures, and most of these patients also had exclusively unilateral MRI abnormality (Franck et al. 1992; Henry et al. 1999a). Further, ictal scalp-sphenoidal EEG recordings are much more likely than are MRI or PET images to show evidence of bilateral TLE among patients who subsequently have intracranial recording of bilateral independent hippocampal ictal onsets (Henry et al. 1999a). Alternatively, some patients who had bilateral independent temporal ictal onsets on extracranial EEG, with unilateral temporal abnormalities on MRI and PET or on PET only, have been shown to have exclusively unilateral hippocampal intracranial EEG onsets that were on the side of the imaging abnormality (and of efficacious temporal lobectomy). On the other hand, bilateral hippocampal atrophy on MRI sometimes is observed in patients who have unilateral temporal hypometabolism interictally, unilateral hippocampal ictal onsets, and good surgical outcome (Knowlton et al. 1997). All focal ictal onset patterns on extracranial EEG, all focal cerebral gray matter lesions on MRI, and all regions of cortical hypometabolism on PET should be considered when planning intracranial electrode placements.

Imaging of ictal CBF with SPECT and of interictal cerebral glucose metabolism with PET have similar roles in evaluations for epilepsy surgery in that both can detect definite abnormalities when structural imaging is normal or nonspecifically altered (Ho et al. 1995;

Hong et al. 2002; Kim SK et al. 2001; Ryvlin et al. 1991, 1992; Spencer et al. 2000; Sturm et al. 2000; Won et al. 1999). Overall sensitivity and specificity of ictal SPECT and interictal FDG PET are similar in large series of partial epilepsies; studies of the two techniques, in the same sets of patients, report sensitivity to functional abnormality in excess of 70% (and usually much greater than 70%), with specificity to the ictal onset zone above 90% (Bouilleret et al. 2002b; Ho et al. 1995; Hwang et al. 2001). In fact, a relatively greater sensitivity of ictal SPECT (over FDG PET) in detecting extratemporal epileptogenic zones may be obscured in series that include all forms of partial epilepsy, due to the predominance of TLE over other partial epilepsies and to the profound glucose metabolic dysfunctions of TLE. Quantitative statistical image analysis may significantly increase the sensitivity and specificity of FDG PET in detecting evidence of neocortical (lateral) temporal and extratemporal ictal onset zones, compared with standard clinical (visual) interpretation (Kim YK et al. 2003).

Interictal regional hypometabolism also is useful in predicting the outcome of temporal lobe resection with respect to seizures. Greater severity of preoperative hypometabolism of the resected temporal lobe is associated with significantly better postoperative seizure control, using either qualitative or quantitative definitions of severity of hypometabolism (Boling et al. 2008; Delbeke et al. 1996; Dupont et al. 2000; Lin et al. 2007; Manno et al. 1994; O'Brien et al. 2001; Radtke et al. 1993; Salanova et al. 1998; Theodore et al. 1992b, 1997; Wong et al. 1996). This strong correlation is independent of the pathologic diagnosis. Uncal or temporal pole metabolism, analyzed quantitatively, may provide the most accurate correlation with seizure outcome (Dupont et al. 2000; Manno et al. 1994). Temporal lobe resections that included more of the significantly hypometabolic zone were more efficacious in eliminating seizures, in a study that analyzed interictal FDG PET with statistical parametric mapping (Vinton et al. 2007). Qualitatively severe *extra*temporal cortical or thalamic hypometabolism, however, is associated with a higher incidence of postoperative seizures (Newberg et al. 2000; Swartz et al. 1992b). Symmetric, severe, bilateral temporal hypometabolism also is associated with a higher incidence of postoperative seizures, even when other data suggest that all seizures originate in one temporal lobe (Blum et al. 1998). A site of reduced FDG activity that is distinct and non-contiguous with a cavernous angioma is highly associated with recurrent seizures after lesionectomy (Kraemer et al 1998; Ryvlin et al. 1995). Temporal lobe hypometabolism contralateral to intracranially recorded ictal onsets also is reportedly associated with recurrent seizures after resections of the electrophysiologically defined focus (Benbadis

et al.1995), although individual cases with good outcome of resection contralateral to temporal lobe hypometabolism have been reported (Nagarajan et al.1996). While most studies of FDG PET in surgical prognostication have focused on mesial TLE, one series of 80 surgically treated neocortical TLE patients found that hypometabolism restricted to the subsequent resection site predicted postoperative seizure freedom, independently of MRI and EEG prognostic data (Yun et al. 2006).

Cognitive activation CBF PET or FDG PET studies might be useful in predicting the outcome of temporal lobe resection with respect to language and memory function, although fMRI has the potential to do so without exposure to ionizing radiation (see Chapter 5). Both activation PET and fMRI appear likely to be able to lateralize hemispheric language specialization (Fried 2000; Henry et al. 1998; Votaw et al. 1999). Specific deficits of delayed recall are variably reported to be associated or unassociated with the distribution and severity of glucose hypometabolism interictally in TLE (Griffith et al 2004; Hong et al. 2000; Rausch et al. 1994; Salanova et al. 2001). These "resting" FDG PET abnormalities have not been used to provide the presurgical memory prognostication afforded by the Wada test (Griffith et al. 2000; Hong et al. 2002; Salanova et al. 2001). Executive dysfunctions were associated with prefrontal cortical hypometabolism in refractory mesial TLE (Takaya et al. 2006). Depression was associated with orbitofrontal hypometabolism ipsilateral to an epileptogenic temporal lobe (Salzberg et al. 2006). Full application of activation PET or fMRI in presurgical evaluation will require many studies to determine the answers to many areas of uncertainty, including (1) whether fMRI techniques can be developed to permit speech-related cranial motion during imaging, and whether it is essential to assess patient effort with analysis of verbal responses (given that patients may not comply with instructions during silent cognitive task performance, as apparently do paid, healthy volunteers in studies of normal cognitive activation); (2) how results of activation PET and fMRI compare with current clinical tools such as the Wada test and direct cortical electrical stimulation mapping; and (3) whether modification of resection based on functional imaging results actually improves functional outcome of surgery. These issues have been discussed in some detail in Chapter 5.

SUMMARY

PET permits in vivo measurement and whole-brain anatomical mapping of a wide variety of brain functions in healthy and in epileptic individuals. Glucose metabolic imaging has revealed unexpected patterns of interictal cerebral dysfunction in most forms of epilepsy. In mesial and neocortical TLE, the zone of interictal metabolic dysfunction is often more lateralized than is interictal electrophysiological dysfunction, but it is typically much larger than the electrophysiologically determined ictal onset zone and larger than any associated structural lesion. The pathophysiology of temporal lobe and extratemporal glucose hypometabolism in TLE remains unclear. Nonetheless, the robust associations of interictally hypometabolic regions with sites of ictal onset and propagation support clinical applications in presurgical evaluations of refractory seizures. Interictal FDG PET is used in correlation with ictal electrophysiological and structural magnetic resonance findings for the purposes of:

1. Increasing certainty that the ictal onset zone has been accurately determined by noninvasive studies prior to anterior temporal lobectomy or amygdalo-hippocampectomy
2. Optimizing selection of intracranial electrode placement sites for ictal monitoring
3. Prognostication with regard to seizure control

REFERENCES

Abou-Khalil, B. W., G. J. Siegel, J. C. Sackellares, et al. 1987. Positron emission tomography studies of cerebral glucose metabolism in chronic partial epilepsy. *Annals of Neurology* 22: 480–6.

Achten, E., P. B. Santens, P. Boon, et al. 1998. Single-voxel MR spectroscopy and positron emission tomography for lateralization of refractory temporal lobe epilepsy. *American Journal of Neuroradiology* 19: 1–9.

Arnold, S., G. Schlaug, H. Niemann, et al. 1996. Topography of interictal glucose hypometabolism in unilateral mesiotemporal epilepsy. *Neurology* 46: 1422–30.

Baete, K., J. Nuyts, K. Van Laere, et al. 2004a. Evaluation of anatomy based reconstruction for partial volume correction in brain FDG-PET. *Neuroimage* 23: 305–17.

Baete, K., J. Nuyts, W. Van Paesschen, et al. 2004b. Anatomical-based FDG-PET reconstruction for the detection of hypo-metabolic regions in epilepsy. *IEEE Transactions Medical Imaging* 23: 510–9.

Banati, R. B., G. W. Goerres, R. Myers, et al. 1999. [^{11}C] (R)-PK11195 positron emission tomography imaging of activated microglia in vivo in Rasmussen's encephalitis. *Neurology* 53: 2199–203.

Baron, J. C., D. Roeda, C. Munari, et al. 1983. Brain regional pharmacokinetics of ^{11}C-labeled diphenylhydantoin positron emission tomography in humans. *Neurology* 33: 580–5.

Barrington, S. F., M. Koutroumanidis, A. Agathonikou, et al. 1998. Clinical value of "ictal" FDG-positron emission tomography and the routine use of simultaneous scalp EEG studies in patients with intractable partial epilepsies. *Epilepsia* 39: 753–66.

Benbadis, S. R., N. K. So, M. A. Antar, et al. 1995. The value of PET scan (and MRI and Wada test) in patients with bitemporal epileptiform abnormalities. *Archives of Neurology* 52: 1062–8.

Benedek, K., C. Juhasz, D. C. Chugani, et al. 2006. Longitudinal changes of cortical glucose hypometabolism in children with intractable epilepsy. *Journal of Child Neurology* 21: 26–31.

Blodgett, T. M., C. C. Meltzer, and D. W. Townsend. 2007. PET/CT: form and function. *Radiology* 242: 360–85.

Blum, D. E., T. Ehsan, D. Dungan, et al. 1998. Bilateral temporal hypometabolism in epilepsy. *Epilepsia* 39: 651–9.

Boling, W. W., M. Lancaster, M. Kraszpulski, et al. 2008. Fluorodeoxyglucose-positron emission tomographic imaging for the diagnosis of mesial temporal lobe epilepsy. *Neurosurgery* 63: 1130–8.

Bouilleret, V., S. Dupont, L. Spelle, et al. 2002a. Insular cortex involvement in mesiotemporal lobe epilepsy: a positron emission tomography study. *Annals of Neurology* 51: 202–8.

Bouilleret, V., F. Semah, F. Chassoux, et al. 2008. Basal ganglia involvement in temporal lobe epilepsy: a functional and morphologic study. *Neurology* 70: 177–84.

Bouilleret, V., M. P. Valenti, E. Hirsch, et al. 2002b. Correlation between PET and SISCOM in temporal lobe epilepsy. *Journal of Nuclear Medicine* 43: 991–8.

Bouvard, S., N. Costes, F. Bonnefoi, et al. 2005. Seizure-related short-term plasticity of benzodiazepine receptors in partial epilepsy: a [11C]flumazenil-PET study. *Brain* 128: 1330–43.

Carne, R. P., T. J. O'Brien, C. J. Kilpatrick, et al. 2004. MRI-negative PET-positive temporal lobe epilepsy: a distinct surgically remediable syndrome. *Brain* 127: 2276–85.

Carne, R. P., T. J. O'Brien, C. J. Kilpatrick, et al. 2007. 'MRI-negative PET-positive' temporal lobe epilepsy (TLE) and mesial TLE differ with quantitative MRI and PET: a case control study. *BMC Neurology* 7: 16.

Chassoux, F., F. Semah, V. Bouilleret, et al. 2004. Metabolic changes and electro-clinical patterns in mesio-temporal lobe epilepsy: a correlative study. *Brain* 127: 164–74.

Chugani, D. C., H. T. Chugani, O. Muzik, et al. 1998. Imaging epileptogenic tubers in children with tuberous sclerosis complex using alpha-[11C]methyl-L-tryptophan positron emission tomography. *Annals of Neurology* 44: 858–66.

Chugani, H. T., D. A. Shewmon, S. Khanna, et al. 1993a. Interictal and postictal focal hypermetabolism on positron emission tomography. *Pediatric Neurology* 9: 10–5.

Debets, R. M., B. Sadzot, J. W. van Isselt, et al. 1997. Is ^{11}C-flumazenil PET superior to ^{18}FDG PET and ^{123}I-iomazenil SPECT in presurgical evaluation of temporal lobe epilepsy? *Journal of Neurology Neurosurgery & Psychiatry* 62(2): 141–50.

Dedeurwaerdere, S., B. Jupp, and T. J. O'Brien. 2007. Positron emission tomography in basic epilepsy research: a view of the epileptic brain. *Epilepsia* 48 Suppl 4: 56–64.

Delbeke, D., S. K. Lawrence, B. W. Abou-Khalil, et al. 1996. Postsurgical outcome of patients with uncontrolled complex partial seizures and temporal lobe hypometabolism on 18FDG-positron emission tomography. *Investigative Radiology* 31: 261–6.

DeLong, G. R., and E. R. Heinz. 1997. The clinical syndrome of early-life bilateral hippocampal sclerosis. *Annals of Neurology* 42: 11–7.

Diehl, B., E. LaPresto, I. Najm, et al. 2003. Neocortical temporal FDG-PET hypometabolism correlates with temporal lobe atrophy in hippocampal sclerosis associated with microscopic cortical dysplasia. *Epilepsia* 44: 559–64.

Dlugos, D. J., J. Jaggi, W. M. O'Connor, et al. 1999. Hippocampal cell density and subcortical metabolism in temporal lobe epilepsy. *Epilepsia* 40: 408–13.

Drzezga, A., S. Arnold, S. Minoshima, et al. 1999. 18F-FDG PET studies in patients with extratemporal and temporal epilepsy: evaluation of an observer-independent analysis. *Journal of Nuclear Medicine* 40: 737–46.

Dupont, S., A. C. Croize, F. Semah, et al. 2001. Is amygdalo-hippocampectomy really selective in medial temporal lobe epilepsy? A study using positron emission tomography with (18)fluorodeoxyglucose. *Epilepsia* 42: 731–40.

Dupont, S., F. Semah, S. Clemenceau, et al. 2000. Accurate prediction of postoperative outcome in mesial temporal lobe epilepsy: a study using positron emission tomography with 18fluorodeoxyglucose. *Archives of Neurology* 57: 1331–6.

Engel, J. Jr., W. J. Brown, D. E. Kuhl, et al. 1982a. Pathological findings underlying focal temporal lobe hypometabolism in partial epilepsy. *Annals of Neurology* 12: 518–28.

Engel, J. Jr., T. R. Henry, M. W. Risinger, et al. 1990. Presurgical evaluation for partial epilepsy: Relative contributions of chronic depth electrode recordings versus FDG-PET and scalp-sphenoidal ictal EEG. *Neurology* 40: 1670–7.

Engel, J. Jr., D. E. Kuhl, M. E. Phelps, et al. 1982c. Comparative localization of epileptic foci in partial epilepsy by PCT and EEG. *Annals of Neurology* 12: 529–37.

Engel, J. Jr., D. E. Kuhl, M. E. Phelps, et al. 1982d. Interictal cerebral glucose metabolism in partial epilepsy and its relation to EEG changes. *Annals of Neurology* 12: 510–7.

Engel, J. Jr., D. E. Kuhl, M. E. Phelps, et al. 1983. Local cerebral metabolism during partial seizures. *Neurology* 33: 400–13.

Engel, J. Jr., D. E. Kuhl, and M. E. Phelps. 1982b. Patterns of human local cerebral glucose metabolism during epileptic seizures. *Science* 218: 64–6.

Engel, J. Jr., P. Lubens, D. E. KuhlE, et al. 1985. Local cerebral metabolic rate for glucose during petit mal absences. *Annals of Neurology* 17: 121–8.

Erbayat Altay, E., A. J. Fessler, M. Gallagher, et al. 2005. Correlation of severity of FDG-PET hypometabolism and interictal regional delta slowing in temporal lobe epilepsy. *Epilepsia* 46: 573–6.

Foldvary, N., N. Lee, M. W. Hanson, et al. 1999. Correlation of hippocampal neuronal density and FDG-PET in mesial temporal lobe epilepsy. *Epilepsia* 40: 26–9.

Franck, G., B. Sadzot, E. Salmon, et al. 1985. Regional cerebral blood flow and metabolic rates in human focal epilepsy and status epilepticus. In A. V. Delgado-Escueta, A. A. Ward Jr., D. M. Woodbury, et al., eds. *Basic mechanisms of the epilepsies: Molecular and cellular approaches.* New York: Raven Press, 935–48.

Frey, K. A. 2000. Radiotracers and analytical approaches in positron and single-photon emission tomography.

In T. R. Henry, S. F. Berkovic, and J. S. Duncan, eds. *Functional imaging in the epilepsies.* Philadelphia: Lippincott Williams & Wilkins, 61–8.

Frey, K. A. 1999. Positron emission tomography. In G. J. Siegel, B. W. Agranoff, R. W. Albers, et al., eds. *Basic neurochemistry: Molecular, cellular, and medical aspects,* 6th ed. Philadelphia: Lippincott-Raven, 1109–31.

Fried, I. 2000. Functional neuroimaging in presurgical localization of essential cortical processing zones. In T. R. Henry, S. F. Berkovic, and J. S. Duncan, eds. *Functional imaging in the epilepsies.* Philadelphia: Lippincott Williams & Wilkins, 297–304.

Frost, J. J., H. S. Mayberg, R. S. Fisher, et al. 1988. Mu-opiate receptors measured by positron emission tomography are increased in temporal lobe epilepsy. *Annals of Neurology* 23: 231–7.

Gaillard, W. D., S. Bhatia, S. Y. Bookheimer, et al. 1995. FDG-PET and volumetric MRI in the evaluation of patients with partial epilepsy. *Neurology* 45: 123–6.

Gaillard, W. D., S. Fazilat, S. White, et al. 1995. Interictal metabolism and blood flow are uncoupled in temporal cortex of patients with complex partial epilepsy. *Neurology* 45: 1841–7.

Gaillard, W. D., L. Kopylev, S. Weinstein, et al. 2002. Low incidence of abnormal (18)FDG-PET in children with new-onset partial epilepsy: a prospective study. *Neurology* 58: 717–22.

Gaillard, W. D., T. Zeffiro, S. Fazilat, et al. 1996. Effect of valproate on cerebral metabolism and blood flow: an ^{18}F-2-deoxyglucose and ^{15}O water positron emission tomography study. *Epilepsia* 37: 515–21.

Griffith, H. R., S. B. Perlman, A. R. Woodard, et al. 2000. Preoperative FDG-PET temporal lobe hypometabolism and verbal memory after temporal lobectomy. *Neurology* 54: 1161–65.

Griffith, H. R., R. W. Pyzalski, M. Seidenberg, et al. 2004. Memory relationships between MRI volumes and resting PET metabolism of medial temporal lobe structures. *Epilepsy & Behavior* 5: 669–76.

Hajek, M., A. Antonini, K. L. Leenders, et al. 1991. Epilepsia partialis continua studied with PET. *Epilepsy Research* 9: 44–8.

Hajek, M., A. Antonini, K. L. Leenders, et al. 1993. Mesiobasal versus lateral temporal lobe epilepsy: metabolic differences in the temporal lobe shown by interictal ^{18}F-FDG positron emission tomography. *Neurology* 43: 79–86.

Hajek, M., H-G. Wieser, N. Khan, et al. 1994. Preoperative and postoperative glucose consumption in mesiobasal and lateral temporal lobe epilepsy. *Neurology* 44: 2125–32.

Hammers, A., M. J. Koepp, R. Hurlemann, et al. 2002. Abnormalities of grey and white matter [11C]flumazenil binding in temporal lobe epilepsy with normal MRI. *Brain* 125: 2257–71.

Henry, T. R., T. L. Babb, J. Engel Jr., et al. 1994. Hippocampal neuronal loss and regional metabolism in temporal lobe epilepsy. *Annals of Neurology* 36: 925–7.

Henry, T. R., H. A. Buchtel, R. A. Koeppe, et al. 1998. Absence of normal activation of the left anterior fusiform gyrus during naming in left temporal lobe epilepsy. *Neurology* 50: 787–90.

Henry, T. R., H. T. Chugani, B. W. Abou-Khalil, et al. 1993a. Positron emission tomography in presurgical evaluation of epilepsy. In J. Engel Jr., ed. *Surgical treatment of the epilepsies*, 2nd ed. New York: Raven Press, 211–32.

Henry, T. R., J. Engel Jr., and J. C. Mazziotta. 1993b. Clinical evaluation of interictal fluorine–18-fluorodeoxyglucose PET in partial epilepsy. *Journal of Nuclear Medicine* 34: 1892–8.

Henry, T. R., K. A. Frey, J. C. Sackellares, et al. 1993c. In vivo cerebral metabolism and central benzodiazepine-receptor binding in temporal lobe epilepsy. *Neurology* 43: 1998–2006.

Henry, T. R., J. C. Mazziotta, J. Engel Jr., et al. 1990. Quantifying interictal metabolic activity in human temporal lobe epilepsy. *Journal of Cerebral Blood Flow Metabolism* 10: 748–57.

Henry, T. R., J. C. Mazziotta, and J. Engel Jr. 1993d. Interictal metabolic anatomy of mesial temporal lobe epilepsy. *Archives of Neurology* 50: 582–9.

Henry, T. R., E. Rohren, and B. P. Mullan. 2005. Positron emission tomography and single photon emission computed tomography in the epilepsies. In R. E. Latchaw, J. Kucharczyk, and M. E. Moseley, eds. *Diagnostic and therapeutic imaging of the nervous system*. Philadlephia: Lippincott Williams & Wilkins, 1211–24.

Henry, T. R., D. A. Ross, L. A. Schuh, et al. 1999. Indications and outcome of ictal recording with intracerebral and subdural electrodes in refractory complex partial seizures. *Journal of Clinical Neurophysiology* 16: 426–38.

Henry, T. R., W. W. Sutherling, J. Engel Jr., et al. 1991. Interictal cerebral metabolism in partial epilepsies of neocortical origin. *Epilepsy Research* 10: 174–82.

Ho, S. S., S. F. Berkovic, S. U. Berlangieri, et al. 1995. Comparison of ictal SPECT and interictal PET in the presurgical evaluation of temporal lobe epilepsy. *Annals of Neurology* 37: 738–45.

Hong, K. S., S. K. Lee, J. Y. Kim, et al. 2002. Pre-surgical evaluation and surgical outcome of 41 patients with non-lesional neocortical epilepsy. *Seizure* 11: 184–92.

Hong, S. B., S. Y. Roh, S. E. Kim, et al. 2000. Correlation of temporal lobe glucose metabolism with the Wada memory test. *Epilepsia* 41: 1554–9.

Hwang, S. I., J. H. Kim, S. W. Park, et al. 2001. Comparative analysis of MR imaging, positron emission tomography, and ictal single-photon emission CT in patients with neocortical epilepsy. *AJNR American Journal of Neuroradiology* 22: 937–46.

Joo, E. Y., S. B. Hong, H. J. Han, et al. 2005. Postoperative alteration of cerebral glucose metabolism in mesial temporal lobe epilepsy. *Brain* 128: 1802–10.

Joo, E. Y., W. S. Tae, and S. B. Hong. 2006. Regional effects of lamotrigine on cerebral glucose metabolism in idiopathic generalized epilepsy. *Archives of Neurology* 63: 1282–6.

Juhasz, C., D. C. Chugani, O. Muzik, et al. 2003. Alpha-methyl-L-tryptophan PET detects epileptogenic cortex in children with intractable epilepsy. *Neurology* 60: 960–8.

Juhasz, C., F. Nagy, O. Muzik, et al. 1999. [11C]Flumazenil PET in patients with epilepsy with dual pathology. *Epilepsia* 40: 566–74.

Kang, K. W., D. S. Lee, J. H. Cho, et al. 2001. Quantification of F-18-FDG PET images in temporal lobe epilepsy patients using probabilistic brain atlas. *Neuroimage* 14: 1–6.

Kim, M. A., K. Heo, M. K. Choo, et al. 2006. Relationship between bilateral temporal hypometabolism and EEG findings for mesial temporal lobe epilepsy: Analysis of 18F-FDG PET using SPM. *Seizure* 15: 56–63.

Kim, Y. K., D. S. Lee, S. K. Lee, et al. 2003. Differential features of metabolic abnormalities between medial and lateral temporal lobe epilepsy: quantitative analysis of (18)F-FDG PET using SPM. *Journal of Nuclear Medicine* 44: 1006–12.

Knowlton, R. C., B. Abou-Khalil, S. M. Sawrie, et al. 2002. In vivo hippocampal metabolic dysfunction in human temporal lobe epilepsy. *Archives of Neurology* 59: 1882–6.

Knowlton, R. C., K. D. Laxer, G. Ende, et al. 1997. Presurgical multimodality neuroimaging in electroencephalographic lateralized temporal lobe epilepsy. *Annals of Neurology* 42: 829–37.

Knowlton, R. C., K. D. Laxer, G. Klein, et al. 2001. In vivo hippocampal glucose metabolism in mesial temporal lobe epilepsy. *Neurology* 57: 1184–90.

Koepp, M. J., C. Labbe, M. P. Richardson, et al. 1997. Regional hippocampal [11C]flumazenil PET in temporal lobe epilepsy with unilateral and bilateral hippocampal sclerosis. *Brain* 120: 1865–76.

Koepp, M. J., K. S. Hand, C. Labbe, et al. 1998. In vivo [11C] flumazenil-PET correlates with ex vivo [3H]flumazenil autoradiography in hippocampal sclerosis. *Annals of Neurology* 43(5): 618–26.

Koutroumanidis, M., C. D. Binnie, R. D. Elwes, et al. 1998. Interictal regional slow activity in temporal lobe epilepsy correlates with lateral temporal hypometabolism as imaged with ^{18}FDG PET: neurophysiological and metabolic implications. *Journal of Neurology Neurosurgery & Psychiatry* 65: 170–6.

Koutroumanidis, M., M. J. Hennessy, P. T. Seed, et al. 2000. Significance of interictal bilateral temporal hypometabolism in temporal lobe epilepsy. *Neurology* 54: 1811–21.

Kraemer, D. L., M. L. Griebel, N. Lee, et al. 1998. Surgical outcome in patients with epilepsy with occult vascular malformations treated with lesionectomy. *Epilepsia* 39: 600–7.

Kuhl, D. E., J. Engel Jr., M. E. Phelps, et al. 1980. Epileptic patterns of local cerebral metabolism and perfusion in humans determined by emission computed tomography of ^{18}FDG and ^{13}NH$_3$. *Annals of Neurology* 18: 348–60.

Kumar, A., H. T. Chugani, A. Luat, et al. 2008. Epilepsy surgery in a case of encephalitis: use of ^{11}C-PK11195 positron emission tomography. *Pediatric Neurology* 38: 439–442.

Kumlien, E., M. Bergström, A. Lilja, et al. 1995. Positron emission tomography with [^{11}C]deuterium-deprenyl in temporal lobe epilepsy. *Epilepsia* 36: 712–21.

Kumlien, E., P. Hartvig, S. Valind, et al. 1999. NMDA-receptor activity visualized with (S)-[N-methyl–11C]ketamine and positron emission tomography in patients with medial temporal lobe epilepsy. *Epilepsia* 40: 30–37.

Kuzniecky, R. I., and G. D. JacksonD. 2005. *Magnetic resonance in epilepsy: neuroimaging techniques*, 2nd ed. Amsterdam: Academic Press.

Lamusuo, S., L. Jutila, A. Ylinen, et al. 2001. [18F]FDG-PET reveals temporal hypometabolism in patients with temporal lobe epilepsy even when quantitative MRI and histopathological analysis show only mild hippocampal damage. *Archives of Neurology* 58: 933–9.

Lee, D. S., J. S. Lee, K. W. Kang, et al. 2001. Disparity of perfusion and glucose metabolism of epileptogenic zones in temporal lobe epilepsy demonstrated by SPM/SPAM analysis on 15O water PET, [18F]FDG-PET, and [99mTc]-HMPAO SPECT. *Epilepsia* 42: 1515–22.

Lee, E. M., K. C. Im, J. H. Kim, et al. 2009. Relationship between hypometabolic patterns and ictal scalp EEG patterns in patients with unilateral hippocampal sclerosis: An FDG-PET study. *Epilepsy Research* 84: 187–93.

Leiderman, D. B., P. Albert, M. Balish, et al. 1994. The dynamics of metabolic change following seizures as measured by positron emission tomography with fluorodeoxyglucose F 18. *Archives of Neurology* 51: 932–6.

Leiderman, D. B., M. Balish, S. Sato, et al. 1992. Comparison of PET measurements of cerebral blood flow and glucose metabolism for the localization of human epileptic foci. *Epilepsy Research* 13: 153–7.

Leiderman, D. B., M. B. Balish, E. B. Bromfield, et al. 1901. The effect of valproic acid on human cerebral glucose metabolism. *Epilepsia* 32: 417–22.

Lin, T. W., M. A. de Aburto, M. Dahlbom, et al. 2007. Predicting seizure-free status for temporal lobe epilepsy patients undergoing surgery: prognostic value of quantifying maximal metabolic asymmetry extending over a specified proportion of the temporal lobe. *Journal of Nuclear Medicine* 48: 776–82.

Leveque, P., S. Sanabria-Bohorquez, A. Bol, et al. 2003. Quantification of human brain benzodiazepine receptors using [18F]fluoroethylflumazenil: a first report in volunteers and epileptic patients. *European Journal of Nuclear Medicine Molecular Imaging* 30: 1630–6.

Manno, E. M., M. R. Sperling, X. Ding, et al. 1994. Predictors of outcome after anterior temporal lobectomy: positron emission tomography. *Neurology* 44: 2331–6.

Matheja, P., T. Kuwert, P. Ludemann, et al. 2001. Temporal hypometabolism at the onset of cryptogenic temporal lobe epilepsy. *European Journal of Nuclear Medicine* 28: 625–32.

Mayberg, H. S., B. Sadzot, C. C. Meltzer, et al. 1991. Quantification of mu and non-mu opiate receptors in temporal lobe epilepsy using positron emission tomography. *Annals of Neurology* 30: 3–11.

Mazziotta, J. C., M. E. Phelps, D. Plummer, et al. 1981. Quantitation in positron emission computed tomography: 5. Physical-anatomical effects. *Journal of Computer Assisted Tomography* 5: 734–43.

Meltzer, C. C., P. D. Adelson, R. P. Brenner, et al. 2000. Planned ictal FDG PET imaging for localization of extratemporal epileptic foci. *Epilepsia* 41: 193–200.

Merlet, I., K. Ostrowsky, N. Costes, et al. 2004. 5-HT1A receptor binding and intracerebral activity in temporal lobe epilepsy: an [18F]MPPF-PET study. *Brain* 127: 900–13.

Mirrione, M. M., W. K. Schiffer, M. Siddiq, et al. 2006. PET imaging of glucose metabolism in a mouse model of temporal lobe epilepsy. *Synapse* 59: 119–21.

Nagarajan, L., N. Schaul, D. Eidelberg, et al. 1996. Contralateral temporal hypometabolism on positron emission tomography in temporal lobe epilepsy. *Acta Neurologica Scandinavica* 93: 81–4.

Natsume, J., Y. Kumakura, N. Bernasconi, et al. 2003. Alpha-[11C] methyl-L-tryptophan and glucose metabolism in patients with temporal lobe epilepsy. *Neurology* 60: 756–61.

Nelissen, N., W. Van Paesschen, K. Baete, et al. 2006. Correlations of interictal FDG-PET metabolism and ictal SPECT perfusion changes in human temporal lobe epilepsy with hippocampal sclerosis. *Neuroimage* 32: 684–95.

Newberg, A. B., A. Alavi, J. Berlin, et al. 2000. Ipsilateral and contralateral thalamic hypometabolism as a predictor of outcome after temporal lobectomy for seizures. *Journal of Nuclear Medicine* 41: 1964–8.

Nickel, J., H. Jokeit, G. Wunderlich, et al. 2003. Gender-specific differences of hypometabolism in mTLE: implication for cognitive impairments. *Epilepsia* 44: 1551–61.

O'Brien, T. J., R. J. Hicks, R. Ware, et al. 2001. The utility of a 3-dimensional, large-field-of-view, sodium iodide crystal-based PET scanner in the presurgical evaluation of partial epilepsy. *Journal of Nuclear Medicine* 42: 1158–65.

O'Brien, T. J., M. R. Newton, M. J. Cook, et al. 1997. Hippocampal atrophy is not a major determinant of regional hypometabolism in temporal lobe epilepsy. *Epilepsia* 38: 74–80.

Olson, D. M., H. T. Chugani, D. A. Shewmon, et al. 1990. Electrocorticographic confirmation of focal positron emission tomographic abnormalities in children with intractable epilepsy. *Epilepsia* 31: 731–9.

Palmini, A., W. Van Paesschen, P. Dupont, et al. 2005. Status gelasticus after temporal lobectomy: ictal FDG-PET findings and the question of dual pathology involving hypothalamic hamartomas. *Epilepsia* 46: 1313–6.

Pascual, J. M., R. L. Van Heertum, D. Wang, et al. 2002. Imaging the metabolic footprint of Glut1 deficiency on the brain. *Annals of Neurology* 52: 458–64.

Pennell, P. B., D. E. Burdette, D. A. Ross, et al. 1999. Muscarinic receptor loss with preservation of cholinergic terminals in mesial temporal sclerosis. *Epilepsia* 40: 38–46.

Pfund, Z., D. C. Chugani, C. Juhasz, et al. 2000. Evidence for coupling between glucose metabolism and glutamate cycling using FDG PET and 1H magnetic resonance spectroscopy in patients with epilepsy. *Journal of Cerebral Blood Flow Metabolism* 20: 871–8.

Phelps, M. E., S-C. Huang, E. J. Hoffman, et al. 1979. Tomographic measurement of local cerebral glucose metabolic rate in humans with (F–18) 2-fluoro–2-deoxy-D-glucose: validation of method. *Annals of Neurology* 6: 371–88.

Radtke, R. A., M. W. Hanson, J. M. Hoffman, et al. 1994. Positron emission tomography: comparison of clinical utility in temporal lobe and extratemporal epilepsy. *Journal of Epilepsy* 7: 27–33.

Radtke, R. A., M. W. Hanson, J. M. Hoffman, et al. 1993. Temporal lobe hypometabolism on PET: predictor of seizure control after temporal lobectomy. *Neurology* 43: 1088–92.

Ramsay, R. E. 1983. Valproate brain tissue kinetics determined by PET. *Neurology* 33 (Suppl 2): 147.

Rausch, R., T. R. Henry, C. M. Ary, et al. 1994. Asymmetric interictal glucose hypometabolism and cognitive performance in epileptic patients. *Archives of Neurology* 51: 139–44.

Reutens, D. C., A. H. Gjedde, and E. Meyer. 1998. Regional lumped constant differences and asymmetry in fluorine–18-FDG uptake in temporal lobe epilepsy. *Journal of Nuclear Medicine* 39: 176–80.

Richardson, M. P., M. J. Koepp, D. J. Brooks, et al. 1996. Benzodiazepine receptors in focal epilepsy with cortical dysgenesis: an 11C-flumazenil PET study. *Annals of Neurology* 40(2): 188–98.

Rusu, V., F. Chassoux, E. Landre, et al. 2005. Dystonic posturing in seizures of mesial temporal origin: electroclinical and metabolic patterns. *Neurology* 65: 1612–9.

Ryvlin, P., S. Bouvard, D. Le Bars, et al. 1999. Transient and falsely lateralizing flumazenil-PET asymmetries in temporal lobe epilepsy. *Neurology* 53(8): 1882–5.

Ryvlin, P., S. Bouvard, D. Le Bars, et al. 1998. Clinical utility of flumazenil-PET versus [18F]fluorodeoxyglucose-PET and MRI in refractory partial epilepsy. A prospective study in 100 patients. *Brain* 121: 2067–81.

Ryvlin, P., L. Cinotti, J. C. Froment, et al. 1991. Metabolic patterns associated with non-specific magnetic resonance imaging abnormalities in temporal lobe epilepsy. *Brain* 114: 2363–83.

Ryvlin, P., F. Mauguiere, M. Sindou, et al. 1995. Interictal cerebral metabolism and epilepsy in cavernous angiomas. *Brain* 118: 677–87.

Ryvlin, P., B. Philippon, L. Cinotti, et al. 1992. Functional neuroimaging strategy in temporal lobe epilepsy: a comparative study of ^{18}FDG-PET and ^{99m}Tc-HMPAO-SPECT. *Annals of Neurology* 31: 650–6.

Sackellares, J. C., G. J. Siegel, B. W. Abou-Khalil, et al. 1990. Differences between lateral and mesial temporal metabolism interictally in epilepsy of mesial temporal origin. *Neurology* 40: 1420–6.

Sadzot, B., R. Debets, P. Maguet, et al. 1992. Regional brain glucose metabolism in patients with complex partial seizures investigated by intracranial EEG. *Epilepsy Research* 12: 121–9.

Salanova, V., O. Markand, R. Worth, et al. 1998. FDG-PET and MRI in temporal lobe epilepsy: relationship to febrile seizures, hippocampal sclerosis and outcome. *Acta Neurologica Scandinavica* 97: 146–53.

Salanova, V., O. Markand, and R. Worth. 2001. Focal functional deficits in temporal lobe epilepsy on PET scans and the intracarotid amobarbital procedure: comparison of patients with unitemporal epilepsy with those requiring intracranial recordings. *Epilepsia* 42: 198–203.

Salzberg, M., T. Taher, M. Davie, et al. 2006. Depression in temporal lobe epilepsy surgery patients: an FDG-PET study. *Epilepsia* 47: 2125–30.

Savic, I., L. Altshuler, L. Baxter, et al. 1997. Pattern of interictal hypometabolism in PET scans with fluorodeoxyglucose F 18 reflects prior seizure types in patients with mesial temporal lobe seizures. *Archives of Neurology* 54: 129–36.

Savic, I., P. Lindstrom, B. Gulyas, et al. 2004. Limbic reductions of 5-HT1A receptor binding in human temporal lobe epilepsy. *Neurology* 62: 1343–51.

Savic, I., A. Persson, P. Roland, et al. 1988. In-vivo demonstration of reduced benzodiazepine receptor binding in human epileptic foci. *Lancet* 8616: 863–6.

Schlemmer, H. P., B. J. Pichler, M. Schmand, et al. 2008. Simultaneous MR/PET imaging of the human brain: feasibility study. *Radiology* 248: 1028–35.

Seitz, R. J., S. Piel, S. Arnold, et al. 1996. Cerebellar hypometabolism in focal epilepsy is related to age of onset and drug intoxication. *Epilepsia* 37: 1194–9.

So, E. L., T. J. O'Brien, B. H. Brinkmann, et al. 2000. The EEG evaluation of single photon emission computed tomography abnormalities in epilepsy. *Journal of Clinical Neurophysiology* 17: 10–28.

Spanaki, M. V., L. Kopylev, C. DeCarli, et al. 2000. Postoperative changes in cerebral metabolism in temporal lobe epilepsy. *Archives of Neurology* 57: 1447–52.

Spencer, S. S., and R. E. D. Bautista. 2000. Functional neuroimaging in localization of the ictal onset zone. In T. R. Henry, S. F. Berkovic, and J. S. Duncan, eds. *Functional imaging in the epilepsies.* Philadelphia: Lippincott Williams & Wilkins, 285–96.

Sperling, M. R., A. Alavi, M. Reivich, et al. 1995. False lateralization of temporal lobe epilepsy with FDG positron emission tomography. *Epilepsia* 36: 722–7.

Sperling, M. R., R. C. Gur, A. Alavi, et al. 1990. Subcortical metabolic alterations in partial epilepsy. *Epilepsia* 31: 145–55.

Stefan, H., G. Pawlik, H. G. Bocher-Schwarz, et al. 1987. Functional and morphological abnormalities in temporal lobe epilepsy: a comparison of interictal and ictal EEG, CT, MRI, SPECT and PET. *Journal of Neurology* 234: 377–84.

Swartz, B. E., U. Tomiyasu, A. V. Delgado-Escueta, et al. 1992. Neuroimaging in temporal lobe epilepsy: test sensitivity and relationships to pathology and post-surgical outcome. *Epilepsia* 33: 624–34.

Szelies, B., G. Weber-Luxenburger, G. Pawlik, et al. 1996. MRI-guided flumazenil- and FDG-PET in temporal lobe epilepsy. *Neuroimage* 3(2): 109–18.

Tai, Y. C., H. Wu, D. Pal, et al. 2008. Virtual-pinhole PET. *Journal of Nuclear Medicine* 49: 471–9.

Takaya, S., T. Hanakawa, K. Hashikawa, et al. 2006. Prefrontal hypofunction in patients with intractable mesial temporal lobe epilepsy. *Neurology* 67: 1674–6.

Theodore, W. H., D. Bairamian, M. E. Newmark, et al. 1986a. Effect of phenytoin on human cerebral glucose metabolism. *Journal of Cerebral Blood Flow Metabolism* 6: 315–20.

Theodore, W. H., E. Bromfield, and L. Onorati. 1989. The effect of carbamazepine on cerebral glucose metabolism. *Annals of Neurology* 25: 516–20.

Theodore, W. H., R. Carson, P. Andreasen, et al. 1992a. PET imaging of opiate receptor binding in human epilepsy using [^{18}F]cyclofoxy. *Epilepsy Research* 13: 129–39.

Theodore, W. H., G. DiChiro, R. Margolin, et al. 1986b. Barbiturates reduce human cerebral glucose metabolism. *Neurology* 36: 60–4.

Theodore, W. H., D. Fishbein, M. Deitz, et al. 1987a. Complex partial seizures: cerebellar metabolism. *Epilepsia* 28: 319–23.

Theodore, W. H., D. Fishbein, R. Dubinsky. 1988. Patterns of cerebral glucose metabolism in patients with partial seizures. *Neurology* 38: 1201–6.

Theodore, W. H., W. D. Gaillard, C. DeCarli, et al. 2001. Hippocampal volume and glucose metabolism in temporal lobe epileptic foci. *Epilepsia* 42: 130–2.

Theodore, W. H., G. Giovacchini, R. Bonwetsch, et al. 2006. The effect of antiepileptic drugs on 5-HT-receptor binding measured by positron emission tomography. *Epilepsia* 47: 499–503.

Theodore, W. H., D. Katz, C. Kufta, et al. 1990. Pathology of temporal lobe foci: correlation with CT, MRI and PET. *Neurology* 40: 797–803.

Theodore, W. H., K. Kelley, M. T. Toczek, et al. 2004. Epilepsy duration, febrile seizures, and cerebral glucose metabolism. *Epilepsia* 45: 276–9.

Theodore, W. H., S. Sato, C. Kufta, et al. 1992b. Temporal lobectomy for uncontrolled seizures: the role of positron emission tomography. *Annals of Neurology* 32: 789–94.

Theodore, W. H., S. Sato, C. V. Kufta, et al. 1997. FDG-positron emission tomography and invasive EEG: seizure focus detection and surgical outcome. *Epilepsia* 38: 81–6.

Theodore, W. H. 1988. Antiepileptic drugs and cerebral glucose metabolism. *Epilepsia* 29(Suppl 2): S48–S55.

Theodore, W. H., R. Dorwart, M. Holmes, et al. 1986. Neuroimaging in refractory partial seizures: comparison of PET, CT, and MRI. *Neurology* 36: 750–9.

Theodore, W. H., M. E. Newmark, S. Sato, et al. 1983. [^{18}F] Fluorodeoxyglucose positron emission tomography in refractory complex partial seizures. *Annals of Neurology* 14: 429–37.

Toczek, M. T., R. E. Carson, L. Lang, et al. 2003. PET imaging of 5-HT1A receptor binding in patients with temporal lobe epilepsy. *Neurology* 60: 749–56.

Turkheimer, F. E., N. Boussion, A. N. Anderson, et al. 2008. PET image denoising using a synergistic multiresolution analysis of structural (MRI/CT) and functional datasets. *Journal of Nuclear Medicine* 49: 657–66.

Uijl, S. G., F. S. Leijten, J. B. Arends, et al. 2007. The added value of [18F]-fluoro-D-deoxyglucose positron emission tomography in screening for temporal lobe epilepsy surgery. *Epilepsia* 48: 2121–9.

Valk, P. E., K. D. Laxer, N. M. Barbero, et al. 1993. High-resolution (2.6-mm) PET in partial complex epilepsy associated with mesial temporal sclerosis. *Radiology* 186: 55–8.

Van Bogaert, P., N. Massager, P. Tugendhaft, et al. 2000. Statistical parametric mapping of regional glucose metabolism in mesial temporal lobe epilepsy. *Neuroimage* 12: 129–38.

Vielhaber, S., J. H. Von Oertzen, A. F. Kudin, et al. 2003. Correlation of hippocampal glucose oxidation capacity and interictal FDG-PET in temporal lobe epilepsy. *Epilepsia* 44: 193–9.

Vinton, A. B., R. Carne, R. J. Hicks, et al. 2007. The extent of resection of FDG-PET hypometabolism relates to outcome of temporal lobectomy. *Brain* 130: 548–60.

Volkow, N. D., G. J. Wang, R. Hitzemann, et al. 1995. Depression of thalamic metabolism by lorazepam is associated with sleepiness. *Neuropsychopharmacology* 12: 123–32.

Votaw, J. R. 2000. PET image acquisition and analysis. In T. R. Henry, S. F. Berkovic, and J. S. Duncan, eds. *Functional imaging in the epilepsies.* Philadelphia: Lippincott Williams & Wilkins, 69–86.

Votaw, J. R. 1995. Physics of PET. *Radiographics* 15: 1179–90.

Votaw, J. R., T. L. Faber, T. R. Henry, et al. 1999. A confrontational naming task produces congruent increases and decreases in PET and MRI. *Neuroimage* 10: 347–56.

Wahl, R. L., ed. 2009. *Principles and practice of PET and PET/CT,* 2nd ed. Philadelphia: Lippincott Williams & Wilkins.

Wang, G. J., N. D. Volkow, J. Overall, et al. 1996. Reproducibility of regional brain metabolic responses to lorazepam. *Journal of Nuclear Medicine* 37: 1609–13.

Werhahn, K. J., C. Landvogt, S. Klimpe, et al. 2006. Decreased dopamine D2/D3-receptor binding in temporal lobe epilepsy: an [^{18}F]fallypride PET study. *Epilepsia* 47: 1392–6.

Willmann, O., R. Wennberg, T. May, et al. 2007. The contribution of 18F-FDG PET in preoperative epilepsy surgery evaluation for patients with temporal lobe epilepsy. A meta-analysis. *Seizure* 16: 509–20.

Won, H. J., K. H. Chang, J. E. Cheon, et al. 1999. Comparison of MR imaging with PET and ictal SPECT in 118 patients with intractable epilepsy. *American Journal of Neuroradiology* 20: 593–9.

Wong, C. Y., E. B. Geller, E. Q. Chen, et al. 1996. Outcome of temporal lobe epilepsy surgery predicted by statistical parametric PET imaging. *Journal of Nuclear Medicine* 37: 1094–100.

Witte, O. W., C. Bruehl, G. Schlaug, et al. 1994. Dynamic changes of focal hypometabolism in relation to epileptic activity. *Journal of Neurologic Science* 124: 188–97.

Yun, C. H., S. K. Lee, S. Y. Lee, et al. 2006. Prognostic factors in neocortical epilepsy surgery: multivariate analysis. *Epilepsia* 47: 574–9.

Zubal, I. G., R. A. Avery, R. Stokking, et al. 2000. Ratio-images calculated from interictal positron emission tomography and single-photon emission computed tomography for quantification of the uncoupling of brain metabolism and perfusion in epilepsy. *Epilepsia* 41: 1560–6.

Chapter 9

POSITRON EMISSION TOMOGRAPHY: GLUCOSE METABOLISM IN EXTRATEMPORAL LOBE EPILEPSY

Csaba Juhász and Harry T. Chugani

The most common clinical application of positron emission tomography (PET) with 2-deoxy–2-[^{18}F]fluoro-D-glucose (FDG) in epilepsy is to localize epileptic foci when structural imaging shows no focal lesion. In adult patients and in older children, the application of FDG PET in temporal lobe epilepsy has become routine in some epilepsy surgery centers. The role of FDG PET in temporal lobe epilepsy has been discussed in detail in the preceding chapter. The present chapter focuses on a more challenging group of patients, with extratemporal lobe epilepsy, where surgical success is not nearly as good as in temporal lobe epilepsy, and how FDG PET may contribute to improved surgical outcome.

LOCALIZING VALUE OF FDG PET IN EXTRATEMPORAL LOBE EPILEPSY

Defining the epileptic focus or epileptogenic region in non-lesional cases of extratemporal lobe epilepsy is particularly challenging because of the high interindividual variability in the site and extent of the foci. Unlike in temporal lobe epilepsy, where "standard" resections have been developed, there is no standard surgical procedure for extratemporal lobe epilepsy. Rather, the type and extent of resection are typically tailored to the individual patient and based on data from scalp electroencephalogram (EEG), intracranial EEG (icEEG), seizure semiology, and various neuroimaging modalities. In addition, neocortical epileptic foci are commonly located adjacent to or may even involve eloquent cortex (sensorimotor, language, visual), and therefore exact delineation of the borders of epileptogenic cortex is of paramount clinical importance prior to surgery.

Early PET studies in extratemporal lobe epilepsy, employing mostly low-resolution PET scanners, showed hypometabolism in structural lesions visualized by CT and/or MRI, but also noted hypometabolism in a subgroup of patients with normal structural imaging (Henry et al. 1991; Swartz et al. 1989, 1990). For example, one study of 22 patients with suspected frontal lobe epilepsy revealed focal hypometabolism in about two thirds of the patients, while both CT and MRI were localizing in less than half of the cases (Swartz et al. 1989). These early studies also demonstrated a good correlation between the general area of cortical glucose hypometabolism and electroclinical localization of epileptic foci. Subsequent PET studies in frontal lobe epilepsy also found a good correspondence between the location of frontal hypometabolism and the presumed region of seizure onset, as assessed by analysis of seizure semiology and scalp EEG (da Silva et al. 1997; Schlaug et al. 1997). However, hypometabolic areas varied in their extent from being quite focal in some cases to multilobar and even subcortical involvement in others (Figs. 9.1 and 9.2). In a study of a large, unselected epilepsy patient population (n = 462, one of the largest PET cohorts reported thus far), which included both surgical and nonsurgical subgroups, Swartz et al. (2002) reported PET abnormalities to be more common in the

surgical than in the nonsurgical group. In this large series, only 32% of patients with normal MRI showed focal PET abnormalities, and PET was useful (with >90% accuracy) in identifying patients with non-epileptic seizures and primary generalized epilepsies: these patients showed no focal metabolic abnormalities. Most other series included exclusively surgical populations, and the localizing value of FDG PET, usually assessed as PET findings concordant with the epileptic focus (defined by ictal EEG or surgical resection site), exceeded 50% in most reports; however, sensitivity varied widely across studies.

In Table 9.1, PET findings from 11 studies on patients with extratemporal lobe epilepsy and normal MRI are summarized (only studies with at least 10 subjects are included). In several studies, patients with temporal and extratemporal lobe seizure foci were combined and these groups were not evaluated separately. As the table demonstrates, the presence of localized

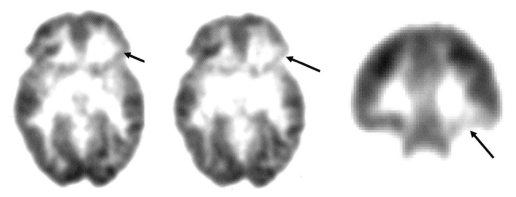

Figure 9.1 A very focal region of cortical glucose hypometabolism (*arrows*) affecting the left inferior frontal cortex in a 6-year-old girl with intractable frontal lobe epilepsy. MRI was normal. The child became and remained seizure-free for more than 2 years after left inferior frontal resection. Pathology showed focal cortical dysplasia.

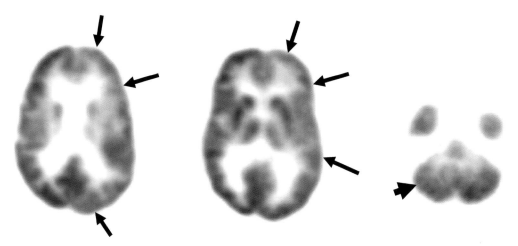

Figure 9.2 Left hemispheric neocortical epilepsy with extensive multilobar cortical hypometabolism (*arrows*). Also note hypometabolism in the ipsilateral thalamus and contralateral cerebellum (*arrowhead*); this latter is most common in frontal lobe foci due to diaschisis resulting from disruption of the fronto-ponto-cerebellar pathways.

Table 9.1 Summary of Studies Evaluating the Localization Value of FDG PET in Non-lesional (Normal MRI) Predominantly Extratemporal Lobe Epilepsy (ETLE)

Author	Journal	Year	Epilepsy Type Included	Outcome Measure	Analytic Approach	No. of Patients with PET	PET Correctly localizing	% PET
Kurian	*Epileptic Disorders*	2007	TLE+ETLE	Resection site	Visual	49	38	78%
Chapman	*Journal of Neurology Neurosurgery & Psychiatry*	2005	TLE+ETLE	Resection site	Visual	24	16	67%
Lee	*Annals of Neurology*	2005	ETLE	Resection site	Obj. [SPM]	79	35	44%
Hader	*Journal of Neurosurgery*	2004	TLE+ETLE (all had FCD)	Resection site	Visual	13	10	77%
Juhasz	*Neurology*	2003	ETLE	Ictal EEG	Obj. [asymm]	27	25	93%
Hong	*Seizure*	2002a	ETLE	Ictal EEG/res.	Visual	28	12	43%
Kim	*Child's Nervous System*	2000	TLE+ETLE	Ictal EEG	Visual	30	26	87%
da Silva	*Epilepsia*	1997	FLE	Ictal EEG	Obj. [asymm]	13	8	62%
Snead	*Pediatric Neurology*	1996	TLE+ETLE	EEG	Visual	14	5	36%
Fois	*Child's Nervous System*	1995	TLE+ETLE	EEG	Visual	14	12	86%
Gaillard	*Epilepsy Research*	1995	TLE+ETLE	Ictal EEG	Obj. [asymm]	13	9	69%
Total						**276**	**196**	**71%**

ETLE = extratemporal lobe epilepsy; TLE = temporal lobe epilepsy; FLE = frontal lobe epilepsy; FCD = focal cortical dysplasia; obj. = objective (analysis); asymm = asymmetry (-based analysis); SPM = statistical parametric mapping; res. = resection site. Seven of the 11 studies also included TLE patients.

FDG PET abnormalities, concordant with ictal EEG or resection site, varied between 36% and 93% (overall 71% when all studies were combined). This wide range reflects interstudy differences in patient selection bias, methods of PET image analysis, and use of different outcome measures. Interestingly, the sensitivity of FDG PET remains very similar regardless of whether or not studies including lesional cases are also considered. This by itself suggests that FDG PET does not simply detect an underlying MRI-detectable lesion; rather, FDG PET can be just as sensitive in identifying potentially epileptogenic cortical abnormalities in patients with non-localizing MRI. Indeed, in many of these cases, histologic examination of resected tissues revealed small cortical dysplasias or microdysgenesis as the pathologic substrate underlying the PET abnormality. Recent studies have demonstrated that FDG PET could indeed detect 70% to 90% of cortical dysplasias, although type II cortical dysplasia (often abnormal on MRI) shows more severe hypometabolism than mild type I cortical dysplasia (Lerner et al. 2009; Salamon et al. 2008) (Fig. 9.3). Thus, PET provides localizing information complementary to MRI findings in extratemporal lobe epilepsies. This is also reflected by studies demonstrating that correct seizure focus localization by FDG PET is an independent predictor of seizure-free outcome after resective epilepsy surgery (see section below on epilepsy surgery outcome).

SIGNIFICANCE OF EXTRATEMPORAL LOBE *HYPER*METABOLISM

Although focal cortical hypometabolism is the most commonly observed interictal finding when FDG PET is used for presurgical localization of epileptic foci, occasionally focal cortical *hyper*metabolism is seen and needs to be interpreted with caution. One potential reason for focal increase of FDG uptake is the presence of a malformation of cortical development. This is most apparent in the case of subcortical or periventricular heterotopias, when the heterotopic tissue is detected as a *relatively* hypermetabolic region surrounded by white matter, which normally shows very low FDG uptake (Bairamian et al. 1985; Conrad et al. 2005; Lee et al. 1994) (Fig. 9.4). These malformations demonstrate FDG uptake similar to or lower than that of normal cortex, while the cortex overlying the heterotopia is often hypometabolic, presumably due to the decreased number of neurons and/or synapses as a result of incomplete neuronal migration. True hypermetabolism (i.e., glucose uptake values *above* normal cortical levels) has been also reported in a few cases with heterotopias and focal cortical dysplasia (Poduri et al. 2007); in two of these cases, increased metabolism could not readily be explained by ictal scan or frequent interictal spiking and, therefore, may be related to other factors intrinsic to the heterotopia, such as its cytoarchitecture or physiologic characteristics. In a

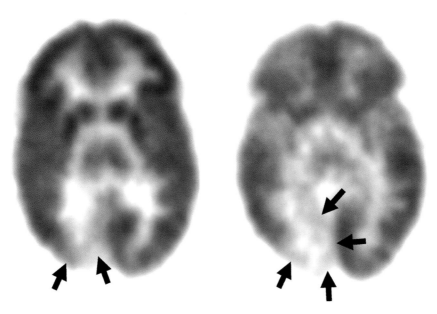

Figure 9.3 Severe right occipital hypometabolism (indicated by arrows) in a 9-year-old boy with intractable epilepsy. MRI showed abnormal signal intensity and blurred gray–white matter interface in the same region; histology of the resected specimen demonstrated type II(A) cortical dysplasia.

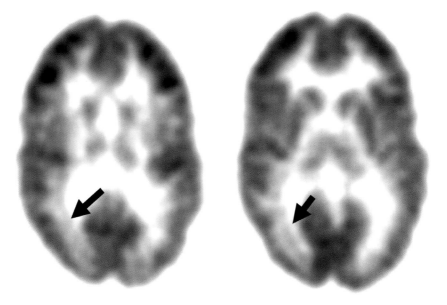

Figure 9.4 FDG PET showing subcortical band heterotopia (*arrows*) in the right temporal-occipital white matter in a 15-year-old boy with intractable epilepsy. The heterotopic band has higher glucose uptake than the adjacent white matter but lower uptake than the cortex.

third case, a 10-month-old boy with infantile spasms, focal hypermetabolism was associated with frequent interictal spiking, and this may have accounted for focally increased metabolism. In fact, focal cortical increase of glucose uptake on PET was first reported in a small group of children with infantile spasms and, in these patients, cortical hypermetabolism appeared in conjunction with activation of the lenticular nuclei (Chugani et al. 1992, see also Chapter 10 on pediatric epilepsy syndromes). Statistically, however, cortical hypermetabolism is most likely to indicate an ictal FDG

PET scan, which is almost always incidental (Chugani et al. 1994); planned ictal FDG PET is feasible only in rare cases where partial seizures, especially simple partial seizures, are very frequent (Meltzer et al. 2000). This problem is not unique to PET and is also encountered when contemplating ictal studies using functional MRI (Chapter 5), magnetic source imaging (Chapter 7), and, to some extent, ictal SPECT (Chapter 14). The pattern of ictal PET hypermetabolism due to complex partial seizures may be difficult to interpret due to metabolic changes seen also at various sites of seizure propagation, including both cortical and subcortical structures. On the other hand, brief, single seizures may not have a significant impact on the overall FDG tracer uptake (which is summed over 45 minutes) and therefore may not induce a detectable hypermetabolism on the PET images (Barrington et al. 1998).

Interictal cortical hypermetabolism can be seen occasionally as a result of active spiking during the FDG uptake period (0 to 40 minutes after injection) even without a clinical seizure, or in the immediate postictal period (Bittar et al. 1999; Chugani et al. 1994). Interictal hypermetabolism can be suspected when a cortical region appears as a focal area clearly different from the surrounding cortex, and shows increased FDG uptake relative to most cortical and subcortical structures, with the exception, perhaps, of the primary visual cortex, which normally has high uptake. This can be confirmed when there is concordance between the cortical area of increased uptake and the localization of frequent spiking recorded on scalp EEG during the FDG uptake period; often the hypermetabolic focus may be surrounded by hypometabolic cortex (Fig. 9.5). Such cases argue for the need to record the EEG during FDG tracer uptake, especially in patients whose EEGs are known to show active epileptiform activity, commonly the case in children. In some instances, a mild hypometabolism may no longer be apparent (i.e., becomes normalized) when there is repetitive spiking in the seizure focus during the FDG uptake. In such cases, the localizing value of the PET scan becomes diminished and, if such a false negative is suspected based on the EEG and seizure semiology, the PET should be repeated in the hope of acquiring a true interictal metabolic pattern.

Statistically, however, actively spiking cortex is more likely to show hypometabolism, which is far more common than hypermetabolism, perhaps due to the relatively long uptake period of FDG (Fig. 9.6). In addition, from a mechanistic perspective, the slow wave

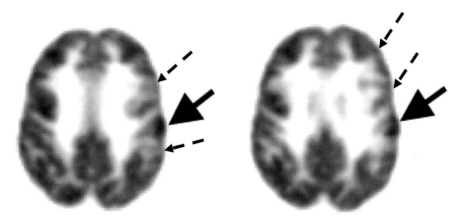

Figure 9.5 Interictal cortical hypermetabolism associated with frequent spiking on EEG recorded during the FDG uptake period. The EEG showed frequent spiking in the left central region, most pronounced in the left posterior frontal cortex where intense glucose uptake (*solid arrow*) was seen on the PET images. Note also the hypometabolism (*dotted arrows*) surrounding the focus of hypermetabolism.

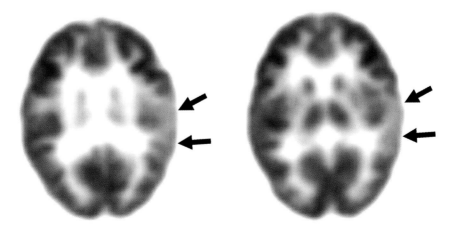

Figure 9.6 Focal cortical hypometabolism in the left central and superior temporal region (*arrows*) associated with interictal left-sided spiking and intermittent slowing recorded on scalp EEG during the FDG uptake period. Subsequent electrocorticography confirmed interictal spiking in the same cortical region.

components following spikes are more relevant to the overall pattern of hypometabolism than the spikes themselves, which contribute to hypermetabolism (Hong et al. 2002b; Nishida et al. 2008). Indeed, in a study that directly compared glucose PET metabolism with intracranial EEG data obtained from non-lesional epileptogenic cortex, our group found that spike frequency is negatively correlated with relative FDG uptake in patients with interictal epileptiform discharges consisting of a spike followed by a slow (delta) wave (Nishida et al. 2008). In contrast, high spike frequency was associated with higher glucose metabolism when the discharges were predominantly spike bursts without much of a slow wave component. This study also suggested that interictal FDG uptake, in general, is related more to high-frequency gamma oscillations (>32 Hz), arising from physiologic or epileptiform neuronal activity, than to interictal epileptiform discharges of low-frequency range. In another study, interictal regional slow wave activity on scalp EEG was strongly related to focal hypometabolism in the temporal neocortex (Koutroumanidis et al. 1998). Nevertheless, interictal hypermetabolism should at the very least always be considered in cases when frequent interictal spiking is seen on EEG during the FDG uptake period to avoid false lateralization.

LOCALIZATION VALUE OF FDG PET IN LESIONAL EPILEPSY

In patients with partial epilepsy associated with an MRI-visible lesion, the epileptogenic cortex is often *adjacent* to the lesion and normal-appearing on MRI (Engel 1993; Pilcher et al. 1993; Tran et al. 1997). Presurgical identification of the location and extent of such perilesional epileptic cortex is important, particularly when it lies in the vicinity of eloquent cortical areas, where precise tailoring of the resection is required to preserve important functions while removing as much epileptogenic tissue as possible. Several PET studies have demonstrated that hypometabolic areas commonly extend beyond the anatomical lesion visualized by MRI, thus presumably encompassing some of the perilesional epileptic cortical regions (Chassoux et al. 2008; Juhasz et al. 2000a; Ryvlin et al. 1995). Our studies with PET/MRI co-registration and objective delineation of hypometabolic regions on the three-dimensional brain surface have suggested that hypometabolic cortical areas may include the lesion, some perilesional epileptic cortex, as well as wider areas that represent a functionally altered zone but do not generate seizures (Juhasz et al. 2000a). Interestingly, extensive perilesional hypometabolism was seen in patients with large seizure number, suggesting that some of this hypometabolism may be related to frequent seizures. It is likely that perilesional hypometabolism may expand progressively as a result of chronic epilepsy; however, this should be confirmed with longitudinal studies. Further studies have found that PET scanning of GABA$_A$ receptor binding using ^{11}C-flumazenil (see Chapter 11) shows greater specificity than FDG PET for perilesional cortex with interictal spiking (Juhasz et al. 2000a). The perilesional epileptogenic cortex shows decreased ^{11}C-flumazenil binding.

In addition to perilesional hypometabolism, FDG PET may also show hypometabolic regions *remote* from the epileptogenic lesional area. These findings are consistent with previous studies using intracranial electrocorticography, which have demonstrated the existence of remote spiking areas, noncontiguous with a lesion (Awad et al. 1991). In our series of 17 patients with lesional epilepsy (including children and adults with temporal or extratemporal epileptic foci), 8 showed at least one area of remote hypometabolism in the hemisphere ipsilateral to the lesion (Juhasz et al. 2000a). These regions did not appear to be random, but were in cortical areas with known cortico-cortical connections to the primary epileptic focus. On intracranial electrocorticography, some of these remote areas were indeed involved in rapid seizure propagation or showed interictal spiking. Whether these remote hypometabolic areas represent secondary epileptic foci in various stages of formation needs to be further investigated.

LOCALIZING VALUE OF SUBCORTICAL AND CEREBELLAR METABOLIC ABNORMALITIES

Although PET evaluation in patients with intractable partial epilepsies is aimed at detecting cortical abnormalities, additional focal PET abnormalities in subcortical structures or cerebellum may also be observed. Such abnormalities are presumably due to involvement of these structures in seizure propagation or indicate remote metabolic effects, referred to as *diaschisis*, resulting from an acute or chronic cerebral injury or lesion. Although the term *diaschisis* implies functional reversibility following functional deafferentation, the remotely affected structures subsequently may undergo permanent damage due to degeneration leading to atrophy (e.g., as in postoperative atrophy of subcortical structures after temporal lobectomy) (Shedlack et al. 1994). Therefore, the term *diaschisis* should be reserved for instances when a remote metabolic effect, such as hypometabolism (or hypoperfusion), is observed while no structural damage (such as atrophy) at the remote site is seen on MRI. Since diaschisis occurs in remote brain regions synaptically connected to the cortical area encompassing the epileptogenic lesion or a non-lesional epileptic focus, diaschisis may provide important clues for localization of the primary epileptic focus (e.g., when the area of diaschisis is better visualized on the images than the epileptic focus itself).

The most commonly seen and reported diaschisis phenomenon is crossed cerebellar diaschisis (see example in Fig. 9.2), which is a common finding on brain perfusion studies in patients with unilateral hemispheric strokes (Liu et al. 2007; Meneghetti et al. 1984). In the context of partial epilepsy and FDG PET, crossed cerebellar diaschisis, manifested by crossed cerebellar hypometabolism, is most commonly seen in patients with frontal lobe epileptic foci (Savic et al. 1996). It is assumed that these contralateral cerebellar metabolic changes are due to the disruption of crossed connections between the frontal lobe and contralateral cerebellum (fronto-ponto-cerebellar connections). In contrast, connections between medial temporal structures and cerebellum are less abundant, with some ipsilateral predominance (Ito 1984). Therefore, temporal lobe epilepsy is not accompanied by crossed cerebellar diaschisis (Savic et al. 1996), although bilateral cerebellar hypometabolism has been described (Theodore et al. 1987); however, this could have been due to chronic phenytoin effects. Thus, in the presence of unilateral cerebellar hypometabolism the contralateral frontal lobe should be carefully evaluated for focal metabolic abnormalities. Furthermore, when unilateral cerebellar hypometabolism is encountered in patients with apparent temporal lobe epilepsy, a frontal-temporal epileptic focus should be considered.

Ipsilateral decrease of glucose metabolism in the thalamus is often seen in patients with temporal lobe epilepsy (Benedek et al. 2004; Henry et al.; Sperling et al. 1990), but this is not a specific finding, since the thalamus is also widely connected with other lobes. Indeed, ipsilateral thalamic hypometabolism can be seen also in frontal lobe epilepsy (Benedek et al. 2004). However, focal hypometabolism confined to the dorsal thalamus (dorsal-medial nucleus) is more specific and a valuable sign for medial temporal lobe epilepsy (Juhasz et al. 1999), since medial temporal structures are strongly connected to this thalamic nucleus. Occasionally, hypometabolism in the dorsal-medial thalamic nucleus may be the only finding on FDG PET; in such cases, there is often medial temporal involvement, but the extent of the epileptogenic region cannot be predicted on this finding alone. Interestingly, patients with longstanding temporal or frontal lobe epilepsy, particularly those with secondary generalization, show more severe thalamic hypometabolism (Benedek et al. 2004), suggesting progressive involvement of thalamus as a result of chronic seizures. Furthermore, in patients with chronic, intractable

epilepsy, the thalamus may show volume loss, suggesting degeneration (Juhasz et al. 1999). Although this is more often ipsilateral to the epileptic focus, recent objective volumetric and morphometric studies have demonstrated *bilateral* thalamic volume loss in unilateral temporal lobe epilepsy (McDonald et al. 2008; Seidenberg et al. 2008). Thalamic atrophy in chronic temporal lobe epilepsy may contribute to cognitive dysfunction (Seidenberg et al. 2008). Importantly, the side of thalamic hypometabolism appears to be a strong predictor of temporal lobe epilepsy surgery outcome: temporal lobectomy contralateral to thalamic hypometabolism has a high likelihood of seizures continuing after surgery (Newberg et al. 2000). No similar data are available for extratemporal epilepsies, which have been much less studied than temporal lobe epilepsy in terms of remote metabolic or volume changes. However, a few studies evaluating subcortical volume changes in extratemporal lobe epilepsies found no significant thalamic volume loss (Gärtner et al. 2004; Natsume et al. 2003).

In addition to cerebellum and thalamus, subcortical hypometabolism can be seen occasionally in the putamen, usually ipsilateral to temporal lobe epileptic foci, and is associated with contralateral dystonic posturing during seizures (Dupont et al. 1998; Lee et al. 2009; Rusu et al. 2005). This association is reviewed in more detail in Chapter 8. However, hypometabolism of putamen is not typically seen in patients with extratemporal lobe epilepsy.

IS CORTICAL HYPOMETABOLISM A CONSEQUENCE OF CHRONIC EPILEPSY?

Longitudinal FDG PET studies in children with both lesional and non-lesional partial epilepsy have demonstrated that an enlargement or expansion of the cortical area showing glucose hypometabolism often occurs in patients with persistent seizures (Benedek et al. 2006; Juhasz et al. 2007). In contrast, patients with no or very few seizures may show no change between scans or even normalization of the hypometabolic area. These findings strongly support the notion that at least one contributory factor for cortical hypometabolism is the presence of chronic seizures and that the hypometabolism actually can be reversible if the seizures come under control. This is also consistent with FDG PET findings of patients with new-onset focal epilepsy, who have a low incidence (25% or less) of focal hypometabolism (Gaillard et al. 2002, 2007), as opposed to patients with chronic "medically controlled" epilepsy (48% abnormal PET; Weitemeyer et al. 2005) and those with chronic *intractable* epilepsy, where focal hypometabolism is present in the majority of cases (see details above). The surgical implications of these findings are clear: FDG PET findings cannot be used in isolation to make a case for surgical treatment but require careful correlation with electrophysiologic and clinical (seizure semiology) data as well as other imaging findings to decide optimal tailoring of extratemporal lobe resections; this is particularly true in patients with longstanding epilepsy who have developed extensive areas of cortical hypometabolism. Complete removal of the primary epileptic focus in fact can result in postsurgical recovery of hypometabolic neocortex in remote projection areas of the affected hemisphere. This has been shown mostly in patients with temporal lobe epilepsy, who underwent temporal lobectomy (Akimura et al. 1999; Joo et al. 2005; Spanaki et al. 2000) or selective amygdalo-hippocampectomy (Takaya et al. 2009), where remote frontal projection areas appear to recover most commonly; however, it is likely that the same principle applies to extratemporal lobe epilepsies. In fact, as alluded to above, reversal of hypometabolic regions to normal metabolism has been demonstrated following successful control of previously uncontrolled seizures by antiepileptic drugs in human neocortical epilepsy (Benedek et al. 2006; Matheja et al. 2000).

SIGNIFICANCE OF ABNORMAL FDG PET FOR EXTRATEMPORAL EPILEPSY SURGERY OUTCOME

The most useful clinical studies to evaluate the contribution of FDG PET in extratemporal lobe epilepsy surgery would include both EEG and multimodal imaging techniques (such as MRI, PET, SPECT, magnetic source imaging) to identify the epileptic focus prior to surgery. In such studies, multivariate analyses are able to determine if each modality provides independent information to predict seizure-free outcome; however, only large series can have adequate statistical power to obtain meaningful results, and such series are difficult to gather from single centers. Various approaches to multimodality neuroimaging in epilepsy are discussed in Chapter 15. In this section, we will limit the discussion to data directly relevant for FDG PET in extratemporal lobe epilepsy.

In one of the largest neocortical epilepsy surgery series to date, Yun et al. (2006) reported on the results of FDG PET in 179 patients, where PET images were analyzed both visually and by statistical parametric mapping (SPM), and the surgical resection site was used as the gold standard for comparing location of epileptic foci to PET findings. In this series, FDG PET abnormalities concordant with the site of surgical resection was an independent predictor of seizure-free outcome, together with a focal lesion on MRI and localized ictal onset on EEG. Using a similar analytic approach, Lee et al. (2005) reported on FDG PET findings in 79 patients with neocortical epilepsy and non-localizing MRI. Although the correct localizing rate of the epileptic focus was relatively low in this study (44%, one of the lowest recently reported), localizing FDG PET, along with interictal EEG, predicted seizure-free outcome. Both of these latter studies employed an objective, voxel-by-voxel analytic approach (SPM), combined with visual assessment, to identify focal hypometabolism. It has been reported previously that SPM results showed similar concordance with the results of ictal EEG as compared to visual assessment and/or a region of interest (ROI) approach (Kim et al. 2002; Plotkin et al. 2003). Nevertheless, SPM includes transformation of native images to a common image template as well as image smoothing, and this invariably leads to loss of spatial resolution; thus, small focal regions with abnormal metabolism may remain undetected with this technique. Each analytic approach has its own advantages and limitations, and results of different studies are often difficult to compare due to different analytic approaches and variable designs.

To further address this difficult issue, in a recent study we compared the sensitivity and specificity of PET abnormalities identified by visual assessment versus SPM in children who underwent resective epilepsy surgery following FDG PET (Kumar et al. 2009). The findings showed complementary contributions from the visual and objective analytic approaches. SPM was most useful to identify difficult-to-detect medial frontal epileptogenic cortex, which was occasionally missed by visual evaluation. Epileptic foci in the medial frontal (and also medial parietal) cortex are often associated with generalized epileptiform activity on scalp EEG due to secondary bilateral synchrony, and these foci may be very difficult to lateralize without corresponding imaging abnormalities. Therefore, medial cortex should be carefully evaluated on PET coronal images, particularly in refractory patients with generalized epileptiform activity on EEG and seizure semiology suggestive of partial epilepsy, and intracranial EEG monitoring should include interhemispheric strip electrodes (Fig. 9.7).

A recent, large study (62 patients included), employing a multimodal imaging approach, has confirmed independently that correctly localizing FDG PET is associated with increased odds for a seizure-free surgical outcome (Knowlton et al. 2008). The results also strongly suggested that PET and other imaging modalities (SPECT and magnetic source imaging) often yielded complementary information regarding the epileptogenic cortex to be resected. This issue is still far from settled: even a very recent study (Kim et al. 2009), including 151 patients with interictal FDG PET, showed that localizing PET (along with localizing MRI and scalp EEG) results were not significant

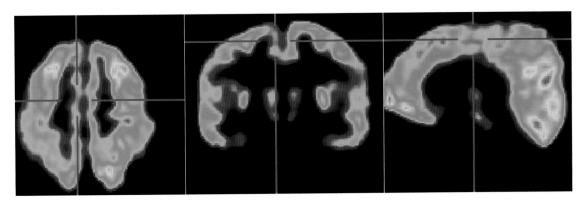

Figure 9.7 Right medial frontal hypometabolism (light blue regions in the crossbars) in a 1-year-old girl with medically refractory infantile spasms. Additional hypometabolic regions were also seen in the right temporal and parietal cortex. Electrocorticography showed frequent spike-and-wave activity in these cortical regions. The child became seizure-free after multifocal resection including portions of the frontal lobe.

predictors of surgical outcome. However, in this latter study, incomplete resection of the epileptogenic area was a strong predictor of poor surgical outcome, and FDG PET can assist in the optimal identification of the epileptogenic region if other imaging modalities fail to localize the epileptic focus.

Overall, the studies discussed above provide evidence that localizing FDG PET, especially when concordant with ictal EEG and/or resection site, represents a clinically valuable prognostic indicator for a seizure-free outcome. However, most of the PET studies in extratemporal lobe epilepsy have not addressed the question of whether *complete* resection of hypometabolic cortex is related to an excellent surgical outcome. Since many previous studies have suggested that cortical hypometabolism can overestimate epileptogenic regions, it should be expected that some patients can achieve seizure freedom even if non-epileptogenic hypometabolic regions remain unresected. This notion is supported by our study of 15 young patients with neocortical, mostly extratemporal lobe epilepsy, where the extent of nonresected cortex with preoperative hypometabolism (defined objectively) was measured by co-registering preoperative FDG PET scans with post-resection MRI images (Juhasz et al. 2001a). In this study, no significant correlations were found between pre- or postoperative (nonresected) cortical hypometabolic cortex and surgical outcome. The findings of this study are at odds with those from a more recent study performed in patients with non-lesional temporal lobe epilepsy (Vinton et al. 2007), which found that the extent of resection of *temporal lobe* hypometabolic region was predictive of surgical outcome. Thus, completeness of resection of hypometabolic cortex may be more important in temporal lobe than in extratemporal lobe epilepsy; in the latter, FDG PET findings are used to identify the general vicinity of the epileptogenic region and guide subdural electrode

placements, but the final tailoring of resection is made based on ictal and interictal intracranial EEG data.

POTENTIAL MECHANISMS OF NECORTICAL HYPOMETABOLISM IN EPILEPSY

After three decades of clinical PET scanning in epilepsy, the exact mechanisms underlying interictal hypometabolism in and around the epileptic neocortex remain elusive. A number of hypotheses have been proposed to explain interictal hypometabolism in epilepsy patients, and some of these are summarized below.

In the brain, both neurons and astrocytes obtain the majority of ATP utilized for cellular processes from glucose oxidation. Glucose is transported through the blood–brain barrier via glucose transporter 1 (GLUT1) (Cornford et al. 1994, 1998), which is expressed in endothelial cells. GLUT1 deficiency syndrome is accompanied by impaired transport of glucose across the blood–brain barrier, leading to developmental delay and refractory seizures (De Vivo et al. 1991, 2002). GLUT1 downregulation in endothelial cells may be implicated in hypometabolism seen in and around seizure foci in subjects who are not GLUT1 deficient. Indeed, Cornford et al. (1999) demonstrated that the PET-detected hypometabolic zone corresponds to a region of decreased glucose transporter activity. Under normal conditions, in the resting awake state, approximately 80% of the energy derived from glucose metabolism goes towards fueling processes related to neuronal firing as well as cycling of GABA and glutamate (Shulman et al. 2004), the two major neurotransmitters that support neurotransmission in about 90% of cortical synapses (Peters & Jones, 1984). GABAergic inhibition, a key mechanism for preventing excessive simultaneous neuronal firing, is costly in terms of metabolic consumption. A potential link between glucose metabolism and epileptogenicity has been proposed via the glycolytic enzyme, glyceraldehyde–3-phosphate dehydrogenase (GADPH) (Laschet et al. 2004; 2007; Pumain & Laschet, 2006; Pumain et al. 2008). GADPH is not only a glycolytic dehydrogenase but also a kinase involved in the endogenous phosphorylation of the alpha1-subunit of the GABA$_A$ receptor, and this is a key mechanism for maintaining GABA$_A$ function. A functional instability of the GABA$_A$ receptor induced by a deficiency in phosphorylation can account for transient GABAergic disinhibition favoring seizure initiation and propagation. In other words, GABAergic function depends on locally produced glycolytic ATP, which provides a direct functional link to regional cerebral glucose hypometabolism observed in patients with partial epilepsy. The authors also proposed that the antiepileptic effects of the ketogenic diet may be mediated by the subsequent rise in the NADH/NAD(+) index, which favors endogenous phosphorylation of the GABA$_A$ receptor, thus contributing to restoration of GABAergic inhibition in the epileptogenic zone (Pumain et al. 2008).

Decreased cortical glucose metabolism also could simply reflect neuronal loss leading to a decrease of active synapses. This is certainly an important component of hypometabolism in atrophic cortex with or without gliosis. Impaired synaptic density, indicated by reduced immunoreactivity for synapsin I, is likely the underlying mechanism of the typically low metabolic rates in cortical tubers in patients with tuberous sclerosis (Lippa et al. Rintahaka & Chugani 1997; Szelies et al. 1983). However, decreased neuronal number and/or reduced synaptic density are not necessarily associated with epileptogenicity. In addition, cortical hypometabolism in neocortical epilepsies commonly extends beyond atrophic or lesional areas, involving cortical areas with no apparent structural abnormalities on MRI or histology. A potential mechanism to account for this hypometabolism is the presence of "surround inhibition" (Collins 1978; Prince & Wilder 1967), an electrophysiologic phenomenon detected in cortical areas around the epileptic focus and manifesting increased inhibitory properties due to tonic hyperpolarization. Indeed, tonic hyperpolarization can be associated with decreased metabolism, as has been shown in an acute seizure model in rats, where reduction of ^{14}C–2-deoxyglucose uptake below normal values was associated with reduced synaptic activity and tonic hyperpolarization (Bruehl & Witte, 1995). Consistent with these observations, in focal penicillin-induced epilepsy in rats, hypermetabolic epileptic foci were surrounded by hypometabolic cortex, and the size of these regions changed dynamically depending on the activity of the epileptic focus (Witte et al. 1994).

Perifocal hypometabolism representing an inhibitory surround may play an important role in limiting seizure spread in cortical areas adjacent to epileptogenic regions. Indeed, this has been demonstrated in human neocortical foci, not associated with any MRI lesion, using co-registration of high-resolution MRI, FDG PET, and subdural electrodes implanted for chronic intracranial monitoring (Alkonyi et al. 2009; Juhasz et al. 2000b, 2008). In these studies, seizure onset electrodes were most commonly found to be located at the edge of hypometabolic cortical zones or in adjacent normometabolic areas (Fig. 9.8), while rapid seizure propagation preferentially involved normometabolic cortex. These findings provide preliminary evidence in human neocortical epilepsy to indicate that most hypometabolic regions are in fact *not* involved in (or even appear to be protected from) early seizure involvement. This is further supported by ictal SPECT studies combined with interictal PET in patients with temporal lobe epilepsy, where interictal hypometabolism was present in the same frontal lobe regions that showed ictal hypoperfusion consistent with ictal inhibition (Nelissen et al. 2006). Although these data do not contradict a close spatial relationship between cortical hypometabolism and epileptogenic zones, they do suggest that the location and extent of hypometabolic cortex in itself would be an imperfect guide for

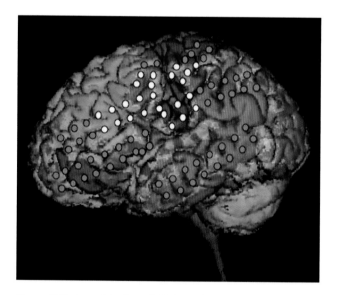

Figure 9.8 Co-registration of high-resolution 3D MRI, FDG PET, and subdural electrode locations to demonstrate cortical surface location of seizure onset (white electrodes) and the location of hypometabolism (red areas) in a patient who underwent two-stage epilepsy surgery due to left fronto-parietal epilepsy. Note that most of the seizure onset electrodes were located *adjacent* to hypometabolic cortex. On the other hand, more than 20 electrodes directly overlying hypometabolic cortex were actually not involved in seizure onset.

tailoring cortical resections in extratemporal lobe epilepsy. In addition, these findings provide a potential explanation as to why hypometabolism commonly extends beyond electrographic seizure foci and also why the extent of resected hypometabolic neocortex is not a good predictor of surgical outcome (Juhasz et al. 2001a). Instead, FDG PET should be used to define the *general area* of the epileptic focus, and then intracranial electrode coverage should include normometabolic cortex *surrounding* the area of hypometabolism in order to optimize the sampling of epileptogenic cortex for resection.

NEUROCOGNITIVE AND BEHAVIORAL CORRELATES OF EXTRATEMPORAL HYPOMETABOLISM

As discussed above, glucose hypometabolism on FDG PET commonly extends beyond the presumed epileptogenic zone in both temporal and extratemporal lobe epilepsies. These non-epileptogenic dysfunctional areas are of clinical interest because they often have important neuropsychological correlates. The frontal lobe is one of the most commonly implicated brain regions when studying the cognitive or behavioral correlates of glucose hypometabolism. For example, patients with temporal lobe epilepsy often show impairment of verbal and performance intelligence measures when they have additional prefrontal hypometabolism on PET (Jokeit et al. 1997). Consistent with this, a more recent study in patients with mesial temporal lobe epilepsy found that hypometabolism in the prefrontal cortex is related to frequent seizures and prefrontal hypofunction (characterized by poor performance on the Wisconsin Card Sorting test) (Takaya et al. 2006). In a study of 32 children with epileptic encephalopathy, Ferrie et al. (1997) reported that adaptive and maladaptive behavior was not related to the presence or absence of focal cortical PET abnormalities. However, adaptive behavior scores showed an inverse correlation with the *degree* of metabolic abnormality in the frontal lobes. In yet another study of 23 patients with complex partial seizures, depressive symptoms were associated with a bilateral reduction of glucose metabolism in inferior frontal cortex, compared with patients without depressive symptoms and normal control subjects (Bromfield et al. 1992). Further, presence of medial prefrontal hypometabolism was related to interictal aggression in children with temporal lobe epilepsy (Juhász et al. 2001b). In these cases, bifrontal hypometabolism was associated with bitemporal neocortical hypometabolism, indicating a widespread dysfunction of neocortical areas. The findings above strongly support that frontal lobe hypometabolism is related to cognitive functioning and behavior, thus suggesting a

lower quality of life even when the epileptic focus is located outside the frontal lobe. As discussed earlier in this chapter, complete resection of the epileptogenic temporal lobe can result in recovery of frontal lobe hypometabolism (Akimura et al. 1999; Joo et al. 2005; Spanaki et al. 2000; Takaya et al. 2009); this metabolic and functional improvement likely reflects a postsurgical improvement of cognitive and/or behavioral abnormalities (Helmstaedter et al. 2003; Hermann & Seidenberg, Reuber et al. 2004), ultimately contributing to a better quality of life in these patients (Wiebe et al. 2001).

CONCLUSIONS

In summary, we have seen in this chapter that interictal FDG PET often shows focal cortical hypometabolism in patients with extratemporal epilepsy and can correctly regionalize neocortical epileptic foci in more than two thirds of the cases, even if MRI is non-localizing. In some cases, however, FDG PET overestimates the epileptogenic region, and hypometabolism may extend progressively to involve remote cortical and subcortical regions, thus establishing an epileptic network in chronic epilepsy. On the other hand, hypometabolism can occur adjacent to, rather than completely overlap with, ictal seizure onset zones. Therefore, FDG PET is best used for presurgical evaluation in combination with other clinical, electrophysiologic, and imaging data to guide intracranial grid placement and optimize tailored neocortical resection. When applied in this manner, the use of FDG PET can improve the outcome of extratemporal lobe epilepsy surgery.

REFERENCES

Akimura, T., H. S. Yeh, J. C. Mantil, et al. 1999. Cerebral metabolism of the remote area after epilepsy surgery. *Neurologia Medico-Chirurgica (Tokyo)* 39: 16–25.

Alkonyi, B., C. Juhász, O. Muzik, et al. 2009. Quantitative brain surface mapping of an electrophysiologic/metabolic mismatch in human neocortical epilepsy. *Epilepsy Research* 87: 77–87.

Awad, I. A., J. Rosenfeld, J. Ahl, et al. 1991. Intractable epilepsy and structural lesions of the brain: mapping, resection strategies, and seizure outcome. *Epilepsia* 32: 179–86.

Bairamian, D., G. Di Chiro, W. Theodore, et al. 1985. MR imaging and positron emission tomography of cortical heterotopia. *Journal of Computer Assisted Tomography* 9: 1137–9.

Barrington, S. F., M. Koutroumanidis, A. Agathonikou, et al. 1998. Clinical value of "ictal" FDG-positron emission tomography and the routine use of simultaneous scalp EEG studies in patients with intractable partial epilepsies. *Epilepsia* 39: 753–66.

Benedek, K., C. Juhász, O. Muzik, et al. 2004. Metabolic changes of subcortical structures in intractable focal epilepsy. *Epilepsia* 45: 1100–5.

Benedek, K., C. Juhász, D. C. Chugani, et al. 2006. Longitudinal changes of cortical glucose hypometabolism in children with intractable epilepsy. *Journal of Child Neurology* 21: 26–30.

Bittar, R. G., F. Andermann, A. Olivier, et al. 1999. Interictal spikes increase cerebral glucose metabolism and blood flow: a PET study. *Epilepsia* 40: 170–8.

Bromfield, E. B., L. Altshuler, D. B. Leiderman, et al. 1992. Cerebral metabolism and depression in patients with complex partial seizures. *Archives of Neurology* 49: 617–23.

Bruehl, C., and O. W. Witte. 1995. Cellular activity underlying altered brain metabolism during focal epileptic activity. *Annals of Neurology* 38: 414–20.

Chapman, K., E. Wyllie, I. Najm, et al. 2005. Seizure outcome after epilepsy surgery in patients with normal preoperative MRI. *Journal of Neurology Neurosurgery Psychiatry* 76: 710–3.

Chassoux, F., E. Landre, S. Rodrigo, et al. 2008. Intralesional recordings and epileptogenic zone in focal polymicrogyria. *Epilepsia* 49: 51–64.

Chugani, H. T., D. A. Shewmon, R. Sankar, et al. 1992. Infantile spasms: II. Lenticular nuclei and brain stem activation on positron emission tomography. *Annals of Neurology* 31: 212–9.

Chugani, H. T., D. A. Shewmon, S. Khanna, et al. 1993. Interictal and postictal focal hypermetabolism on positron emission tomography. *Pediatric Neurology* 9: 10–15.

Chugani, H. T., P. J. Rintahaka, and D. A. Shewmon. 1994. Ictal patterns of cerebral glucose utilization in children with epilepsy. *Epilepsia* 35: 813–22.

Collins, R. C. 1978. Use of cortical circuits during focal penicillin seizures: an autoradiographic study with [^{14}C] deoxyglucose. *Brain Research* 1978;150: 487–501.

Conrad, G. R, and P. Sinha. 2005. FDG PET imaging of subependymal gray matter heterotopia. *Clinical Nuclear Medicine* 30: 35–6.

Cornford, E. M., S. Hyman, and B. E. Swartz. 1994. The human brain GLUT1 glucose transporter: ultrastructural localization to the blood-brain-barrier endothelia. *Journal of Cerebral Blood Flow Metabolism* 14: 106–12.

Cornford, E. M., S. Hyman, M. E. Cornfor, et al. 1998. Interictal seizure resections show two configurations of endothelial Glut1 glucose transporter in the human blood-brain barrier. *Journal of Cerebral Blood Flow Metabolism* 18: 26–42.

Cornford, E. M. 1999. Epilepsy and the blood brain barrier: endothelial cell responses to seizures. *Advances in Neurology* 79: 845–62.

da Silva, E. A., D. C. Chugani, O. Muzik, et al. 1997. Identification of frontal lobe epileptic foci in children using positron emission tomography. *Epilepsia* 38: 1198–208.

Dupont, S., F. Semah, M. Baulac, et al. 1998. The underlying pathophysiology of ictal dystonia in temporal lobe epilepsy: an FDG-PET study. *Neurology* 51: 1289–92.

de Jong, B. M., J. H. van de Hoeven, J. Pruim, et al. 2008. Cortico-thalamic activation in generalized status epilepticus, a PET study. *Clin Neurology Neurosurgery* 110: 182–5.

De Vivo, D. C., R. R. Trifiletti, R. I. Jacobson, et al. 1991. Defective glucose transport across the blood-brain barrier as a cause of persitent hypoglycorrhachia, seizures, and developmental delay. *New England Journal of Medicine* 325: 703–9.

De Vivo, D. C., L. Leary, and D. Wang. 2002. Glucose transporter 1 deficiency syndrome and other glycolytic defects. *Journal of Child Neurology* 17 (suppl 3): 3S15–3S23.

Engel, J., Jr. 1993. Intracerebral recordings: organization of the human epileptogenic region. *Journal of Clinical Neurophysiology* 10: 90–8.

Ferrie, C. D., C. Madigan, K. Tilling, et al. 1997. Adaptive and maladaptive behaviour in children with epileptic encephalopathies: correlation with cerebral glucose metabolism. *Developmental Medicine & Child Neurology* 39: 588–95.

Fois, A., M. A. Farnetani, P. Balestri, et al. 1995. EEG, PET, SPET and MRI in intractable childhood epilepsies: possible surgical correlations. *Childs Nervous System* 11: 672–8.

Gaillard, W. D., S. White, B. Malow, et al. 1995. FDG-PET in children and adolescents with partial seizures: role in epilepsy surgery evaluation. *Epilepsy Research* 20: 77–84.

Gaillard, W. D., L. Kopylev, S. Weinstein, et al. 2002. Low incidence of abnormal (18)FDG-PET in children with new-onset partial epilepsy: a prospective study. *Neurology* 58: 717–22.

Gaillard, W. D., S. Weinstein, J. Conry, et al. 2007. Prognosis of children with partial epilepsy: MRI and serial 18FDG-PET. *Neurology* 68: 655–9.

Gärtner, B., M. Seeck, C. M. Michel, et al. 2004. Patients with extratemporal lobe epilepsy do not differ from healthy subjects with respect to subcortical volumes. *Journal of Neurology Neurosurgery Psychiatry* 75: 588–92.

Hader, W. J., M. Mackay, H. Otsubo, et al. 2004. Cortical dysplastic lesions in children with intractable epilepsy: role of complete resection. *Journal of Neurosurgery* 100(2 Suppl Pediatrics): 110–7.

Helmstaedter, C., M. Kurthen, S. Lux, et al. 2003. Chronic epilepsy and cognition: a longitudinal study in temporal lobe epilepsy. *Annals of Neurology* 54: 425–32.

Henry, T. R., J. C. Mazziotta, J. Engel Jr., et al. 1990. Quantifying interictal metabolic activity in human temporal lobe epilepsy. *Journal of Cerebral Blood Flow Metabolism* 10: 748–57.

Henry, T. R., W. W. Sutherling, J. Engel Jr., et al. 1991. Interictal cerebral metabolism in partial epilepsies of neocortical origin. *Epilepsy Research* 10: 174–82.

Hermann, B., and M. Seidenberg. 1995. Executive system dysfunction in temporal lobe epilepsy: effects of nociferous cortex versus hippocampal pathology. *Journal of Clinical & Experimental Neuropsychology* 17: 809–19.

Hong, K. S., S. K. Lee, J. Y. Kim, et al. 2002a. Pre-surgical evaluation and surgical outcome of 41 patients with non-lesional neocortical epilepsy. *Seizure* 11: 184–92.

Hong, S. B., H. J. Han, S. Y. Roh, et al. 2002b. Hypometabolism and interictal spikes during positron emission tomography scanning in temporal lobe epilepsy. *European Neurology* 48: 65–70.

Ito, M. 1984. *The cerebellum and neural control.* New York: Raven Press, 14–5.

Jokeit, H., R. J. Seitz, H. J. Markowitsch, et al. 1997. Prefrontal asymmetric interictal glucose hypometabolism and cognitive impairment in patients with temporal lobe epilepsy. *Brain* 120: 2283–94.

Joo, E. Y., S. B. Hong, H. J. Han, et al. 2005. Postoperative alteration of cerebral glucose metabolism in mesial temporal lobe epilepsy. *Brain* 128: 1802–10.

Juhász, C., F. Nagy, C. Watson, et al. 1999. Glucose and [^{11}C] flumazenil positron emission tomography abnormalities of thalamic nuclei in temporal lobe epilepsy. *Neurology* 53: 2037–45.

Juhász, C., D. C. Chugani, O. Muzik, et al. 2000a. Electroclinical correlates of flumazenil and fluorodeoxyglucose PET abnormalities in lesional epilepsy. *Neurology* 55: 825–34.

Juhász, C., D. C. Chugani, O. Muzik, et al. 2000b. Is epileptogenic cortex truly hypometabolic on interictal positron emission tomography? *Annals of Neurology* 48: 88–96.

Juhász, C., D. C. Chugani, O. Muzik, et al. 2001a. Relationship of flumazenil and glucose PET abnormalities to neocortical epilepsy surgery outcome. *Neurology* 56: 1650–8.

Juhász, C., M. E. Behen, O. Muzik, et al. 2001b. Bilateral prefrontal and temporal neocortical hypometabolism in children with epilepsy and aggression. *Epilepsia* 42: 991–1001.

Juhász, C., D. C. Chugani, O. Muzik, et al. 2003. Alpha-methyl-L-tryptophan PET detects epileptogenic cortex in children with intractable epilepsy. *Neurology* 60: 960–8.

Juhász, C., E. A. Batista, D. C. Chugani, et al. 2007. Evolution of cortical metabolic abnormalities and their clinical correlates in Sturge-Weber syndrome. *European Journal of Paediatric Neurology* 11: 277–84.

Juhász, C., E. Asano, C. Batista, et al. 2008. Cortical seizure foci and hypometabolism on PET: When do they not match well? [abstract] *Epilepsia* 49(suppl 7): 416–7.

Kim, S. K., K. C. Wang, Y. S. Hwang, et al. 2000. Pediatric intractable epilepsy: the role of presurgical evaluation and seizure outcome. *Childs Nervous System* 16: 278–85.

Kim, Y. K., D. S. Lee, S. K. Lee, et al. 2002. (18)F-FDG PET in localization of frontal lobe epilepsy: comparison of visual and SPM analysis. *Journal of Nuclear Medicine* 43: 1167–74.

Kim, D. W., S. K. Lee, K. Chu, et al. 2009. Predictors of surgical outcome and pathologic considerations in focal cortical dysplasia. *Neurology* 72: 211–6.

Knowlton, R. C., R. A. Elgavish, A. Bartolucci, et al. 2008. Functional imaging: II. Prediction of epilepsy surgery outcome. *Annals of Neurology* 64: 35–41.

Koutroumanidis, M., C. D. Binnie, R. D. Elwes, et al. 1998. Interictal regional slow activity in temporal lobe epilepsy correlates with lateral temporal hypometabolism as imaged with ^{18}FDG PET: neurophysiological and metabolic implications. *Journal of Neurology Neurosurgery Psychiatry* 65: 170–6.

Kumar, A., C. Juhasz, and H. T. Chugani. 2009. Objective lateralization and localization of epileptic foci by FDG

PET using voxel-based analysis in children with intractable epilepsy undergoing surgery [abstract]. *Journal of Nuclear Medicine* 50(suppl. 2): 95P.

Kurian, M., L. Spinelli, J. Delavelle, et al. 2007. Multimodality imaging for focus localization in pediatric pharmacoresistant epilepsy. *Epileptic Disorders* 9: 20–31.

Laschet, J. J., F. Minier, I. Kurcewicz, et al. 2004. Glyceraldehyde–3-phosphate dehydrogenase is a GABAA receptor kinase linking glycolysis to neuronal inhibition. *Journal of Neuroscience* 24: 7614–22.

Laschet, J. J., I. Kurcewicz, F. Minier, et al. 2007. Dysfunction of GABA$_A$ receptor glycolysis-dependent modulation in human partial epilepsy. *Proceedings of the National Academy of Sciences U S A* 104: 3472–7.

Lee, E. M., K. C. Im, and J. H. Kim. 2009. Relationship between hypometabolic patterns and ictal scalp EEG patterns in patients with unilateral hippocampal sclerosis: An FDG-PET study. *Epilepsy Research* 84: 187–93.

Lee, N., R. A. Radtke, L. Gray, et al. 1994. Neuronal migration disorders: positron emission tomography correlations. *Annals of Neurology* 35: 290–7.

Lee, S. K., S. Y. Lee, K. K. Kim, et al. 2005. Surgical outcome and prognostic factors of cryptogenic neocortical epilepsy. *Annals of Neurology* 58: 525–32.

Lerner, J. T., N. Salamon, J. S. Hauptman, et al. 2009. Assessment and surgical outcomes for mild type I and severe type II cortical dysplasia: A critical review and the UCLA experience. *Epilepsia* 50: 1310–35.

Lippa, C. F., D. Pearson, and T. W. Smith. 1993. Cortical tubers demonstrate reduced immunoreactivity for synapsin I. *Acta Neuropathologica* 85: 449–51.

Liu, Y., J. O. Karonen, J. Nuutinen, et al. 2007. Crossed cerebellar diaschisis in acute ischemic stroke: a study with serial SPECT and MRI. *Journal of Cerebral Blood Flow Metabolism* 27: 1724–32.

Luat, A. F., E. Asano, R. Rothermel, et al. 2008. Psychosis as a manifestation of frontal lobe epilepsy. *Epilepsy & Behavior* 12: 200–4.

McDonald, C. R., D. J. Hagler Jr., M. E. Ahmadi, et al. 2008. Subcortical and cerebellar atrophy in mesial temporal lobe epilepsy revealed by automatic segmentation. *Epilepsy Research* 79: 130–8.

Magistretti, P. J., and L. Pellerin. 1996. The contribution of astrocytes to the ^{18}F–2-deoxyglucose signal in PET activation studies. *Molecular Psychiatry* 1(6): 445–52.

Magistretti, P. J., and L. Pellerin. 1999. Cellular mechanisms of brain energy metabolism and their relevance to functional brain imaging. *Philosophical Transactions of the Royal Society of London B Biological Sciences* 354: 1155–63.

Matheja, P., M. Weckesser, O. Debus, et al. 2000. Drug-induced changes in cerebral glucose consumption in bifrontal epilepsy. *Epilepsia* 41: 588–93.

Meltzer, C. C., P. D. Adelson, R. P. Brenner, et al. 2000. Planned ictal FDG PET imaging for localization of extratemporal epileptic foci. *Epilepsia* 41: 193–200.

Meneghetti, G., S. Vorstrup, B. Mickey, et al. 1984. Crossed cerebellar diaschisis in ischemic stroke: a study of regional cerebral blood flow by ^{133}Xe inhalation and single photon emission computerized tomography. *Journal of Cerebral Blood Flow Metabolism* 4: 235–40.

Natsume, J., N. Bernasconi, F. Andermann, et al. 2003. MRI volumetry of the thalamus in temporal, extratemporal, and idiopathic generalized epilepsy. *Neurology* 60: 1296–300.

Newberg, A. B., A. Alavi, J. Berlin, et al. 2000. Ipsilateral and contralateral thalamic hypometabolism as a predictor of outcome after temporal lobectomy for seizures. *Journal of Nuclear Medicine* 41: 1964–8.

Nishida, M., E. Asano, C. Juhász, et al. 2008. Cortical glucose metabolism correlates negatively with delta-slowing and spike-frequency in epilepsy associated with tuberous sclerosis. *Human Brain Mapping* 29: 1255–64.

Palmini, A., I. Najm, G. Avanzini, et al. 2004. Terminology and classification of the cortical dysplasias. *Neurology* 62: S2–S8.

Peters, A., and E. G. Jones. 1984. *Cerebral Cortex: Cellular Components of the Cerebral Cortex.* New York: Plenum.

Pilcher, W. H., D. L. Silbergeld, M. S. Berger, et al. 1993. Intraoperative electrocorticography during tumor resection: impact on seizure outcome in patients with gangliogliomas. *Journal of Neurosurgery* 78: 891–902.

Plotkin, M., H. Amthauer, M. Merschhemke, et al. 2003. Use of statistical parametric mapping of (18) F-FDG-PET in frontal lobe epilepsy. *Nuklearmedizin* 42: 190–6.

Poduri, A., A. Golja, M. Takeoka, et al. 2007. Focal cortical malformations can show asymmetrically higher uptake on interictal fluorine–18 fluorodeoxyglucose positron emission tomography (PET). *Journal of Child Neurology* 22: 232–7.

Prince, D. A., and B. J. Wilder. 1967. Control mechanisms in cortical epileptogenic foci. "Surround" inhibition. *Archives of Neurology* 16: 194–202.

Pumain, R., and J. Laschet. 2006. A key glycolytic enzyme plays a dual role in GABAergic neurotransmission and in human epilepsy. *Critical Reviews in Neurobiology* 18: 197–203.

Pumain, R., M. S. Ahmed, I. Kurcewicz, et al. 2008. Lability of GABAA receptor function in human partial epilepsy: possible relationship to hypometabolism. *Epilepsia* 49 (Suppl 8): 87–90.

Reuber, M., B. Andersen, C. E. Elger, et al. 2004. Depression and anxiety before and after temporal lobe epilepsy surgery. *Seizure* 13: 129–35.

Rintahaka, P. J., and H. T. Chugani. 1997. Clinical role of positron emission tomography in children with tuberous sclerosis complex. *Journal of Child Neurology* 12: 42–52.

Rusu, V., F. Chassoux, E. Landré, et al. 2005. Dystonic posturing in seizures of mesial temporal origin: electroclinical and metabolic patterns. *Neurology* 65: 1612–9.

Ryvlin, P., F. Mauguière, M. Sindou, et al. 1995. Interictal cerebral metabolism and epilepsy in cavernous angiomas. *Brain* 118: 677–87.

Salamon, N., J. Kung, S. J. Shaw, et al. 2008. FDG-PET/MRI coregistration improves detection of cortical dysplasia in patients with epilepsy. *Neurology* 71: 1594–601.

Savic, I., L. Altshuler, E. Passaro, et al. 1996. Localized cerebellar hypometabolism in patients with complex partial seizures. *Epilepsia* 37: 781–7.

Savic, I., L. Altshuler, L. Baxter, et al. 1997. Pattern of interictal hypometabolism in PET scans with fludeoxyglucose F 18 reflects prior seizure types in patients with mesial temporal lobe seizures. *Archives of Neurology* 54: 129–36.

Schlaug, G., C. Antke, H. Holthausen, et al. 1997. Ictal motor signs and interictal regional cerebral hypometabolism. *Neurology* 49: 341–50.

Shedlack, K. J., E. K. Lee, R. A. Radtke, et al. 1994. Ipsilateral subcortical atrophy associated with temporal lobectomy. *Psychiatry Research* 54: 295–304.

Shulman, R. G., D. L. Rothman, K. L. Behar, et al. 2004. Energetic basis of brain activity: implications for neuroimaging. *Trends in Neuroscience* 27: 489–95.

Seidenberg, M., B. Hermann, D. Pulsipher, et al. 2008. Thalamic atrophy and cognition in unilateral temporal lobe epilepsy. *Journal of the International Neuropsychology Society* 14: 384–93.

Snead, O. C. 3rd, L. S. Chen, W. G. Mitchell, et al. 1996. Usefulness of [^{18}F]fluorodeoxyglucose positron emission tomography in pediatric epilepsy surgery. *Pediatric Neurology* 14: 98–107.

Spanaki, M. V., L. Kopylev, C. DeCarli, et al. 2000. Postoperative changes in cerebral metabolism in temporal lobe epilepsy. *Archives of Neurology* 57: 1447–52.

Sperling, M. R., R. C. Gur, A. Alavi, et al. 1990. Subcortical metabolic alterations in partial epilepsy. *Epilepsia* 31: 145–55.

Swartz, B. E., E. Halgren, A. V. Delgado-Escueta, et al. 1989. Neuroimaging in patients with seizures of probable frontal lobe origin. *Epilepsia* 30: 547–58.

Swartz, B. E., E. Halgren, A. V. Delgado-Escueta, et al. 1990. Multidisciplinary analysis of patients with extratemporal complex partial seizures. I. Intertest agreement. *Epilepsy Research* 5: 61–73.

Swartz, B. E., C. Brown, M. A. Mandelkern, et al. 2002. The use of 2-deoxy–2-[^{18}F]fluoro-D-glucose (FDG-PET) positron emission tomography in the routine diagnosis of epilepsy. *Molecular Imaging Biology* 4: 245–52.

Szelies, B., K. Herholz, W. D. Heiss, et al. 1983. Hypometabolic cortical lesions in tuberous sclerosis with epilepsy: demonstration by positron emission tomography. *Journal of Computer Assisted Tomography* 7: 946–53.

Takaya, S., T. Hanakawa, K. Hashikawa, et al. 2006. Prefrontal hypofunction in patients with intractable mesial temporal lobe epilepsy. *Neurology* 67: 1674–6.

Takaya, S., N. Mikuni, T. Mitsueda, et al. 2009. Improved cerebral function in mesial temporal lobe epilepsy after subtemporal amygdalohippocampectomy. *Brain* 132: 185–94.

Theodore, W. H., D. Fishbein, M. Dietz, et al. 1987. Complex partial seizures: cerebellar metabolism. *Epilepsia* 28: 319–23.

Tran, T. A., S. S. Spencer, M. Javidan, et al. 1997. Significance of spikes recorded on intraoperative electrocorticography in patients with brain tumor and epilepsy. *Epilepsia* 38: 1132–9.

Vinton, A. B., R. Carne, R. J. Hicks, et al. 2007. The extent of resection of FDG-PET hypometabolism relates to outcome of temporal lobectomy. *Brain* 130: 548–60.

Weitemeyer, L., C. Kellinghaus, M. Weckesser, et al. 2005. The prognostic value of [F]FDG-PET in nonrefractory partial epilepsy. *Epilepsia* 46: 1654–60.

Wiebe, S., W. T. Blume, J. P. Girvin, et al. 2001. A randomized, controlled trial of surgery for temporal-lobe epilepsy. *New England Journal of Medicine* 345: 311–8.

Witte, O. W., C. Bruehl, G. Schlaug, et al. 1994. Dynamic changes of focal hypometabolism in relation to epileptic activity. *Journal of the Neurological Sciences* 124: 188–97.

Yun, C. H., S. K. Lee, S. Y. Lee, et al. 2006. Prognostic factors in neocortical epilepsy surgery: multivariate analysis. *Epilepsia* 47: 574–9.

Chapter 10

POSITRON EMISSION TOMOGRAPHY: BRAIN GLUCOSE METABOLISM IN PEDIATRIC EPILEPSY SYNDROMES

Aimee F. Luat and Harry T. Chugani

INTRODUCTION

Epilepsy syndrome is defined by the International League Against Epilepsy (ILAE) as a complex of signs and symptoms that characterize a unique epilepsy condition with different etiologies (Engel 2001). Syndrome classification of epilepsy is based on the cluster of clinical features, including age of onset, seizure types, and interictal as well as ictal electroencephalography (EEG) findings. Structural imaging, particularly magnetic resonance imaging (MRI), is the primary neuroimaging modality used in the evaluation and management of epilepsy, and this has been reviewed elsewhere in this volume. However, there are several epilepsy syndromes where MRI is normal, is nonspecific, or provides limited information, and in these instances functional neuroimaging assumes an important role.

The measurement of cerebral glucose metabolism using 2-deoxy-2- [^{18}F]fluoro-D-glucose (FDG) with positron emission tomography (PET) has dramatically altered our understanding and management approach to some childhood epilepsy syndromes. Indeed, in infants and children with intractable epilepsy, glucose metabolism PET scanning has assumed an important role in localizing epileptogenic cortex for surgical resection even in syndromes where the epilepsy was previously believed to be primary generalized and not amenable to cortical resection. When localization of the epileptogenic zone is apparent, FDG PET can also assess the functional integrity of brain regions outside of the suspected epileptogenic zone as well as the contralateral hemisphere, thereby providing useful prognostic information. Conversely, glucose metabolism PET studies may suggest the presence of an underlying neurogenetic or metabolic condition and preclude further epilepsy surgery evaluation. This chapter reviews the role of cerebral glucose metabolism PET imaging in various childhood epilepsy syndromes with respect to patterns of glucose utilization to provide a better understanding of underlying mechanisms, surgical treatment, and prognostic implications. PET applications of temporal lobe epilepsy (Chapter 8) and extratemporal lobe epilepsy (Chapter 9) are discussed elsewhere in this volume and will not be included in the present chapter.

NEONATAL SEIZURES

The incidence of neonatal seizures has been reported to range from 1.8 to 3.5 per 1,000 live births (Lanska et al. 1995; Saliba et al. 1999). Premature and low birth weight infants have a much higher rate of neonatal seizures compared to full-term and normal birth weight infants (Lanska et al. 1995). The etiologies of seizures in the neonatal period are diverse and are usually due to symptomatic causes, which include hypoxic ischemic encephalopathy, stroke, infection, cerebral malformations, and neurocutaneous and neurometabolic disorders. The recognition of the underlying etiology of neonatal seizures is important because some etiologies indicate specific treatments that when implemented early in the course may improve neurologic outcome.

Neuroradiologic investigations are an integral part of the diagnostic approach to uncover the causes of neonatal seizures. Neuroimaging is routinely performed to exclude the presence of brain pathology or lesions such as cortical malformations and stroke. Cranial ultrasound, MRI, and computed tomography (CT) scanning are among the most frequently used neuroimaging tests in neonates. Cranial ultrasound is readily available in most neonatal intensive care units (NICUs) and has been used as a first-line neuroimaging tool in the evaluation. However, it is not sensitive enough to detect certain brain lesions such as stroke and cortical malformations. In addition, the test tends to be somewhat dependent on the skill of the technologist performing the test. If the cranial ultrasound is normal, further testing using cranial CT or MRI should be performed. However, in neonates, certain brain malformations (e.g., some cortical dysplasias) may still not be detectable even when using high-resolution MRI.

Glucose metabolism PET studies in neonates and infants can provide important localizing information in cases of intractable seizures by detecting subtle malformations of cortical development at a time when they are not yet apparent on the MRI scan because of the relatively low state of myelination. However, due to the normal developmental changes of brain glucose metabolism in the first year of life (Chugani et al. 1987), these changes must be taken into account and the PET scans cautiously interpreted (Fig. 10.1).

At Children's Hospital of Michigan, a microPET scanner originally intended for scanning monkeys was adapted for human use and placed in the NICU. This microPET Focus 220 positron emission tomograph (Concorde Microsystems, Knoxville, TN) (Fig. 10.2)

ONTOGENY OF BRAIN GLUCOSE METABOLISM IN HUMANS

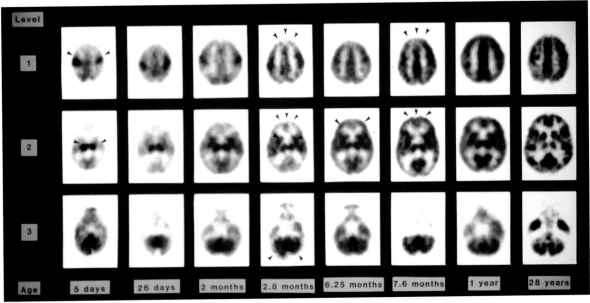

Figure 10.1 Patterns of cerebral glucose utilization during neonatal and infancy periods shown on PET scans. In the neonate, glucose metabolism is highest in sensorimotor cortex, thalamus, brain stem, and cerebellar vermis. In higher-resolution scans, medial temporal lobe regions also show relatively high glucose metabolism. Note the relatively low glucose metabolic rates in most of the cerebral and cerebellar cortex at this stage. By 3 months, there is increased glucose utilization in parietal, temporal, and occipital cortex, as well as cerebellar hemispheres. By 8 months, glucose utilization has increased in the lateral portion of frontal cortex much more than in the medial portion. The pattern of cerebral glucose utilization in a 1-year-old infant resembles that of an adult.

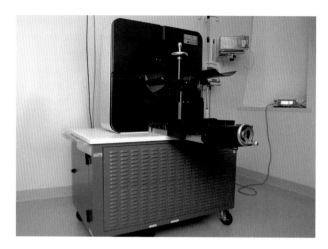

Figure 10.2 The Focus 220 microPET scanner located inside the neonatal intensive care unit at Hutzel Women's Hospital in the Detroit Medical Center, Wayne State University. This scanner can also be used to scan larger infants weighing less than 15 kilograms.

FDG PET IN A NEWBORN

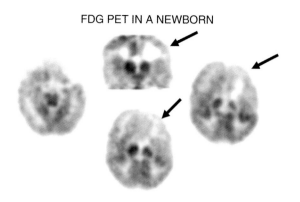

Figure 10.3 FDG PET scan using the Focus 220 microPET scanner from a 36-week gestational age newborn showing left frontal hypometabolism (*arrows*) following intracranial hemorrhage. Note the high spatial resolution capable of identifying even brain stem nuclei. Note also functional activity in medial temporal regions.

operates exclusively in 3D mode and produces images with a reconstructed isotropic resolution of $2 \times 2 \times 2$ mm at full-width-half-maximum. The port diameter of this system is 22 cm, with an axial field-of-view of 8 cm. The gantry is connected to a Pentium PC for data reconstruction, display, and archiving. Because the scanner is housed in the NICU, minimal transport of the newborn is necessary and the NICU nurse continues to care for the infant during the study. If necessary, the infant is fed 2 hours prior to the PET scan. A venous catheter is typically already in place in these infants and provides the route of radiotracer administration. We do not sedate these babies during the time required to acquire the images since they typically lie quite still after being wrapped in a blanket. After reconstruction of the raw data, images are transferred to the main PET Center using the local area network for further processing.

The PET studies of cerebral glucose metabolism in neonates using the microPET scanner have replicated our previous findings indicating the very early functional maturation of sensorimotor cortex, thalamus, brain stem, and cerebellar vermis (Chugani et al. 2005). However, in addition to these, increased glucose metabolism can also be noted in limbic structures such as amygdala, even in prematurely born babies (Fig. 10.3) (Chugani et al. 2005). As indicated above, these maturational changes must be taken into account when interpreting potential abnormalities. For example, a frontal lobe epileptic focus might be missed when an interictal glucose metabolism PET scan is performed prior to about 8 to 12 months of age, since frontal lobe glucose metabolic activity is still undergoing a maturational increase. In fact, in the neonatal period, interictal glucose metabolism PET studies are of limited value in seizure patients because of the

normally very low glucose metabolism in most of the cerebral cortex at this age. In contrast, ictal scans are often highly localizing and may even reveal areas of seizure propagation in newborns.

OHTAHARA SYNDROME

Ohtahara syndrome, also called early infantile epileptic encephalopathy with suppression bursts, is the earliest form of epileptic encephalopathy (Ohtahara 1978). The syndrome is characterized by the onset in early infancy (within the first 3 months, mainly in the first 10 days of life) of intractable epilepsy, particularly tonic spasms, and a diffuse burst suppression pattern on the EEG. In addition to tonic seizures, partial seizures and hemiconvulsions are observed in between a third and a half of these infants. Although the majority of cases of Ohtahara syndrome are associated with structural brain abnormalities, infants with various other underlying disorders can also meet the criteria for Ohtahara syndrome. Indeed, Ohtahara's series included cases of Aicardi syndrome, porencephaly, hydrocephalus, hemimegalencephaly, and lissencephaly.

There is no specific pattern of abnormal glucose metabolism on PET scans for Ohtahara syndrome. Figure 10.4 shows the MRI and FDG PET findings of an 8-day-old infant who presented with Ohtahara syndrome. MRI showed bilateral perisylvian and perirolandic polymicrogyria, left more involved than right. Ictal FDG PET showed increased glucose metabolism in the left frontal and left medial temporal areas, as well as retrosplenial portion of the cingulate cortex. Hmaimess et al. (2005) have reported a case of Ohtahara syndrome associated with left parietooccipital hemimegalencephaly. Glucose metabolism PET scan showed left posterior hypermetabolism.

ICTAL FDG PET SCAN IN 8 DAY OLD TERM INFANT WITH OHTAHARA SYNDROME

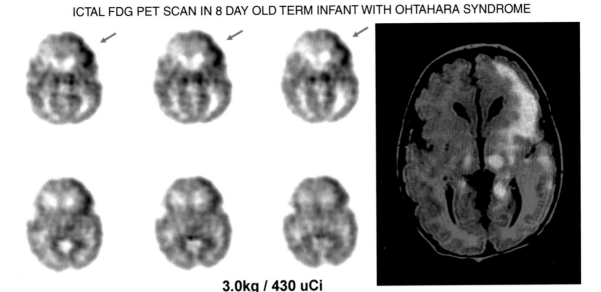

3.0kg / 430 uCi

Figure 10.4 An 8-day-old neonate with Ohtahara syndrome whose MRI shows bilateral perisylvian cortical dysplasia (polymicrogyria), which is more extensive on the left side. Ictal FDG PET scan shows increased glucose metabolism in the left frontal cortex (*arrows*), left thalamus, and left retrosplenial cingulate cortex. EEG during the scanning showed frequent sharp and wave activities in the left frontal and temporal areas, and occasionally in the right temporal region. Clusters of tonic spasms were captured, during which the EEG showed lateralization to the left hemisphere.

Left transcortical perisylvian resection led to resolution of the seizures and resulted in developmental progress. The report suggests the need to seek for an underlying unilateral pathology in Ohtahara syndrome since epilepsy surgery may be a promising treatment option in at least some cases.

EPILEPTIC SPASMS

Epileptic spasms are seizures characterized by clusters of short contractions typically involving the head, trunk, and extremities. Previously called infantile spasms, *epileptic spasms* is the preferred term because they can occur or persist beyond infancy. Epileptic spasms can occur in isolation or as part of West syndrome, which is the triad of epileptic spasms, an EEG pattern of hypsarrhythmia, and developmental arrest. When epileptic spasms are associated with an underlying condition (e.g., tuberous sclerosis, Down syndrome, brain injury), they are referred to as *symptomatic*, but when no underlying etiology can be determined, the term *cryptogenic* is applied to signify that there probably is an underlying hidden cause, albeit elusive. Rare cases have been described where there is truly no underlying etiology and the spasms are a transient manifestation of a neurophysiologic immaturity that resolves readily with treatment such as adrenocortical hormone (ACTH) or vigabatrin without any subsequent adverse outcome ("idiopathic" epileptic spasms) (Dulac et al. 1986, 1993).

Epileptic spasms, because of the bilateral and relatively symmetric clinical semiology, have traditionally been classified as a form of generalized seizure. However, following the report of Chugani et al. (1990), it became apparent that in a subset of patients, epileptic spasms may be a form of secondary generalized seizure propagating from cortical lesions not always apparent on MRI but readily appreciated on FDG PET scans. In that report, unilateral cortical areas of glucose hypometabolism were demonstrated in five children with presumed cryptogenic intractable epileptic spasms (normal MRI in 4/5). Four of these five children underwent resection of the cortical areas of glucose hypometabolism, guided by intracranial electrocorticography, resulting in seizure freedom or improvement of seizure control. Neuropathology of the resected brain tissue showed cortical dysplasia. A subsequent study on a large number of patients with spasms (n = 140) found that among the 97 cases classified as cryptogenic, a single cortical focus of abnormal glucose metabolism (unilateral hemispheric or focal) was identified in 30 and multifocal abnormalities were found in 62 (Chugani et al. 1996). These unifocal and unilateral PET abnormalities (Fig. 10.5A,B) are believed to be due to underlying cortical dysplasia. The recognition that a subset of patients with intractable epileptic spasms may harbor potentially resectable focal areas of cortical dysplasia has led to the challenge of pediatric epilepsy surgery centers to identify these surgical candidates to improve their outcome. Indeed, following the original report of Chugani et al. in 1990

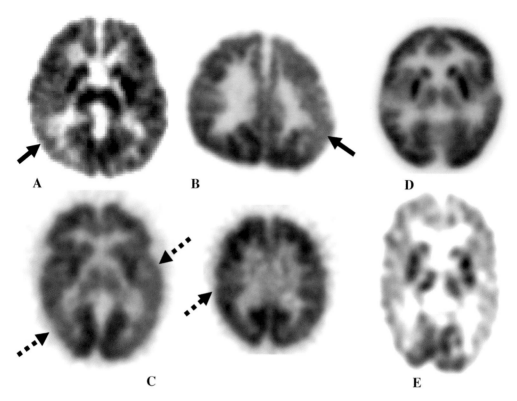

Figure 10.5 Four different patterns of cortical glucose hypometabolism in infants with epileptic spasms. (A) Unifocal and (B) unilateral cortical hypometabolism (surgical candidates), 20% (*black arrows*). (C) Multifocal cortical hypometabolism, 65% (*dotted arrows*). (D) Bitemporal cortical hypometabolism, 10%. (E) Diffuse cortical hypometabolism, 5%.

and a subsequent study in 1993 involving 23 surgical cases (Chugani et al. 1993), several investigators have replicated the finding that surgical resection of the cortical abnormality in selected patients with intractable spasms can provide seizure control (Kramer et al. 1997; Sugimoto et al. 1999; Wyllie et al. 1996, 1998).

Unfortunately, about 65% of children with cryptogenic epileptic spasms demonstrate *multifocal* areas of glucose hypometabolism, an additional 10% show *bitemporal* areas of glucose hypometabolism, and 5% show bilateral *diffuse* cortical hypometabolism (Fig. 10.5C–E). In these infants, epilepsy surgery is usually not an option, although in some multifocal cases we have performed a "palliative" resection to improve the patient's quality of life if the seizures are intractable and very frequent and the vast majority emanate from one general region.

Based on FDG PET studies, our insights on the pathophysiology of epileptic spasms have greatly expanded. Ictal FDG PET scans performed during prolonged clusters of spasms or during frequent interictal spiking on the EEG have shown bilateral symmetric *hypermetabolism* of the lenticular nuclei and brainstem, in addition to focal area of cortical hypo- or hypermetabolism, thus suggesting that the spasms are initiated by a primary cortical epileptic focus that

interacts with subcortical and brainstem structures (Fig. 10.6A) (Chugani et al. 1992). This finding led to the proposal of a neuronal circuitry illustrated in Figure 10.6B. Thus, it is proposed that during a critical stage of brain development (beginning at about 3 months, when cortical maturation becomes evident on FDG PET scans), the primary cortical focus interacts through its epileptic discharges with brainstem structures, particularly the raphe nuclei, which have strong cortical projections. The raphe-cortical and cortico-cortical propagation may be responsible for the EEG feature of hypsarrhythmia. The raphe nuclei also have projections to the striatal region (bilateral putamen), and these pathways may activate descending spinal pathways bilaterally to result in the bilateral and relatively symmetric clinical semiology of epileptic spasms.

As previously mentioned, about 10% of all infants with cryptogenic spasms show bilateral temporal lobe hypometabolism on their PET scans (Fig. 10.5D). These children show a distinct clinical phenotype characterized by severe developmental delay (particularly in the language domain) and autism. The PET scan may also reveal bilateral frontal cortical hypometabolism, and occasionally generalized cortical hypometabolism, with or without associated cerebellar involvement

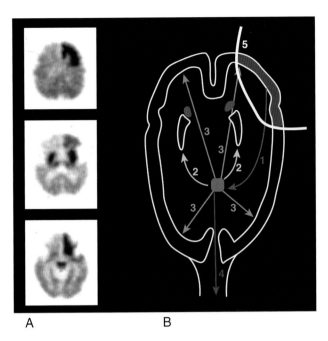

A   B

Figure 10.6 (A) FDG PET (ictal PET) scan obtained during a prolonged cluster of spasms showing bilateral symmetric hypermetabolism of the lenticular and brain stem nuclei in addition to a focal area of cortical hypermetabolism, suggesting that spasms are initiated by a primary cortical epileptic focus that interacts with the subcortical and brain stem structures. (B) Schematic representation of brain pathways hypothesized in infantile spasms, with PET images showing increased glucose metabolism in activated regions (from Chugani et al. 1992). **Pathway 1 (green).** "Nociferous" influence of abnormal cortical region (red) on brain stem (raphe area). **Pathway 2 (yellow).** Raphe-striatal pathway, serotonergic ($5HT_{1D}$), under tonic control by corticosteroids. **Pathway 3 (blue).** Generation of hypsarrhythmic pattern. **Pathway 4 (purple).** Spinal cord propagation (direct or indirect) and lenticular nuclei involvement results in the generation of clinical spasms. **Pathway 5 (white).** Surgical resection of the primary cortical abnormality abolishes activation of the circuitry.

(Fig. 10.5E). This type of pattern is not suggestive of an underlying lesional etiology but, rather, may indicate an underlying genetic/metabolic condition and represents a heterogeneous group. When this pattern is encountered, more detailed metabolic and genetic studies (e.g., chromosomal microarray analysis) should be performed and the idea of cortical resection should be abandoned. Thus, in patients with cryptogenic epileptic spasms, FDG PET scans are a useful guide into optimal clinical management.

TUBEROUS SCLEROSIS COMPLEX

Tuberous sclerosis complex (TSC) is a multisystem autosomal dominant disorder characterized by the presence of multiple hamartomas in various organs of the body, including the brain. It is caused by mutation

of one of two tumor suppressor genes: TSC 1 on chromosome 9q34 (Fryer et al. 1987; van Slegtenhorst et al. 1997) or TSC 2 on chromosome 16p13.3 (Kandt et al. 1992); these genes encode for hamartin and tuberin, respectively. Epilepsy is its most common neurologic presentation, occurring in 80% to 90% of TSC patients, and seizures in TSC often become refractory to medical treatment. Cortical tubers have been implicated as the sites of epileptogenesis in TSC (Curatolo and Cusmai 1988; Cusmai et al. 1990). However, not all tubers are epileptogenic, as indicated by surgical outcome studies showing good seizure outcome following resection of the suspected epileptogenic tubers and leaving the non-epileptogenic ones in place (Jansen et al. 2007; Kagawa et al. 2005; Lachwani et al. 2005; Madhavan et al. 2007; Teutonico et al. 2008; Weiner et al. 2006). Over the past several years, epilepsy surgery in TSC has become an important treatment option, although the identification of the epileptogenic tuber can be a challenge because it may be difficult to identify amid the presence of multiple bilateral lesions.

The application of multimodality neuroimaging is important in the presurgical evaluation of TSC patients. FDG PET can detect small cortical tubers that are not visualized on T2-weighted MRI but that can be observed on fluid attenuated inversion recovery (FLAIR) images; however, the area of glucose hypometabolism is usually larger than the lesions seen on MRI (Asano et al. 2000a, Asano et al. 2000b). Furthermore, glucose metabolism PET allows detection of not only the cortical tubers, but also of dysplastic cortex, which may appear normal on MRI. Although FDG PET cannot distinguish between epileptogenic and non-epileptogenic tubers, it can assess the full extent of functional abnormalities in the brain and evaluate the integrity of cortex homotopic to a planned surgical resection (Asano et al. 2003), thereby predicting potential postoperative cognitive deficits. Typically, cortical tubers are depicted as multifocal areas of glucose hypometabolism (Asano et al. 2003; Rintahaka et al. 1997; Szelies et al. 1983), which is hypothesized to be due to the decreased number of neurons and simplified dendritic pattern within the tubers, and hence less requirement for glucose (Mata et al. 1980) (Fig. 10.7).

The application of glucose metabolism PET in TSC has also contributed to our understanding of the neurobehavioral phenotypes of TSC, including autism, attention-deficit/hyperactivity disorder, aggression, and cognitive impairment. Together with alpha[^{11}C]methyl-L-tryptophan (AMT) PET (see Chapter 12 for the role of AMT PET in identifying epileptogenic tubers), these PET studies have expanded our understanding of the pathophysiology of autism in TSC, pointing to both cortical and subcortical dysfunction (Asano et al. 2001). The severity of language disturbance has been

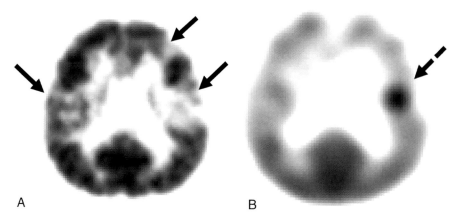

Figure 10.7 (A) FDG PET scan of a 1-year-old boy with TSC 2 gene mutation and intractable epileptic spasms, showing multiple and bilateral areas of glucose hypometabolism (*black arrows*). (B) AMT PET scan of the same patient showing increased AMT uptake in the left frontal-parietal tuber (*dotted arrow*), but no other tubers. Left fronto-parietal resection provided seizure freedom (4 years follow-up).

correlated with bilateral temporal cortex glucose hypometabolism. Autistic features consisting of stereotyped behavior, impaired social interaction, and communication disturbance have been correlated with glucose hypermetabolism in the deep cerebellar nuclei and increased AMT uptake in the caudate nucleus. Furthermore, the presence of right-sided cerebellar lesions was associated with higher social isolation, and communicative and developmental disturbance when compared with left-sided cerebellar lesions (Eluvathingal et al. 2006).

STURGE-WEBER SYNDROME

Sturge-Weber syndrome (SWS) is a rare sporadic neurocutaneous syndrome characterized by facial cutaneous angioma (unilateral or bilateral "port-wine stains") typically located in the distributions of the trigeminal nerve, associated with ipsilateral leptomeningeal angiomatosis, and congenital glaucoma. The angiomatous changes in SWS have been attributed to the failure of regression of the primitive embryonal vascular plexus on the cephalic portion of the neural tube (Di Rocco and Tamburrini 2006). Although the precise etiology of the dysregulated angiogenesis in SWS is still poorly understood, somatic mutation has been implicated based on cytogenetic and karyotype analyses of tissues from affected individuals (Huq et al. 2002). Similarly, tissue culture studies have demonstrated that fibronectin gene expression in fibroblasts derived from SWS port-wine tissue samples is increased (Comi et al. 2003; Zhou et al. 2009), suggesting that excessive expression of fibronectin may contribute to the dysregulated embryonal angiogenesis in SWS. The angioma may lead to venous stasis and thrombosis, resulting in hypoxia and chronic ischemia in the underlying cortical and subcortical areas with subsequent calcifications.

The clinical course of SWS is variable. It may be clinically static but can be a progressive neurologic condition leading to mental retardation, hemiplegia, visual deficit, and intractable epilepsy. Seizures are the most common feature. Indeed, 75% to 90% of children with SWS develop epilepsy.

Structural neuroimaging using CT and MRI helps to establish the diagnosis of SWS and define the extent of the angioma, which may involve the entire hemisphere or portions of the hemisphere (often posteriorly). CT scan typically shows intracranial dense gyriform calcifications of the affected cortical areas and/or the choroid plexus, diffuse high attenuation of the superficial and deep white matter, gyriform enhancement, brain atrophy and thickening of the calvarium (Fig. 10.8A). Contrast-enhancing leptomeningeal angioma on T1-weighted MRI is the hallmark of intracranial involvement of SWS (Fig. 10.9A). In addition, MRI can demonstrate cortical atrophy, choroid plexus enlargement (Fig. 10.9A), prominence of the deep venous system, and angiomas of the eyes. Susceptibility weighted imaging (SWI), an MRI technique with an exquisite sensitivity for defining the venous vasculature by detecting deoxygenated blood in small veins without contrast administration, has superior sensitivity to conventional T1-weighted gadolinium-enhanced MRI by showing fine details of deep transmedullary and periventricular veins (Hu et al. 2008; Juhász et al. 2007a); SWI can also visualize calcified regions, which may be difficult to appreciate on conventional MRI (Fig. 10.8B).

Functional neuroimaging with FDG PET has been used to aid in the early diagnosis (Reid et al. 1997) and

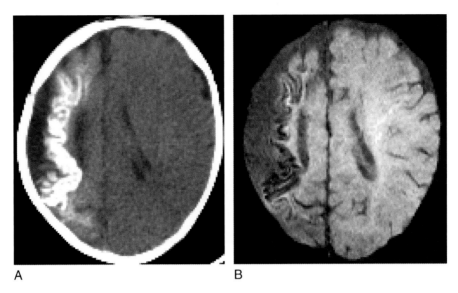

Figure 10.8 CT (A) and MRI (susceptibility weighted imaging [SWI]) (B) of a 3-month-old infant with Sturge-Weber syndrome affecting the right hemisphere. This child had daily seizures starting from the newborn period. Both scans showed severe right hemispheric atrophy with gyriform calcifications on the right side. The child underwent right hemispherectomy and became seizure-free.

assessment of the progression of the disease (Chugani et al. 1989; Juhász et al., 2007b; Lee et al. 2001). FDG PET in SWS often shows widespread unilateral hypometabolism ipsilateral to the facial nevus, and the abnormalities typically extend beyond the structural abnormalities depicted on MRI (Chugani et al., 1989; Juhász et al., 2007a; Lee et al., 2001) (Fig. 10.9B). Interestingly, children with unilateral SWS and early, rapid hemispheric progression, leading to early severe hemispheric hypometabolism, may paradoxically maintain or develop good cognitive functions (Behen et al., 2006; Lee et al., 2001). This observation suggests that functional reorganization occurs more readily when unilateral cortex is severely damaged at an early age. It is very likely that rapid demise of the affected areas, especially at younger ages, can facilitate more effective reorganization. FDG PET studies indeed demonstrated increased metabolism, likely indicating functional reorganization, in the contralateral occipital cortex of children with SWS and severe ipsilateral occipital damage (Batista et al. 2007). In contrast, cortex with mild cortical hypometabolism, which does not progress rapidly, may exert a prolonged nociferous effect on the remainder of the brain.

By studying the longitudinal changes in two consecutive glucose PET scans in 14 children with SWS and unilateral leptomeningeal angiomatosis, and correlating these changes with age, clinical seizure frequency, and hemiparesis, Juhász et al. (2007b) demonstrated that major metabolic progression in SWS occurs prior to 4 years of age, coinciding with a sharp increase of metabolic demand in the developing brain (Chugani et al. 1987). Progressive expansion of glucose hypometabolism correlated with high seizure frequency in these children. On the other hand, metabolic abnormalities may remain limited or may even recover to some extent in children with well-controlled seizures. The extent of cortical hypometabolism also correlated with an increase in hemiparesis. Taken together, these findings suggest that therapeutic interventions aimed at preventing further damage in SWS should be started early, since most of the detrimental metabolic changes occur before 4 years of age. However, children with early, rapid hemispheric progression may be observed and may not need surgery if seizures become controlled and neurocognitive functions reorganize to the opposite hemisphere.

In addition to cortical hypometabolism, a subset of young children with SWS shows a peculiar pattern of interictal *hyper*metabolism on the side of the angioma (Chugani et al. 1989; Juhász and Chugani 2009). This pattern typically occurs in young children (less than 2 years of age), shortly before or after their first seizure(s), and is not related to ongoing seizures or interictal spikes. Follow-up PET studies showed that cortical hypermetabolism in these cases is a transient phenomenon and invariably switches to hypometabolism in older children. It has been hypothesized that interictal hypermetabolism in young children with SWS may reflect a transient increase of metabolic demand in cortex undergoing excitotoxic tissue damage; affected children often (but not always) develop intractable seizures requiring surgical resection (Juhász and Chugani 2009).

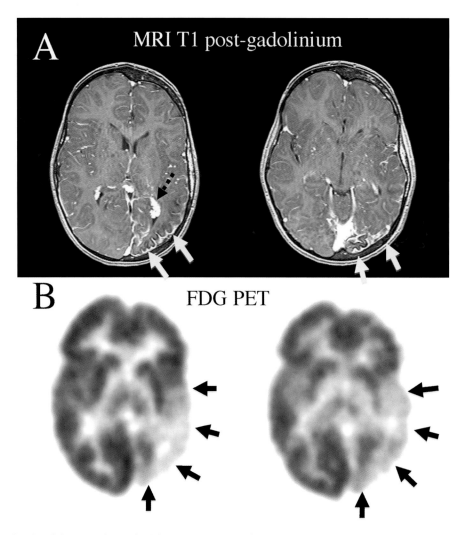

Figure 10.9 T1-weighted gadolinium-enhanced axial MRI images (A) and corresponding planes of FDG PET (B) from a 2-year-old girl with Sturge-Weber syndrome affecting the left posterior region. Contrast-enhancing leptomeningeal angioma (*white arrows*) was confined to the left occipital and parietal regions. The choroid plexus was also enlarged on the left side (*dotted arrow*). However, the FDG PET showed a more widespread hypometabolism, affecting also the entire temporal lobe (*black arrows*).

LANDAU-KLEFFNER SYNDROME AND THE SYNDROME OF CONTINUOUS SPIKE-AND-WAVE DISCHARGES DURING SLOW-WAVE SLEEP

Landau-Kleffner syndrome (LKS) (Landau 1957) or acquired epileptic aphasia is an age-related epileptic encephalopathy associated with language regression after normal development of speech; it is associated with neuropsychological impairment and paroxysmal sleep-activated epileptiform activity, particularly in the bitemporal regions. Seizures in LKS occur in 70% to 85% of cases and may co-occur, precede, or follow the onset of language regression. The syndrome typically manifests at age 3 to 7 years; however, symptoms have been described in children as young as 18 months and as old as 13 years. EEG abnormalities and epileptic

seizures in LKS usually disappear in adolescence, but language disturbances tend to persist in most patients (Duran et al. 2009).

The syndrome of continuous spike-and-wave discharges during slow-wave sleep (CSWS) or electrical status epilepticus of slow-wave sleep (ESES) is also an age-related disorder that occurs between ages 3 and 7 years, and is characterized by variable neuropsychological impairment and epilepsy with different seizure types: partial or generalized, which occur during sleep and atypical absence during wakefulness. The EEG findings consist of intense subcontinuous paroxysmal slow spike-wave complexes during interictal sleep (Patry et al. 1971; Tassinari et al. 1977). During non-REM sleep, the EEG shows continuous generalized spike-and-wave discharges occupying more than 85% of the recording (ESES). It has been proposed that the term *ESES* should be reserved to describe these EEG findings alone, without reference to specific clinical symptoms (Nickels and Wirrell 2008). Compared to children with LKS, children with CSWS tend to have more global neuropsychological dysfunction and more severe epilepsy and their epileptiform EEG abnormalities tend to predominate in the fronto-temporal or fronto-central regions.

Although the ILAE classifies LKS and CSWS as two distinct syndromes, the clinical and EEG phenotypes overlap. The EEG pattern during sleep in LKS may resemble the EEG pattern described in the syndrome of CSWS, suggesting that these two syndromes may lie along the continuum of a single age-related epileptic encephalopathy.

The neurologic substrates associated with both LKS and CSWS remain poorly understood. Structural brain damage as demonstrated by CT and MRI is usually absent, but regional functional abnormalities are often recognized on glucose metabolism PET and single photon emission computed tomography (SPECT) (da Silva et al. 1997; Gaggero et al. 1995; Harbord et al. 1999; Maquet et al. 1990, 1995; O'Tuama et al. 1992; Park et al. 1994; Rintahaka et al. 1995; Sankar et al. 1990). In LKS, the pattern of brain glucose metabolism abnormalities varies but there is a unifying abnormality in the temporal lobes (Fig. 10.10). More recently, using ^{11}C-flumazenil (FMZ) PET scans, Shiraishi et al. (2007) demonstrated diminished FMZ binding at the tip of the left temporal lobe, while FDG PET showed hypometabolism of the bilateral medial temporal regions and left superior temporal cortex in a single 8-year-old patient with LKS.

Most PET studies on CSWS have used FDG and have shown heterogeneous abnormalities: some showed focal or multifocal areas of glucose hypometabolism, whereas others showed focal or multifocal areas of glucose hypermetabolism (De Tiege et al. 2004; Luat et al. 2006; Maquet et al. 1995; Rintahaka et al. 1995) (Fig. 10.11). In the study by da Silva et al. (1997) on 17 children with LKS, FDG PET during the awake state showed bitemporal glucose hypometabolism in the majority, although some cases presented with focal or bilateral hypermetabolism. On the other hand, FDG PET taken during the sleep state in two patients with LKS and ESES showed a relative increase in glucose metabolism in the bilateral temporal cortex compared to the scans performed during the awake state (Rintahaka et al. 1995). Absolute glucose metabolic rates were not measured. The authors hypothesized that the relative increase in glucose metabolism during sleep may be an expression of functional dysregulation. In contrast, the patterns noted by Maquet et al. (1995) on six patients with CSWS were somewhat different. Five of the six showed regional increase in glucose metabolism both in the awake and sleep states. In two patients, during the sleep state, the location of the unilateral continuous spike-and-wave discharges was consistent with the area showing regional hypermetabolism. In three other patients, although the discharges were bilateral, glucose metabolism was increased in a restricted area of one hemisphere, the location of which was in close concordance with the predominant EEG abnormalities. In all of these five patients, regional glucose hypermetabolism was still observed during wakefulness, although the EEG changes were no longer continuous. The authors hypothesized that the underlying etiology of glucose hypermetabolism noted even during the awake state may be related to the disorder itself, associated with outbreak of spike-and-wave discharges, or may represent

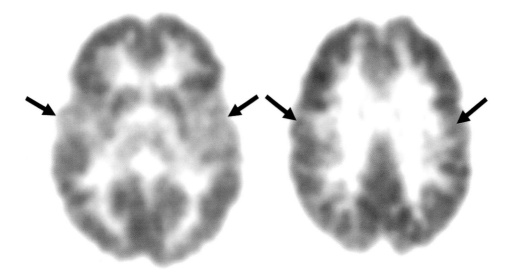

Figure 10.10 FDG PET scan of a 4-year-old girl with Landau-Kleffner syndrome showing hypometabolism of the bilateral superior temporal gyrus (*arrows*).

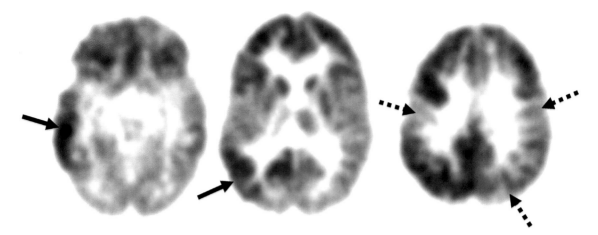

Figure 10.11 FDG PET studies of three different patients with CSWS showing heterogenous abnormalities: some showed focal or multifocal areas of glucose hypometabolism (*dotted arrows*), whereas others showed focal or multifocal areas of glucose hypermetabolism (*black arrows*).

an increased inhibitory drive in an attempt to control the outbreak of epileptic discharges.

Recently, de Tiege et al. (2004) have identified three glucose metabolic patterns in patients whose EEGs show ESES: Group 1, presence of hypermetabolic cortical areas related to epileptic foci and associated with hypometabolic areas; Group 2, presence of one or multiple areas of hypometabolism; and Group 3, absence of significant abnormalities. The association of right parietal hypermetabolism and bifrontal hypometabolism was specific for Group 1, suggesting the presence of altered functional connectivity between the parietal and frontal cortices. The authors speculated that remote functional inhibition may be related to direct intracortical connections from the epileptic focus to the hypometabolic area or polysynaptic pathways involving subcortical structures.

The Commission on Classification and Terminology of the ILAE has categorized the syndrome of CSWS under a group of syndromes undetermined as to whether they are focal or generalized. However, as reviewed here, there are functional neuroimaging and neurophysiologic data suggesting that the generalized spike-and-wave discharges in CSWS are a result of secondary bilateral synchrony. For example, neuroimaging studies have demonstrated focal glucose hypermetabolism on FDG PET (Maquet et al., 1995; Park et al., 1994) and focal decreased (or increased) blood flow on SPECT in patients with continuous spike-and-wave during slow wave sleep (Gaggero et al. 1995). It was reported that the hypermetabolic regions identified by FDG PET correlated with the epileptic focus on EEG (De Tiege et al., 2004; Maquet et al., 1995). Our own group studied the relationships between the brain glucose metabolism patterns and objectively defined EEG parameters in six children

with CSWS (Luat et al. 2005). In five of the six patients, areas of increased glucose metabolism were noted to be either confined to one hemisphere or were highly asymmetric. The origin of the spike-and-wave activity determined by sequential voltage mapping was generally concordant with the brain regions showing increased glucose metabolism. One patient underwent surgical resection of the hypermetabolic region, which was the same area noted to be the origin of generalized spike-and-wave discharges. This child became seizure-free and improved cognitively, suggesting that in at least some subjects with CSWS, resective surgery may be beneficial, provided that there is concordance between the location of focal hypermetabolism and localization of ESES based on sequential voltage mapping.

LENNOX-GASTAUT SYNDROME

Lennox-Gastaut syndrome (LGS) is an epilepsy syndrome characterized by multiple seizure types, including brief tonic, atonic, myoclonic, and atypical absence seizures, associated with intellectual disability and an interictal EEG pattern of diffuse, slow (less than 2.5 Hz) spike-wave complexes. In sleep, bursts of fast rhythmic waves and slow polyspikes, and generalized fast rhythms at about 10 Hz are also seen (Beaumanoir and Blume 2005). Several studies have demonstrated the interictal PET scan patterns in children with LGS (Chugani et al. 1987; Ferrie et al. 1996; Gur et al. 1982; Iinuma et al. 1987, Miyauchi et al. 1988, Theodore et al. 1987). Most cases demonstrated bilateral diffuse glucose hypometabolism (Fig. 10.12). However, there were cases showing focal or unilateral diffuse abnormalities. For example, Gur et al. (1982) reported two

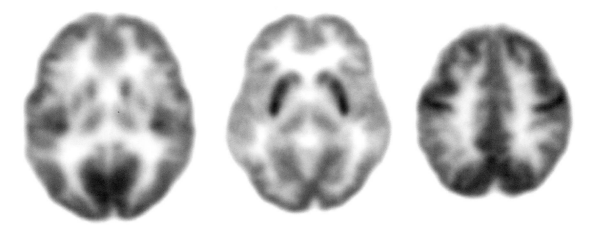

Figure 10.12 FDG PET scan of a 13-year-old girl with Lennox-Gastaut syndrome demonstrating bilateral glucose hypometabolism. EEG during the PET scan showed generalized slow spike-and-wave discharges consistent with Lennox-Gastaut syndrome.

adult patients with LGS who underwent FDG PET study before and after corpus callosotomy. Both preoperative scans showed left temporal hypometabolism compared to the contralateral side. Six weeks postoperatively, repeat FDG PET on the patient who had persistent seizure showed persistence of the left temporal lobe glucose hypometabolism. However, repeat FDG PET of the second patient, whose seizures became controlled after callosotomy, revealed a higher metabolic rate in the previously noted hypometabolic temporal lobe. These findings suggest that a temporal lobe seizure focus could be present in some patients with LGS. Theodore et al. (1987), on the other hand, did not find any focal abnormalities in their study of five children with LGS. Chugani et al. (1987), who studied a larger number of patients (n = 15), identified four metabolic subtypes: unilateral focal, unilateral diffuse, bilateral diffuse hypometabolism, and normal patterns; the most common pattern was bilateral diffuse hypometabolism. They also demonstrated that the focal areas of glucose hypometabolism need not be confined to the temporal lobe but can also be seen in the frontal regions. The finding of focal glucose hypometabolism (whether unilateral diffuse or unilateral focal) implies that surgical resection of these focal areas, if proven by intensive EEG monitoring to be the origin of a substantial number of seizures, may be an alternative treatment option for patients with LGS.

RASMUSSEN ENCEPHALITIS

Rasmussen encephalitis (Rasmussen 1958) is a rare form of chronic focal encephalitis characterized by intractable focal seizures, hemiplegia, and progressive encephalopathy, associated with inflammation and progressive atrophy of a single hemisphere. The pathogenesis of Rasmussen encephalitis is believed to be immune-mediated, involving both humoral autoimmunity and T-cell–mediated cytotoxicity. Autoantibodies to glutamate receptor GluR3 in Rasmussen encephalitis have been implicated in the pathogenesis of this disorder by some investigators (McNamara et al. 1999; Rogers et al. 1994).

Due to the progressive neurologic deterioration that accompanies Rasmussen encephalitis, aggressive treatment is necessary and surgical hemispherectomy is the mainstay of treatment. Thus, early diagnosis is necessary. Progressive, lateralized cerebral hemiatrophy demonstrated by CT and MRI is the characteristic finding in Rasmussen encephalitis. However, during the early stages of the disease, structural imaging may be normal. In this situation, functional neuroimaging using SPECT or PET scanning can detect functional abnormalities (Burke et al. 1992; Kaiboriboon et al. 2000; Lee et al. 2001).

Typically, glucose metabolism PET scanning in children with Rasmussen encephalitis shows unilateral lobar or hemispheric hypometabolism, but within the hypometabolic zone, focal areas of hypermetabolism may be found that represent sites of epileptic activity (Fig. 10.13). Lee et al. (2001) has demonstrated the order of progression of the cerebral glucose metabolism abnormalities during the early and late stages in 15 children with biopsy-proven Rasmussen encephalitis. During the early stages (less than 1 year from seizure onset), abnormal glucose metabolism is typically seen in the frontal and temporal regions and less frequently in parietal areas, whereas the posterior cortex is preserved. In the later stages of the disease (more than 1 year after onset of seizures), FDG PET studies show more extensive hemispheric involvement, including the occipital cortex, but the functional

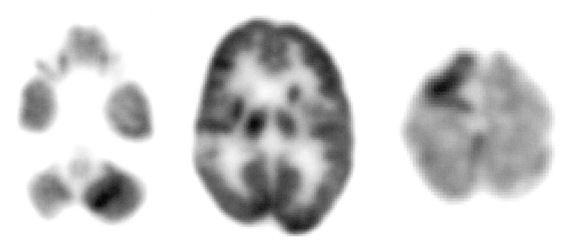

Figure 10.13 A 9-year-old boy with Rasmussen encephalitis who presented with intractable focal motor seizure involving the left body. The FDG PET brain images showed increased glucose metabolism in the right central region, right thalamus, and left cerebellum related to ongoing seizure activity and propagation.

abnormalities remained lateralized. The authors suggested that identification of the most involved areas by PET even during the early stages when MRI is usually normal may serve to guide the site of brain biopsy and may therefore facilitate the diagnosis and early treatment of the disease.

HEMIMEGALENCEPHALY

Hemimegalencephaly is a rare developmental brain malformation characterized by unilateral hemispheric enlargement and ventriculomegaly, arising from abnormalities of neuroglial differentiation and cellular migration involving predominantly one hemisphere. Some investigators believe that hemimegalencephaly results from neuronal migration disturbances between the third and fifth months of gestation, while others believe that it is a primary disorder of cellular lineage, differentiation, and proliferation (Flores-Sarnat 2002) (see also Chapter 3).

Hemimegalencephaly may occur in isolation as a sporadic disorder (without associated hemicorporal hypertrophy or cutaneous or systemic manifestation) or as part of a neurocutaneous syndrome, such as neurofibromatosis, epidermal nevus syndrome, linear nevus sebaceous syndrome, hypomelanosis of Ito, and Klippel-Trenaunay-Weber syndrome. The clinical features of hemimegalencephaly include epilepsy, mental retardation, and hemiparesis.

Epilepsy in hemimegalencephaly often becomes drug-resistant, and cerebral hemispherectomy is the recommended treatment option. The MRI demonstrates cerebral hemisphere hypertrophy, with enlargement of the lateral ventricle, an abnormal gyral pattern with a thick cortex, and gliosis in the white matter of the affected side (Fig. 10.14A) (Barkovich and Chuang 1990). Advanced myelination in the affected hemisphere has been reported. Interictal glucose metabolism PET typically shows hypometabolism in the involved hemisphere (Fig. 10.14B) but may also show intense hypermetabolism associated with continuous seizure activity such that interictal PET scans are difficult to acquire (Rintahaka et al. 1993). In addition, FDG PET may reveal that the apparently normal hemisphere, based on MRI, may in fact not be entirely normal because of focal areas of hypometabolism, suggesting the presence of additional underlying structural abnormalities at the microscopic level. This observation may explain why even after hemispherectomy, children with hemimegalencephaly, as a group, have a relatively poorer developmental outcome compared to children who underwent hemispherectomy for other disorders, such as SWS or Rasmussen encephalitis. Preoperative assessment of the contralateral hemisphere using glucose metabolism PET scanning is therefore useful to assess its integrity, thereby providing important prognostic information (Rintahaka et al. 1993).

SEVERE MYOCLONIC EPILEPSY OF INFANCY (DRAVET SYNDROME) AND GENERALIZED EPILEPSY WITH FEBRILE SEIZURE PLUS

Severe myoclonic epilepsy of infancy or Dravet syndrome (Dravet 1978) is an intractable epilepsy syndrome initially presenting with fever-induced prolonged, generalized or unilateral clonic seizures followed by the development of mixed seizure types: generalized tonic-clonic, myoclonic, atypical absence,

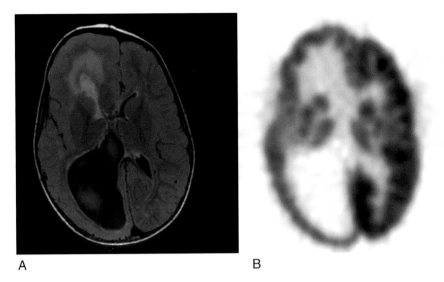

A   B

Figure 10.14 (A) T1-weighted MRI of a 2-year-old boy with intractable left-sided focal motor seizures and hemimegalencephaly showing right cerebral hemisphere hypertrophy, with enlargement of the right lateral ventricle and an abnormal gyral pattern with a thick cortex, and gliosis in the white matter of the affected hemisphere. (B) FDG PET of the same child showing glucose hypometabolism in the involved hemisphere and normal glucose metabolism in the contralateral side.

and focal seizures with or without secondary generalization. Other neurologic features include progressive psychomotor delay and ataxia. Generalized epilepsy with febrile seizure plus (GEFS+) is a childhood-onset epilepsy syndrome of multiple febrile seizures, but unlike the typical febrile convulsion syndrome, attacks with fever continue beyond 6 years of age, or afebrile seizures occur (Scheffer and Berkovic 1997). Both conditions can arise from mutations of the SCN1A gene, the gene encoding the alpha 1 pore-forming subunit of the sodium channel (Claes et al. 2001; Escayg et al. 2000). The majority of patients with Dravet syndrome and GEFS+ have mutations of SCN1A. In addition, GEFS+ is associated with mutation of the beta subunit of the sodium channel, SCN1B (Wallace et al. 1998) and the GABA$_A$ receptor gamma 2 subunit, GABARG2 (Baulac et al. 2001).

Structural neuroimaging is usually nonspecific and does not demonstrate brain lesions. Glucose metabolism PET studies of these children have shown diffuse, bilateral cortical glucose hypometabolism with relative preservation of the basal ganglia (Fig. 10.15). Although some children may show subtle asymmetries in cortical glucose metabolism, the overall pattern is a diffuse, bilateral cortical glucose hypometabolism. Since focal seizures may occur in this condition, genetic testing, if positive, should preclude epilepsy surgery.

GLUCOSE METABOLISM PET STUDIES IN CHILDREN ON KETOGENIC DIET

The ketogenic diet is a high-fat, low-protein, and low-carbohydrate diet that has been used for the treatment of intractable epilepsy. It has been used for various pediatric epilepsy syndromes, including infantile spasms, myoclonic-astatic epilepsy, severe myoclonic epilepsy syndrome of infancy or Dravet syndrome, LGS, TSC, LKS, and glucose transporter protein 1 deficiency (Kosoff et al. 2009).

The mechanism of action of the antiepileptic effects of the ketogenic diet is still controversial, but several mechanisms have been proposed (Bough and Rho 2007). The hallmark feature of ketogenic diet therapy is the achievement of ketosis as a consequence of increased fatty acid oxidation. It has been speculated that ketosis modifies the tricarboxcylic acid cycle to increase brain gamma aminobutyric acid (GABA) synthesis. The ketogenic diet increases the production of polyunsaturated fatty acids, which in turn induce the expression of neuronal uncoupling proteins, causing upregulation of numerous energy metabolism genes, and mitochondrial biogenesis. Others have hypothesized that glucose restriction during the ketogenic diet activates adenosine triphosphate (ATP)-sensitive potassium channels that lead to membrane hyperpolarization. Overall, these changes stabilize synaptic function and increase the resistance to seizure generation.

Since many patients with intractable epilepsy on the ketogenic diet are also referred for PET scanning as part of epilepsy surgery evaluation, it is important to note the effect of the diet on brain glucose metabolism. During starvation and the ketotic state, brain energy metabolism in humans shifts towards oxidation of ketone bodies. Changes in glucose availability during starvation and administration of the ketogenic diet provide the earliest evidence of cerebral metabolic

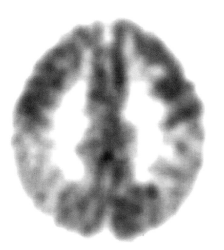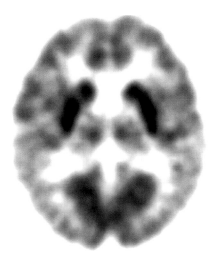

Figure 10.15 FDG PET scan of a 4-year-old boy with generalized epilepsy with febrile seizure plus (GEFS+) and SCN1A gene mutation showing severe bilateral cortical hypometabolism with relative sparing of the primary visual cortex. Prominence of the spared bilateral basal ganglia is noted.

adaptation (Prins 2008). During starvation and administration of the ketogenic diet, plasma glucose diminishes and the availability of plasma ketones increases, as does its transport to the brain. Melo et al. (2006) have shown a decrease in neuronal oxidative metabolism of glucose and an increase in astrocytic oxidative metabolism of acetate in starved rats. During short-term starvation in humans, the presence of ketones decreases brain glucose consumption in the cortex and in the cerebellum (Hasselbach et al. 1994). Using Patlak analysis, it has been demonstrated that the cerebral metabolic rate of glucose consumption in the cortex and cerebellum of ketotic rats is reduced by 10% per mM of plasma ketone bodies (LaManna et al. 2009). Taken together, these observations imply that children on the ketogenic diet will have an expected decrease in global cerebral glucose metabolism. Hence, FDG PET scanning for seizure focus localization while these patients are on the ketogenic diet is not ideal. The few such studies that have been performed have been difficult to interpret. Therefore, our policy has been not to perform FDG PET studies while patients are on the ketogenic diet.

CONCLUSION

We have discussed the value and clinical utility of glucose metabolism PET scanning in various pediatric epilepsy syndromes. As part of the presurgical evaluation for intractable epilepsy in children, FDG PET has an established role not only in the lateralization and localization of the epileptic focus, especially if structural imaging is normal, but also in the assessment of the functional integrity of areas outside the epileptic

zone. FDG PET has provided important insights regarding the pathogenesis and mechanisms of different epilepsy syndromes, particularly cryptogenic epileptic spasms, resulting in altered treatment approaches in these children. In certain other catastrophic epilepsy syndromes like Rasmussen encephalitis, it has provided us with a means of early diagnosis that leads to prompt intervention.

REFERENCES

Asano, E., D. C. Chugani, O. Muzik, et al. 2000a. Multimodality imaging for improved detection of epileptogenic foci in tuberous sclerosis complex. *Neurology* 54: 1976–84.

Asano, E., D. C. Chugani, C. Juhász, et al. 2000b. Epileptogenic zones in tuberous sclerosis complex: subdural EEG versus MRI and FDG PET. *Epilepsia* 41 (suppl 17): 128.

Asano, E., D. C. Chugani, O. Muzik, et al. 2001. Autism in tuberous sclerosis complex is related to both cortical and subcortical dysfunction. *Neurology* 57: 1269–77.

Asano, E., D. C. Chugani, and H. T. Chugani. 2003. Positron emission tomography. In: *Tuberous sclerosis complex: From basic science to clinical phenotypes.* International Review of Child Neurology Series, P. Curatolo (Ed.). London: Mac Keith Press, 124–36.

Barkovich, A.J., and S. H. Chuang. 1990. Unilateral megal-encephaly: correlation of MR imaging and pathologic characteristics. *AJNR American Journal of Neuroradiology* 11: 523–31.

Batista, C. E., C. Juhász, O. Muzik, et al. 2007. Increased visual cortex glucose metabolism contralateral to angioma in children with Sturge-Weber syndrome. *Developmental Medicine Child Neurology* 49: 567–73.

Baulac, S., G. Huberfeld, I. Gourfinkel-An, et al. 2001. First genetic evidence of GABA(A) receptor dysfunction in epilepsy: a mutation in the gamma2-subunit gene. *Nature Genetics* 28: 46–8.

Beaumanoir, A., and W. Blume. 2005. The Lennox-Gastaut syndrome. In J. Roger, M. Bureau, C. Dravet, et al. (Eds.), *Epileptic syndromes in infancy, childhood and adolescence.* John Libbery, 125–41.

Behen, M. E., C. Juhász, E. Helder, et al. 2006. Cognitive function in Sturge-Weber syndrome: Effect of side and extent of severe hypometabolism on PET scanning [abstract]. *Annals of Neurology* 60 (suppl 3): S122.

Bough, K. J., and J. M. Rho. 2007. Anticonvulsant mechanisms of ketogenic diet. *Epilepsia* 48: 43–58.

Burke, G. J., S. A. Fifer, and J. Yoder. 1992. Early detection of Rasmussen's syndrome by brain SPECT imaging. *Clinical Nuclear Medicine* 17: 730–1.

Chugani, H. T., J. C. Mazziotta, J. Engel Jr., et al. 1987. The Lennox-Gastaut syndrome: metabolic subtypes determined by 2-deox-2[18 F] fluoro-D glucose positron emission tomography. *Annals of Neurology* 21: 4–13.

Chugani, H. T., M. E. Phelps, and J. C. Mazziotta. 1987. Positron emission tomography study of human brain functional development. *Annals of Neurology* 22: 487–97.

Chugani, H. T., J. C. Mazziotta, and M. E. Phelps. 1989. Sturge-Weber syndrome: a study of cerebral glucose utilization with positron emission tomography. *Journal of Pediatrics* 114: 244–53.

Chugani, H. T., W. D. Shields, D. A. Shewmon, et al. 1990. Infantile spasms: I. PET identifies focal cortical dysgenesis in cryptogenic cases for surgical treatment. *Annals of Neurology* 27: 406–13.

Chugani, H. T., D. A. Shewmon, R. Sankar, et al. 1992. Infantile spasms: II. Lenticular nuclei and brain stem activation on positron emission tomography. *Annals of Neurology* 31: 212–9.

Chugani, H. T., D. A. Shewmon, W. D. Shields, et al. 1993. Surgery for intractable infantile spasms: neuroimaging perspectives. *Epilepsia* 34: 764–71.

Chugani, H. T., and J. R. Conti. 1996. Etiologic classification of infantile spasms in 140 cases: role of positron emission tomography. *Journal of Child Neurology* 11: 44–8.

Chugani, H. T., A. Pappas, J. Aranda, et al. 2005. MicroPET scanner within the intensive care nursery for evaluation of neonatal seizures [abstract]. *Epilepsia* 46 (suppl 8): S48–9.

Claes, L., J. Del-Favero, B. Ceulemans, et al. 2001. De novo mutations in the sodium-channel gene SCN1A cause severe myoclonic epilepsy of infancy. *American Journal of Human Genetics* 68: 1327–32.

Curatolo, P., and R. Cusmai. 1988. Magnetic resonance imaging in Bourneville's disease: relation to EEG. *Neurophysiology Clinics* 18: 459–67.

Cusmai, R., C. Chiron, P. Curatolo, et al. 1990. Topographic comparative study of magnetic resonance imaging and electroencephalography in 34 children with tuberous sclerosis. *Epilepsia* 31: 747–55.

Comi, A. M., P. Hunt, M. P. Vawter, et al. 2003. Increased fibronectin expression in Sturge-Weber syndrome fibroblasts and brain tissue. *Pediatric Research* 53: 762–9.

da Silva, E. A., D. C. Chugani, O. Muzik, et al. 1997. Landau-Kleffner syndrome: metabolic abnormalities in temporal lobe are a common feature. *Journal of Child Neurology* 12: 489–95.

De Tiege, X., S. Goldman, S. Laureys, et al. 2004. Regional cerebral glucose metabolism in epilepsies with continuous spikes and waves during sleep. *Neurology* 63: 853–7.

Di Rocco, C., and G. Tamburrini. 2006. Sturge-Weber syndrome. *Childs Nervous System* 22: 909–21.

Dravet C. 1978. Les epilepsies graves de l'enfant. *Vie Med* 8: 543–48.

Dulac, O., P. Plouin, I. Jambaque, et al. 1986. Benign epileptic infantile spasms. *Revue d'Electroencephalographique et de Neurophysiologie Clinique* 16: 371–82.

Dulac, O., P. Plouin, and I. Jambaque. 1993. Predicting favorable outcome in idiopathic West syndrome. *Epilepsia* 34: 747–56.

Duran, M. H., C. A. Guimaraes, L. L. Medeiros, et al. 2009. Landau-Kleffner syndrome: long term follow up. *Brain Development* 31: 58–63.

Eluvathingal, T. J., M. E. Behen, H. T. Chugani, et al. 2006. Cerebellar lesions in tuberous sclerosis complex: neurobehavioral and neuroimaging correlates. *Journal of Child Neurology* 21: 846–51.

Engel, J., Jr.; International League Against Epilepsy (ILAE). 2001. A proposed diagnostic scheme for people with epileptic seizures and with epilepsy: report of the ILAE Task Force on Classification and Terminology. *Epilepsia* 42: 796–803.

Escayg, A., B. T. MacDonald, M. H. Meisler, et al. 2000. Mutations of SCN1A encoding a neuronal sodium channel in two families with GEFS+2. *Nature Genetics* 24: 343–5.

Ferrie, C. D., M. Maisey, T. Cox, et al. 1996. Focal abnormalities detected by 18FDG PET in epileptic encephalopathies. *Archives of Disease in Childhood* 75: 102–7.

Flores-Sarnat, L. 2002. Hemimegalencephaly: part 1. Genetic, clinical, and imaging aspects. *Journal of Child Neurology* 17: 373–84.

Fryer, A. E., A. Chalmers, J. M. Connor, et al. 1987. Evidence that the gene for tuberous sclerosis is on chromosome 9. *Lancet* 1: 659–61.

Gaggero, R., M. Caputo, P. Fiorio, et al. 1995. SPECT and epilepsy with continuous spike waves during slow-wave sleep. *Childs Nervous System* 11: 154–60.

Gur, R. C., N. M. Sussman, A. Alavi, et al. 1982. Positron emission tomography in two cases of childhood epileptic encephalopathy (Lennox-Gastaut syndrome). *Neurology* 32: 1191–4.

Harbord, M. G., R. Singh, and S. Morony. 1999. SPECT abnormalities in Landau-Kleffner syndrome. *Journal of Clinical Neuroscience* 6: 9-16.

Hasselbach, S. G., G. M. Knudsen, J. Jakobsen, et al. 1994. Brain metabolism during short-term starvation in humans. *Journal of Cerebral Blood Flow Metabolism* 14: 125–31.

Hmaimess, G., C. Raftopoulos, H. Kadhim, et al. 2005. Impact of early hemispherectomy in a case of Ohtahara syndrome with left parieto-occipital megalencephaly. *Seizure* 14: 439–42.

Hu, J., Y. Yu, C. Juhász, et al. 2008. MR susceptibility weighted imaging (SWI) complements conventional contrast enhanced T1-weighted MRI in characterizing brain abnormalities of Sturge-Weber syndrome. *Journal of Magnetic Resonance Imaging* 28: 300–7.

Huq, A. H., D. C. Chugani, B. Hukku, et al. 2002. Evidence of somatic mosaicism in Sturge-Weber syndrome. *Neurology* 59: 780–2.

Iinuma, K., K. Yanai, T. Yanagisawa, et al. 1987. Cerebral glucose metabolism in five patients with Lennox-Gastaut syndrome. *Pediatric Neurology* 3: 12–8.

Jansen, F. E., A. C. van Huffelen, A. Algra, et al. 2007. Epilepsy surgery in tuberous sclerosis: a systematic review. *Epilepsia* 48: 1477–84.

Juhász, C., E.M. Haacke, J. Hu, et al. 2007a. Multimodality imaging of cortical and white matter abnormalities in Sturge-Weber syndrome. *AJNR American Journal of Neuroradiology* 28: 900–6.

Juhász, C., C.E. Batista, D. C. Chugani, et al. 2007b. Evolution of cortical metabolic abnormalities and their clinical correlates in Sturge-Weber syndrome. *European Journal of Paediatric Neurology* 11: 277–84.

Juhász, C., and H. T. Chugani. 2009. Transient focal increase of interictal glucose metabolism in Sturge-Weber syndrome: Implications for epileptogenesis. *Epilepsia* 50(s11): 430.

Kagawa, K., D. C. Chugani, E. Asano, et al. 2005. Epilepsy surgery outcome in children with tuberous sclerosis complex evaluated with alpha [11C] methyl-L-tryptophan positron emission tomography (PET). *Journal of Child Neurology* 20: 429–38.

Kaiboriboon, K., C. Cortese, and R. E. Hogan. 2000. Magnetic resonance and positron emission tomography changes during the clinical progression of Rasmussen encephalitis. *Journal of Neuroimaging* 10: 122–5.

Kandt, R. S., J. L. Haines, M. Smith, et al. 1992. Linkage of an important gene locus for tuberous sclerosis to a chromosome 16 marker for polycystic kidney disease. *Nature Genetics* 2: 37–41.

Kossoff, E. H., B. A. Zupec-Kania, and J. M. Rho. 2009. Ketogenic diets: an update for child neurologists. *Journal of Child Neurology* 24: 979–88.

Kramer, U., W. C. Sue, and M. A. Mikati. 1997. Focal features in West syndrome indicating candidacy for surgery. *Pediatric Neurology* 16: 213–7.

LaManna, J. C., N. Salem, M. Puchowicz, et al. 2009. Ketones suppress brain glucose consumption. *Advances in Experimental Medicine and Biology* 645: 301–6.

Landau, W.M., and F.R. Kleffner. 1957. Syndrome of acquired aphasia with convulsive disorder in children. *Neurology* 7: 523–30.

Lanska, M. J., D. J. Lanska, R. J. Baumann, et al. 1995. A population-based study of neonatal seizures in Fayette County, Kentucky. *Neurology* 45: 724–32.

Lachwani, D. K., E. Pestana, A. Gupta, et al. 2005. Identification of candidates for epilepsy surgery in patients with tuberous sclerosis complex. *Neurology* 64: 1651–4.

Lee, J. S., E. Asano, O. Muzik, et al. 2001. Sturge-Weber syndrome: correlation between clinical course and FDG PET findings. *Neurology* 57: 189–95.

Lee, J. S., C. Juhász, A.K. Kaddurah, et al. 2001. Patterns of cerebral glucose metabolism in early and late stages of Rasmussen's syndrome. *Journal of Child Neurology* 16: 798–805.

Luat, A. F., E. Asano, C. Juhász, et al. 2005. Relationship between brain glucose metabolism positron emission tomography (PET) and electroencephalography (EEG) in children with continuous spike-and-wave during slow wave sleep. *Journal of Child Neurology* 20: 682–90.

Luat, A. F., H. T. Chugani, E. Asano, et al. 2006. Episodic receptive aphasia in a child with Landau-Kleffner Syndrome: PET correlates. *Brain Development* 28: 592–6.

Madhavan, D., S. Schaffer, A. Yankovsky, et al. 2007. Surgical outcome in tuberous sclerosis complex: a multicenter survey. *Epilepsia* 48: 1625-8.

Maquet, P., E. Hirsch, D. Dive, et al. 1990. Cerebral glucose utilization during sleep in Landau-Kleffner syndrome: A PET study. *Epilepsia* 31: 778–83.

Maquet, P., E. Hirsch, M. N. Metz-Lutz, et al. 1995. Regional cerebral glucose metabolism in children with deterioration of one or more cognitive functions and continuous spike-and-wave discharges during sleep. *Brain* 118: 1497–520.

Mata, M., D. J. Fink, H. Gainer, et al. 1980. Activity-dependent energy metabolism in rat posterior pituitary primarily reflects sodium pump activity. *Journal of Neurochemistry* 34: 213–5.

McNamara, J. O., K. D. Whitney, P. I. Andrews, et al. 1999. Evidence for glutamate receptor autoimmunity in the pathogenesis of Rasmussen encephalitis. *Advances in Neurology* 79: 543–50.

Melo, T. M., A. Nehlig, and U. Sonnewald. 2006. Neuronal-glial interactions in rats fed a ketogenic diet. *Neurochemistry International* 48: 498–507.

Miyauchi, T., Y. Nomura, S. Ohno, et al. 1988. Positron emission tomography in three cases of Lennox-Gastaut syndrome. *Japanese Journal of Psychiatry and Neurology* 42: 795–804.

Nickels, K., and E. Wirrell. 2008. Electrical status epilepticus in sleep. *Seminars in Pediatric Neurology* 15: 50–60.

Ohtahara, S. 1978. Clinico-electrical delineation of epileptic encephalopathies in childhood. *Asian Medical Journal* 21: 499–509.

O'Tuama, L. A., D. K. Urion, M. J. Janicek, et al. 1992. Regional cerebral perfusion in Landau-Kleffner syndrome and related childhood aphasias. *Journal of Nuclear Medicine* 33: 1758–65.

Park, Y. D., J. M. Hoffman, R. A. Radtke, et al. 1994. Focal cerebral metabolic abnormality in a patient with continuous spike waves during slow-wave sleep. *Journal of Child Neurology* 9: 139–43.

Patry, G., S. Lyagoubi, and C. A. Tassinari. 1971. Subclinical"electrical status epilepticus" induced by sleep in children. A clinical and electroencephalographic study of six cases. *Archives of Neurology* 24: 242–52.

Prins, M. L. 2008. Cerebral metabolic adaptation and ketone metabolism after brain injury. *Journal of Cerebral Blood Flow Metabolism* 28: 1–16.

Rasmussen, T., J. Olszewski, and D. Lloydsmith. 1958. Focal seizures due to chronic localized encephalitis. *Neurology* 8: 435–45.

Reid, D. E., B. L. Maria, W. E. Drane, et al. 1997. Central nervous system perfusion and metabolism abnormalities in Sturge-Weber syndrome. *Journal of Child Neurology* 12: 218–22.

Rintahaka, P. J., H. T. Chugani, C. Messa, et al. 1993. Hemimegalencephaly: evaluation with positron emission tomography. *Pediatric Neurology* 9: 21–8.

Rintahaka, P. J., H. T. Chugani, and R. Sankar. 1995. Landau-Kleffner syndrome with continuous spikes and waves during slow wave sleep. *Journal of Child Neurology* 10: 127–33.

Rintahaka, P. J., and H. T. Chugani. 1997. Clinical role of positron emission tomography in children with tuberous sclerosis complex. *Journal of Child Neurology* 12: 42–52.

Rogers, S. W., P. I. Andrews, L. C. Gahring, et al. 1994. Autoantibodies to glutamate receptor 3 GluR3 in Rasmussen's encephalitis. *Science* 265: 648–51.

Saliba, R. M., J. F. Annegers, D. K. Waller, et al. 1999. Incidence of neonatal seizures in Harris County, Texas, 1992–2004. *American Journal of Epidemiology* 150: 763–9.

Sankar, R., H. T. Chugani, P. Lubens, et al. 1990. Heterogeneity in the patterns of cerebral glucose utilization in children with Landau-Kleffner syndrome. *Neurology* 40 (Suppl): 257.

Scheffer, I. E., and S. F. Berkovic. 1997. Generalized epilepsy with febrile seizure plus. A genetic disorder with heterogenous clinical phenotypes. *Brain* 120: 479–90.

Shiraishi, H., K. Takano, T. Shiga, et al. 2007. Possible involvement of the tip of the temporal lobe in Landau-Kleffner syndrome. *Brain Development* 29: 529–33.

Sugimoto, T., H. Otsubo, P. A. Hwang, et al. 1999. Outcome of epilepsy surgery in the first three years of life. *Epilepsia* 40: 560–5.

Szelies, B., K. Herholz, W. D. Heiss, et al. 1983. Hypometabolic cortical lesions in tuberous sclerosis with epilepsy: demonstration by positron emission tomography. *Journal of Computer Assisted Tomography* 7: 946–53.

Tassinari, C. A., G. Terzano, G. Capocchi, et al. 1977. Epileptic seizures during sleep in children. In J. K. Penry (Ed.), *Epilepsy: The Eighth International Symposium.* New York: Raven Press, 345–54.

Teutonico, F., R. Mai, O. Devinsky, et al. 2008. Epilepsy surgery in tuberous sclerosis complex: early predictive elements and outcome. *Childs Nervous System* 24: 1437–45.

Theodore, W. H., D. Rose, N. Patronas, et al. 1987. Cerebral glucose metabolism in the Lennox-Gastaut syndrome. *Annals of Neurology* 21: 14–21.

van Slegtenhorst, M., R. de Hoogt, C. Hermans, et al. 1997. Identification of the tuberous sclerosis gene TSC1 on chromosome 9q34. *Science* 277: 805–8.

Wallace, R. H., D. W. Wang, R. Singh, et al. 1998. Febrile seizures and generalized epilepsy associated with a mutation in the Na+ channel beta 1 subunit gene SCN1B. *Nature Genetics* 19: 366–70.

Weiner, H. L., C. Carlson, E. B. Ridgway, et al. 2006. Epilepsy surgery in young children with tuberous sclerosis: results of a novel approach. *Pediatrics* 117: 1494–502.

Wyllie, E., Y. G. Comair, P. Kotagal, et al. 1996. Epilepsy surgery in infants. *Epilepsia* 37: 625–37.

Wyllie, E., Y. G. Comair, P. Kotagal, et al. 1998. Seizure outcome after epilepsy surgery in children and adolescents. *Annals of Neurology* 44: 740–8.

Zhou, Q., J. W. Zheng, X. J. Yang, et al. 2009. Fibronectin: characterization of somatic mutation in Sturge-Weber syndrome (SWS). *Medical Hypotheses* 73: 199-200.

Chapter *11*

[¹¹C]FLUMAZENIL POSITRON EMISSION TOMOGRAPHY

Matthias J. Koepp

Gamma amino-butyric acid (GABA) is the major inhibitory neurotransmitter in the brain. Flumazenil (FMZ) acts as a specific, reversibly bound antagonist at the benzodiazepine binding sites of $GABA_A$ receptors and its PET analog, [¹¹C]FMZ (Olsen et al. 1990), therefore, acts as a good marker for the $GABA_A$ receptor. As most neurons express $GABA_A$ receptors, FMZ can also, to some extent, be regarded as a neuronal marker. The vast majority of clinical FMZ PET studies have been performed on patients with epilepsy, with very few studies addressing altered $GABA_A$ receptor function in stroke (Heiss et al. 2004), addiction (Linford-Hughes et al. 2005), neurodegenerative disease (Wicks et al. 2008), and hepatic encephalopathies (Jalan et al. 2000).

DATA ACQUISITION AND ANALYSIS: METHODOLOGICAL CONSIDERATIONS

[¹¹C]FMZ binds principally in neocortex, with lower binding in hippocampus, basal ganglia, thalamus, and cerebellum. It has several properties that make it a useful PET tracer, including no metabolism in the brain, polar metabolites that do not cross the blood–brain barrier, suitable kinetics, and relatively low nonspecific binding (unlike labeled benzodiazepine *agonists*).

[¹¹C]FMZ data can be analyzed without a reference (ADD or summed images), or using a reference region from the images themselves (e.g., pons or brain stem [Lamuso et al. 2000]), including those with equilibrium scanning (Szelies et al. 2000) and partial saturation (Delforge et al. 1997), or using an external reference (e.g., an arterial plasma input function). However, the reproducibility of [¹¹C]FMZ measurements is considerably better with analytical measures based on arterial input function than those using pons as the reference tissue (Salmi et al. 2008).

In healthy volunteers, significant linear intra-subject correlations were reported between regional binding values obtained with kinetic modeling (parametric images) versus regional summed activity obtained from integrated (ADD) images, thus alleviating the need for arterial lines (Millet et al. 1995; Mishina et al. 2000; Okazawa et al. 2004). Hammers et al. (2008) formally compared the diagnostic yield of parametric images in patients with histologically confirmed unilateral hippocampal sclerosis. Parametric images were obtained either with a parent tracer arterial plasma input function and spectral analysis (yielding volume-of-distribution [VD] images) or with an image-based input function and the simplified reference tissue model (binding potential images, BP-SRTM), and the diagnostic yield of these "modeled" images was compared with semiquantitative-integrated (ADD) images from 10 to 20 or 20 to 40 minutes (ADD1020 and ADD2040) after [^{11}C]FMZ injection. These particular times were selected because ADD1020 [^{11}C]FMZ PET images (Juhász et al. 1999, 2000, 2001; Muzik et al. 2000; Niimura et al. 1999) and ADD2040 images (Mishina et al. 2000; Ryvlin et al. 1998, 1999) have been widely used in the study of epilepsy. The comparison revealed that VD images showed ipsilateral hippocampal decreases in all 15 patients, while ADD1020 and ADD2040 images had a lower detection rate for decreased FMZ uptake ipsilateral to the epileptogenic hippocampus in 13 and 12 out of 15 cases, respectively. Therefore, it appears that full quantification with an image-independent input should ideally be used in the evaluation of FMZ PET, at least in temporal lobe epilepsy (TLE).

Voxel-based analyses and region-of-interest approaches were found to have similar reproducibility in test–retest studies (Salmi et al. 2008). Voxel-based approaches, such as statistical parametric mapping (SPM) (Friston et al. 1995), have the advantage of increased objectivity compared with hand-drawn or anatomically placed regions, do not assume a specific site or size of the area of changes, and easily allow the investigation of the entire brain volume. They do not, however, lend themselves to absolute quantification. If structural changes are present that affect control and patient populations differently, as for example in hippocampal sclerosis, correction for partial volume effects is mandatory as these are non-linear and therefore more prominent in smaller structures (Hoffman et al. 1979). This requires a correction for partial volume effects caused by the limited spatial resolution of PET, by comparison with higher-resolution MRI data (Labbé et al. 1998; Meltzer et al. 1990, 1996; Rousset et al. 1993). Correction for partial volume effect increased the sensitivity of [^{11}C]FMZ PET for detecting unilateral hippocampal sclerosis from 65% to 100% in 17 patients with MRI-defined hippocampal sclerosis (Koepp et al. 1997c). Further, [^{11}C]FMZ PET was more sensitive than MRI in the detection of contralateral abnormalities, which were found in a third of patients with apparent unilateral hippocampal sclerosis on MRI (Koepp et al. 1997a) and also showed that loss of GABA$_A$ receptor binding was consistently over and above loss of hippocampal volume, indicating that the loss of binding was not simply due to hippocampal atrophy.

[^{11}C]FMZ PET IN TEMPORAL LOBE EPILEPSY

The hallmark of TLE is the area of reduced [^{11}C]FMZ binding. The first study using FMZ PET in focal epilepsies showed an average reduction of [^{11}C]FMZ binding of 30% in the epileptogenic focus. Such results have been replicated by several groups, and comparative studies with [^{18}F]FDG PET have consistently shown the area of reduced [^{11}C]FMZ binding to be more restricted than the area of hypometabolism in TLE (Debets et al. 1997; Henry et al. 1993; Savic et al. 1993; Szelies et al. 1996).

The pathologic basis of reduced [^{11}C]FMZ binding in hippocampal sclerosis has been investigated in some detail (Burdette et al. 1995; Hand et al. 1997; Johnson et al. 1992; Koepp et al. 1998a). Quantitative autoradiographic and neuropathologic studies of surgically removed hippocampi, compared with autopsy controls, showed a reduction of the number of GABA$_A$ receptors bearing benzodiazepine recognition sites over and above neuronal loss in the CA1 subregion, but the loss of receptors paralleled the loss of neurons in other subregions. Also, increases in affinity were noted in the subiculum, hilus, and dentate gyrus (Hand et al. 1997; Koepp et al. 1998a). A direct comparison of quantitative in vivo hippocampal [^{11}C]FMZ binding and quantitative ex vivo [^{3}H]FMZ autoradiography showed a mean 42% reduction in binding in the hippocampal body in ten patients with hippocampal sclerosis, compared with control material, with both methods, and a good correlation between the in vivo and ex vivo measures in individual patients (Koepp et al. 1998a). In the white matter, [^{11}C]FMZ binding was tightly correlated with the number of heterotopic neurons, determined semiquantitatively ex vivo in resected specimens (Hammers et al. 2001a).

The first study applying the voxel-by-voxel analysis of SPM in patients with MRI-detected hippocampal sclerosis found decreases of [^{11}C]FMZ binding to be restricted to the sclerotic hippocampus (Koepp et al. 1996) (Fig. 11.1, left panel). This may have implications for outcome as areas of abnormal [^{11}C]FMZ binding were likely to be part of the epileptogenic zone in a surgical series of patients with neocortical focal epilepsies, while widespread hypometabolism on FDG PET seemed less important surgically (Juhász et al. 2001). Further elaboration of this technique, however, revealed extra-FMZ binding abnormalities not only in the hippocampus, but also in the symptomatic zone, in particular involvement of the insula associated with emotional seizure symptoms (Bouilleret et al. 2002) (Fig. 11.1, right panel).

TEMPORAL LOBE EPILEPSY WITH NORMAL MRI

A successful postoperative outcome is less likely in imaging-negative patients. Indeed, in about 20% of

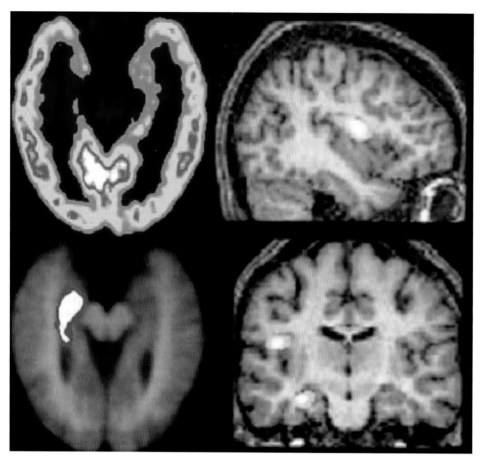

Figure 11.1 SPM of FMZ PET. Left panel shows axial slice of FMZ PET in patients with unilateral hippocampal sclerosis (top) and group results of 12 patients with unilateral hippocampal sclerosis compared to 17 controls. Right panel depicts the late benzodiazepine receptor dependent images in the group of 18 patients compared to the control group of 8 volunteers. Benzodiazepine receptor density abnormalities are localized in the temporo-mesial region and in the ipsilateral insula. (Adapted from Koepp, M. J., M. P. Richardson, D. J. Brooks, et al. 1996. Cerebral benzodiazepine receptors in hippocampal sclerosis. An objective in vivo analysis. *Brain* 119: 1677–87 and Bouilleret, V., S. Dupont, L. Spelle, et al. 2002. Insular cortex involvement in mesiotemporal lobe epilepsy: a positron emission tomography study. *Annals of Neurology* 51(2): 202–8.)

patients with chronic focal epilepsy, high-resolution qualitative and quantitative MRI does not reveal any significant pathology.

Abnormalities of [^{11}C]FMZ binding have repeatedly been demonstrated even when hippocampal volumes were normal (Hammers et al. 2002; Koepp et al. 2000; Lamusuo et al. 2000; Ryvlin et al. 1998; Szelies et al. 2000). In the largest of these series of MRI-negative TLE patients (Hammers et al. 2002), potentially surgically relevant changes (i.e., focal reductions of hippocampal or extrahippocampal FMZ-VD) were found in 7 of 18 patients. Increased FMZ-VD in white matter, representing an increased density of heterotopic white matter neurons (microdysgenesis), was found in 11 of 18 individual patients. Microdysgenesis is not detectable on MRI, and this new finding may represent the

pathophysiologic basis of a proportion of TLE cases with normal MRI.

MALFORMATIONS OF CORTICAL DEVELOPMENT

Malformations of cortical development (MCD) commonly underlie partial seizures and may not be detectable on MRI (Chugani et al. 1990; Desbiens et al. 1993; Hammers et al. 2002). Surgery for seizures is less successful in these patients than in patients with discrete lesions, most likely because of anatomical and functional abnormalities extending beyond the visible lesions. A study using fully quantified [^{11}C]FMZ PET and SPM in 12 patients with MCD and partial seizures found areas of abnormal [¹¹C]FMZ VD in 10 patients. The abnormal regions were frequently more extensive than the abnormality seen with MRI, and were also noted in distant sites that were unremarkable on MRI (Richardson et al. 1996). Only some of the abnormalities could be accounted for by structural changes, as shown by a follow-up study that compared [¹¹C]FMZ binding and gray matter on a voxel basis (Richardson et al. 1997): this study also revealed abnormalities in areas that had appeared normal on PET alone, underlining the need to interpret functional data in the light of structural data. These studies demonstrated, for the first time, focal increases of [¹¹C]FMZ binding in patients with epilepsy that had not been seen in other pathologies. Possible explanations include increased neuronal density, the presence of heterotopic neurons expressing GABA_A receptors, and increased numbers or availability of receptors.

A study examining explicitly areas of MCD as well as the adjacent or overlying cortex found a general pattern of reduced [¹¹C]FMZ VD in areas of abnormal gray matter, and increases in some adjacent or overlying areas (Hammers et al. 2001c). Detailed analysis of invasive EEG recordings and FMZ PET findings in individual patients revealed concordance in about 50% of patients (Fig. 11.2), but also a high degree of false-positive findings due to anatomical variants (Fig. 11.3) (Vollmar and Noachtar 2004).

ACQUIRED LESIONS

Only decreases of [¹¹C]FMZ binding were seen in six patients with acquired lesions (Richardson et al. 1998). Similarly, in another study, eight of nine patients with TLE and mass lesions showed decreases matching the MRI abnormalities; the ninth had a small lesion that was not detected on [¹¹C]FMZ PET, and asymmetry indices were falsely lateralizing (Ryvlin et al. 1998). FMZ PET was felt to be clinically useful in 17 patients with lesional epilepsies (Juhász et al. 2000). Areas of reduced binding included cortex with epileptiform discharges on electrocorticography, and the complete resection of the cortex and the epileptogenic cortex yielded good results in eight of nine patients, while incomplete resection of the lesion or the perilesional epileptogenic cortex led to persistence of seizures in four patients.

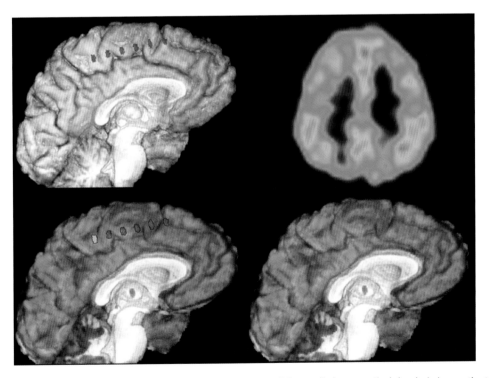

Figure 11.2 FMZ PET in malformations of cortical development. MRI (upper left panel) shows cortical dysplasia in a patient with right frontal lobe epilepsy. FDG PET (upper right panel) of this patient shows widespread hypometabolism in the right frontal lobe. FMZ-PET (lower left panel) shows a more circumscribed reduction of GABA_A receptor binding, which is consistent in its localization with the seizure onset zone (red) as identified by invasive EEG recordings with subdural electrodes (lower right panel). (Courtesy of Dr. Christian Vollmar and adapted from Christian Vollmar and Soheyl Noachtar. 2004. Neuroimaging in epilepsy. *Turkish Journal of Neurology* 10: 185–200.)

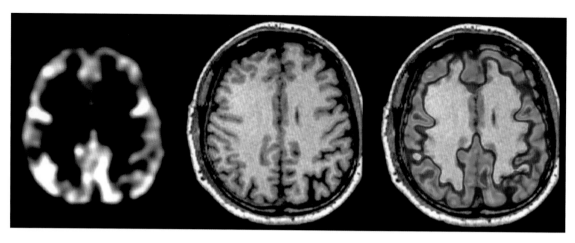

Figure 11.3 False-positive FMZ PET. FMZ PET shows left occipital focal reduction in FMZ binding. Co-registration with MRI reveals anatomical variant with wide sulcus, which explains the PET finding. (Courtesy of Dr. Christian Vollmar)

FOCAL EPILEPSIES OF EXTRATEMPORAL ORIGIN

A limited number of studies have investigated patients with extratemporal seizures. In the first but small series of six patients with frontal lobe epilepsy compared with seven controls, [11C]FMZ PET correctly identified the epileptogenic zone as an area of decreased binding in all, including the five in whom MRI was normal (Savic et al. 1995). The MRI technique, however, was suboptimal, and some of these patients would probably now no longer be classified as "MRI-negative." In ten children with seizures of extratemporal origin who subsequently underwent epilepsy surgery, FMZ PET detected at least part of the epileptogenic focus in all (Muzik et al. 2000).

In 18 patients with normal high-resolution MRI and refractory extratemporal seizures, [11C]FMZ PET showed focal decreases of [11C]FMZ VD in 6 and focal increases in 10 (Richardson et al. 1998). Since focal increases of [11C]FMZ binding had previously been seen only in patients with MCD (Richardson et al. 1996), the implication of these data is that focally increased [11C]FMZ binding may be a marker of MCD and may indicate occult MCD in patients who are MRI-negative. An explanation as to why increases of [11C]FMZ binding were not seen in earlier studies is that most other studies relied on semiquantitative data and/or asymmetry indices, which make the detection of such changes more difficult, and in some studies, visually detected decreases were used for region placement.

In the largest series of MRI-negative patients with seizures of extratemporal origin, abnormalities of [11C]FMZ VD were found in 33 of 44 patients (Hammers et al. 2003). Only patients with normal optimal-quality MRI were included, and patients were not required to be undergoing presurgical evaluation. Relatively few patients had surgically relevant focal decreases of [11C]FMZ binding (Fig. 11.4). Seven of 44 patients, however, had significantly increased [11C] FMZ VD in periventricular areas, compatible with an occult migration disorder, and at a lower threshold 89% of patients showed such changes. The surgical relevance of such findings is still unclear, but the study suggests a prominent role of occult migration disorders in the pathophysiology of cryptogenic focal epilepsies (Fig. 11.5).

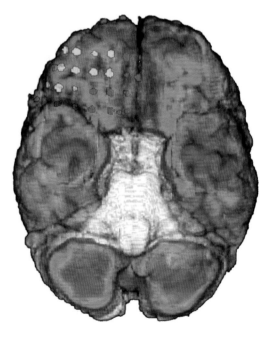

Figure 11.4 FMZ PET in a patient with frontal lobe epilepsy and normal MRI. Good correlation was noted between reduced orbito-frontal FMZ binding (blue) and seizure onset as detected by subdural electrodes (yellow). (Courtesy of Dr. Christian Vollmar)

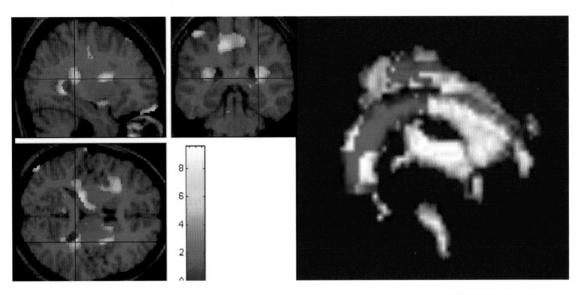

Figure 11.5 White matter changes in a patient with frontal lobe epilepsy. Periventricular increases of [¹¹C]FMZ VD with results of SPM comparison of a single patient against 16 controls (left panel), overlaid onto the individual patient's segmented ventricular system to show spatial relationship (right panel). (Courtesy of Prof. Alexander Hammers and adapted from Alexander Hammers. 2004. Flumazenil PET and other ligands for functional imaging. *Neuroimaging Clinics of North America* 14(3): 537–51.)

CLINICAL UTILITY OF FMZ PET IN FOCAL EPILEPSIES

[¹¹C]FMZ PET has been used for the evaluation of patients with presumed mesial TLE since early 1988, but it has not become part of routine preoperative evaluation. This is due to technical difficulties as well as the proliferation of other, particularly MRI-based, imaging procedures. In MRI-identifiable hippocampal sclerosis, FMZ PET does not currently yield additional information. In hippocampal sclerosis, [¹¹C]FMZ PET abnormalities are often more restricted than [¹⁸F]FDG abnormalities, but no additional information may be obtained from detecting localized abnormalities of [¹¹C]FMZ binding, if standard anterior temporal lobe resections are carried out. In Ryvlin et al.'s large series (1998), [¹¹C]FMZ PET helped to confirm the bilateral origin of seizures in a third of patients with bitemporal epilepsy and identified contralateral abnormalities in a number of cases.

In contrast to these situations, FMZ PET seems to be useful in MRI-negative TLE, and it is likely to be useful in a substantial number of patients with MRI-negative focal epilepsy of extratemporal origin.

The practical utility and significance of the different PET techniques and their findings in MRI-negative patients are difficult to assess, with hardly any studies using different modalities together in large enough samples. Diagnostic methods with a high sensitivity increase the risk of type I errors, the positive identification of false abnormalities. Type I errors could

cause unnecessary explorations using possibly harmful procedures or even resections.

There are only a few studies assessing the significance of contributions from multimodality imaging in this clinically challenging patient population. Comparisons between different techniques are usually biased towards the technique the investigators have the most experience with. "Negativity" with a certain imaging tool very much depends on the level of sophistication of its users. In clinical practice, standard MRI investigations based on axial images and read by radiologists outside of epilepsy centers ("non-experts") failed to detect 57% of focal epileptogenic lesions, thus leading to false "MRI-negativity" (Von Oertzen et al. 2002). When expert assessment of MRI epilepsy protocols failed to depict a lesion in a large study and a subgroup of these MRI-negative patients went to surgery based on electrophysiologic findings, histopathologic findings were often unrevealing (Urbach et al. 2004).

[¹¹C]FMZ-PET had a higher yield than MRI in detecting abnormalities by decreased (and, sometimes, increased) binding, but the overall yield of identifying a clinically relevant focus and aiding in the assessment of possible surgical treatment in refractory epilepsy patients with normal MRI has been low. Out of 45 published patients with TLE and normal MRI, 38 patients (84%) had abnormal [¹¹C]FMZ PET scans, but only in 21 patients (46%) were these abnormalities thought to be surgically useful. In MRI-negative patients with extratemporal seizure origin, this ratio was even lower: out of 102 published, 73 patients (71%) showed abnormalities of FMZ binding, but these findings were surgically useful in only 27 patients (26%).

Why is the yield of [^{11}C]FMZ PET so low in adult patients with refractory epilepsy? Ryvlin et al. (1999) highlighted a total of three patients with TLE and normal MRI in whom FMZ decreases were seen contralateral to the epileptogenic temporal lobe and varied in severity on two separate studies, and the authors proposed that time since last seizure may account for some such false lateralizations. In a controlled follow-up study, a test–retest [^{11}C]FMZ PET study was undertaken in 10 drug-resistant epileptic patients, including 6 patients with mesial TLE and 10 normal controls, to investigate seizure-related short-term plasticity of benzodiazepine receptors. All subjects underwent two FMZ PET scans at a 1-week interval. Patients benefited from a concurrent video-EEG monitoring, which allowed determination of the duration of the interictal period preceding each PET. Five patients (50%), but no controls, demonstrated clinically significant test–retest FMZ PET variations in the mesial temporal region. This was observed in all three patients with mesial TLE and no hippocampal atrophy in whom only the PET study associated with the shortest interictal period correctly identified the epileptogenic zone. Statistical analysis revealed a significant effect of interictal period duration on benzodiazepine receptor B_{max} in TLE patients, suggesting that the shorter the interictal period, the lower the B_{max} in the epileptogenic hippocampus. These findings suggest that FMZ PET ideally should be performed within a few days following a seizure in patients with mesial TLE and a normal MRI.

Presence of multifocal FMZ PET abnormalities may limit the clinical usefulness of this imaging modality for presurgical evaluation unless a more detailed understanding of clinical, electrophysiologic, and neuropathologic correlates of such abnormalities can be achieved. Juhász et al. (2009) analyzed the significance of focal cortical decreases of $GABA_A$ receptor binding using PET in 20 children with non-localizing MRI who underwent resective epilepsy surgery following intracranial EEG monitoring with subdural electrodes because of intractable neocortical epilepsy. Their goal was to determine the clinical (seizure variables, surgical outcome), electrophysiologic (intracranial EEG), and histopathologic correlates (where available) of cortical decreases of $GABA_A$ receptor binding detected in and outside the lobe of the primary epileptic focus. Focal decrease of cortical FMZ binding was detected in the lobe of seizure onset in 17 (85%) patients. Eleven patients (55%) had 17 remote cortical areas with decreased FMZ binding outside the lobe of seizure onset. Thirteen of those 16 (81%) of the 17

remote cortical regions that were covered by subdural EEG were around cortex showing rapid seizure spread on intracranial EEG.

Such multiple cortical regions with decreased $GABA_A$ receptor binding may participate in an epileptic network that includes cortical areas of seizure onset and rapid seizure propagation to remote connected areas detected by intracranial EEG. Presence of such remote PET abnormalities was also associated with high clinical seizure frequency. This is indeed highly relevant clinically, as removal of both perifocal and remote cortex, some of which may be missed by scalp EEG alone or FDG PET, may need to be resected to achieve seizure freedom. A careful evaluation of cortex with decreased $GABA_A$ receptor binding prior to resection using intracranial EEG may facilitate optimal surgical outcome in patients with intractable neocortical epilepsy.

Similar correlations between seizure frequency, seizure propagation areas, and reduced [^{11}C]FMZ binding have been reported also in adults. One study explicitly investigated a correlation between seizure frequency and [^{11}C]FMZ binding in 19 patients with partial seizures and normal MRI, using manually placed regions of interest (Savic et al. 1996). In patients with daily seizures, reductions were also seen in the primary projection areas of the focus. Similarly, the same group reported decreased binding in some but not all of the primary projection areas in four patients with TLE, compared to seven controls. In some of these areas with reduced binding, the FMZ binding increased one year after epilepsy surgery, albeit with a very wide spread (+29 ± 17%).

OUTCOME

Ultimately, only postoperative follow-up studies will provide information about the specificity of the various imaging abnormalities seen. Only one study so far has attempted to correlate preoperative FMZ PET directly with postoperative outcome, and it assessed the significance of periventricular increases of white matter FMZ binding, implying heterotopic neurons in white matter of patients with mesial TLE (Hammers et al 2008). Using SPM, increased periventricular white matter FMZ binding was compared in patients who were not seizure-free compared with those who became seizure-free following surgery. On individual analysis, four of seven patients who were not seizure-free after temporal lobectomy versus three of eight who did become seizure-free demonstrated increased periventricular white matter binding (compared with control values) around the posterior horns of both ventricles ipsilateral and contralateral to the epileptic focus, with some individual variations. Patients who were not seizure-free or those with increased FMZ binding tended to be less likely to have strictly unilateral discharges on video-EEG. FMZ PET might be detecting occult periventricular migration abnormalities, or microdysgenesis. The detection of increased periventricular white matter FMZ binding may be an adverse prognostic factor, even when MRI shows mesial temporal sclerosis, and these subtle malformations may underlie additional seizure foci, leading to persistent postoperative seizures.

FMZ PET IN IDIOPATHIC GENERALIZED EPILEPSIES

Interictal FMZ PET studies in patients with various idiopathic generalized epilepsy syndromes have revealed abnormalities of GABA$_A$ receptor binding. Savic (1990) reported a slight reduction in cortical binding of [¹¹C]FMZ in a heterogenous group of patients with generalized seizures, compared with the non-focus areas of patients with partial seizures. Subsequently, the same author presented data in patients with primary generalized tonic-clonic seizures that showed increased FMZ binding in the cerebellar nuclei and decreased FMZ binding in the thalamus (Savic et al. 1994). While Prevett et al. (1995) found no significant changes in FMZ binding in a large group of patients with childhood absence epilepsy and

juvenile absence epilepsy not taking valproate, FMZ binding was reduced by about 9% in the patients receiving valproate, suggesting that this drug might result in a reduced number of available benzodiazepine receptors. In a longitudinal follow-up study, FMZ binding before valproate addition was significantly increased globally, and was only reduced in those patients after valproate who had obtained benefit from this medication in terms of reduction in seizure frequency (Koepp et al. 1997b).

Further analysis in the subgroup of patients suffering from juvenile myoclonic epilepsy (JME) revealed accentuation of increased FMZ binding bilaterally in the dorsolateral prefrontal cortex and ventral premotor area (Fig. 11.6, left panel) (Koepp and Duncan 2000). These bifrontal areas are close to those areas 45 and 46 in the medial and inferior frontal gyrus, where the most profound increases in neuronal density had been observed in histopathologic examinations of autopsy specimens (Meencke and Janz 1994). Furthermore, JME is associated with a particular personality profile, and behavioral and neuropsychological studies have suggested the possible involvement of frontal lobe dysfunction with quantitative MRI revealing significant abnormalities of cortical gray matter in medial frontal areas (Fig. 11.6, right panel) (Woerman et al. 1999). There is now sufficient evidence from multimodality imaging of multifocal disease mechanisms to suggest that JME is a frontal lobe variant of a multiregional,

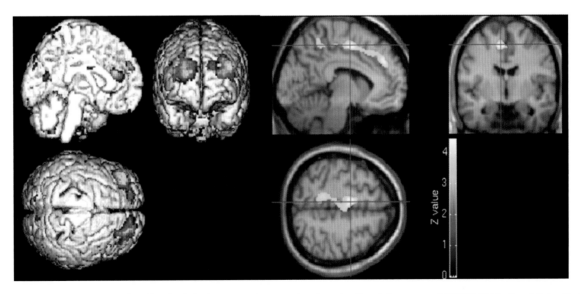

Figure 11.6 FMZ PET and MRI in JME. Statistical parametric map showing significant increases of [¹¹C]FMZ binding bilaterally in the dorsolateral prefrontal cortex of five patients with JME, when compared with 20 healthy normal controls (left panel). Voxel-based statistical parametric mapping of structural MRI data, comparing gray matter of 20 JME patients with that of 30 control subjects, after semiautomated segmentation (right panel). (Adapted from M. J. Koepp and J. S. Duncan. 2000. Positron emission tomography in idiopathic generalized epilepsy: imaging beyond structure. In B. Schmitz and T. Sander (Eds.), *Juvenile myoclonic epilepsy: The Janz syndrome*. London: Wrightson, 91–9, and F. G. Woermann, S. L. Free, M. J. Koepp, et al. 1999. Abnormal cerebral structure in juvenile myoclonic epilepsy demonstrated with voxel-based analysis of MRI. *Brain* 122: 2101–8).

thalamocortical "network" epilepsy rather than a generalized epilepsy syndrome.

FMZ IN GENE MUTATIONS ASSOCIATED WITH EPILEPSY

Understanding the consequences of newly discovered single gene mutations associated with human epilepsy has the potential to yield new insights into the underlying mechanisms of this disorder. A mutation of the gamma2 subunit of the $GABA_A$ receptor, where there is a substitution of glutamine for arginine at position 43 (R43Q), has been found in a familial generalized epilepsy. Individuals affected by the GABRG2(R43Q) mutation had reduced [11C]FMZ binding (Fedi et al. 2006). The greatest change in binding occurred anteriorly, with peak differences in insular and anterior cingulate cortices revealed by SPM. As synaptic inhibition in the human brain is largely mediated by the $GABA_A$ receptor, these findings are likely to represent an important clue to the mechanisms linking this gene defect to the epilepsy phenotype.

Succinic semialdehyde dehydrogenase (SSADH) deficiency is an autosomal recessive disorder of GABA metabolism characterized by elevated levels of GABA and gamma-hydroxybutyric acid (Pearl et al. 2009). Clinical findings include intellectual impairment, hypotonia, hyporeflexia, hallucinations, autistic behaviors, and seizures. Autoradiographic labeling and slice electrophysiology studies in the murine model demonstrate use-dependent downregulation of $GABA_A$ receptors. SSADH-deficient patients showed widespread reduction in FMZ binding compared to parents and controls, in particular affecting the amygdala, hippocampus, cerebellar vermis, and frontal, parietal, and occipital cortex. These findings suggest a potential mechanism for neurologic dysfunction in a serious neurodevelopmental disorder with high endogenous brain GABA levels in SSADH deficiency downregulating $GABA_A$-FMZ binding site availability.

Other PET studies have shown that [11C]FMZ-PET can detect alterations in GABA receptor binding with anticonvulsant use. For example, prolonged vigabatrin treatment is associated with decreased FMZ binding in children with epilepsy (Juhász et al. 2001). Since vigabatrin increases synaptic GABA availability by inhibiting enzymatic degradation, this study supports the concept of receptor downregulation of GABA receptors due to increased GABA levels, potentially exacerbated by elevations of other metabolites (e.g., gamma-hydroxybutyrate). Alternatively, reduced binding could be due to altered receptor properties rather than number.

BENZODIAZEPINE RECEPTOR LIGANDS BEING DEVELOPED

5-(2'-[18F]Fluoroethyl)flumazenil ([18F]FEF) is a fluorine-18-labeled PET tracer for central benzodiazepine receptors. Compared with the established [11C]FMZ, it has the advantage of the longer half-life of the fluorine-18 label. After optimization of its synthesis and determination of its in vitro receptor affinities, the first PET studies were performed in humans with a second PET scan conducted after pretreatment with unlabeled flumazenil (1 mg or 2.5 mg IV, 3 minutes before tracer injection) (Gründer et al. 2001). [18F] FEF uptake followed the known central benzodiazepine receptor distribution in the human brain (occipital cortex > temporal cortex > cerebellum > thalamus > pons). Pretreatment with unlabeled flumazenil resulted in reduced tracer uptake in all brain areas except for receptor-free reference regions like the pons. Parametric images of VD and binding potential generated on a voxel-wise basis revealed two- to three-fold lower in vivo receptor binding of [18F]FEF compared with [11C]FMZ, while relative uptake of [18F] FEF was higher in the cerebellum, most likely owing to its relatively higher affinity for benzodiazepine receptors containing the alpha6 subunit. Although [11C]FMZ had some advantages over [18F]FEF (e.g., higher affinity, slower metabolism, slower kinetics), these results indicate that [18F]FEF is a suitable PET ligand for quantitative assessment of central benzodiazepine receptors, with the advantage that it can be transported to a PET facility without an on-site cyclotron.

[18F]FEF kinetic data were also acquired in two patients suffering from mesial TLE, showing reduced uptake of [18F]FEF in the implicated left hippocampus (Levêque et al. 2003).

SUMMARY

[11C]FMZ PET has an invaluable research role in the basic mechanisms of epilepsies, can in addition be extremely useful in selected clinical situations. It is unlikely that in mesial TLE, [11C]FMZ PET yields information over, above that provided by MRI, but it should be useful in the investigation of patients without MRI signs of hippocampal sclerosis. [11C]FMZ is a good marker of the integrity of neuronal systems in the hippocampus and neocortex, and is probably able to detect occult MCD and microdysgeneses. [11C]FMZ PET can yield information that is complementary to structural MR imaging techniques. The future clinical role of [11C]FMZ PET is likely to be in the presurgical evaluation of patients in whom the epileptogenic area is difficult to define by other means—that is, patients with focal epilepsy and normal high-quality MRI ("MRI-negative") and patients with epilepsy due to malformations of cortical development.

REFERENCES

Bouvard, S., N. Costes, F. Bonnefoi, et al. 2005. Seizure-related short-term plasticity of benzodiazepine receptors in partial epilepsy: a [¹¹C]flumazenil-PET study. *Brain* 128: 1330–43.

Bouilleret, V., S. Dupont, L. Spelle, et al. 2002. Insular cortex involvement in mesiotemporal lobe epilepsy: a positron emission tomography study. *Annals of Neurology* 51(2): 202–8.

Burdette, D. E., S. Y. Sakurai, T. R. Henry, et al. 1995. Temporal lobe central benzodiazepine binding in unilateral mesial temporal lobe epilepsy. *Neurology* 45: 934–941.

Chugani, H. T., W. D. Shields, D. A. Shewmon, et al. 1990. Infantile spasms: I. PET identifies focal cortical dysgenesis in cryptogenic cases for surgical treatment. *Annals of Neurology* 27: 406–13.

Debets, R. M. C., B. Sadzot B, J. W. van Isselt, et al. 1997. Is ¹¹C -flumazenil PET superior to ¹⁸F FDG PET and 123I-iomazenil SPECT in presurgical evaluation of temporal lobe epilepsy? *Journal of Neurology Neurosurgery & Psychiatry* 62: 141–50.

Delforge, J., S. Pappata, P. Millet, et al. 1995. Quantification of benzodiazepine receptors in human brain using PET, [¹¹C]flumazenil, and a single-experiment protocol. *Journal of Cerebral Blood Flow Metabolism* 15: 284–300.

Desbiens, R., S. F. Berkovic, F. Dubeau, et al. 1993. Life-threatening focal status epilepticus due to occult cortical dysplasia. *Archives of Neurology* 50: 695–700.

Fedi, M., S. F. Berkovic, C. Marini, et al. 2006. A GABA_A receptor mutation causing generalized epilepsy reduces benzodiazepine receptor binding. *Neuroimage* 32(3): 995–1000.

Friston, K. J., A. P. Holmes, K. J. Worsley, et al. 1995. Statistical parametric maps in functional imaging: A general linear approach. *Human Brain Mapping* 2: 189–210.

Geuze, E., B. N. van Berckel, A. A. Lammertsma, et al. 2008. Reduced GABA_A benzodiazepine receptor binding in veterans with post-traumatic stress disorder. *Molecular Psychiatry* 13(1): 74–83.

Gründer, G., T. Siessmeier, C. Lange-Asschenfeldt, et al. 2001. [¹⁸F]Fluoroethylflumazenil: a novel tracer for PET imaging of human benzodiazepine receptors. *European Journal of Nuclear Medicine* 28(10): 1463–70.

Hammers, A., M. J. Koepp, C. Labbé, et al. 2001a. Neocortical abnormalites of [¹¹C]-flumazenil PET in mesial temporal lobe epilepsy. *Neurology* 56: 897–906.

Hammers, A., M. J. Koepp, M. P. Richardson, et al. 2001b. [¹¹C]-diprenorphine PET in malformations of cortical development (MCD) [abstract]. *Epilepsia* 42 (Suppl.).

Hammers, A., M. J. Koepp, M. P. Richardson, et al. 2001c. Central benzodiazepine receptors in malformations of cortical development. A quantitative study. *Brain* 124: 1555–65.

Hammers, A., M. J. Koepp, R. Hurlemann, et al. 2002. Abnormalities of grey and white matter [¹¹C]flumazenil binding in temporal lobe epilepsy with normal MRI. *Brain* 125: 2257–71.

Hammers, A., M. J. Koepp, M. P. Richardson, et al. 2003. Grey and white matter flumazenil binding in neocortical epilepsy with normal MRI. A PET study of 44 patients. *Brain* 126: 1300–18.

Hammers, A., M. J. Koepp, D. J. Brooks, et al. 2005. Periventricular white matter flumazenil binding and postoperative outcome in hippocampal sclerosis. *Epilepsia* 46(6): 944–8.

Hammers, A., P. Panagoda, R. A. Heckemann, et al. 2008. [(11)C]Flumazenil PET in temporal lobe epilepsy: do we need an arterial input function or kinetic modeling? *Journal of Cerebral Blood Flow and Metabolism* 79(6): 686–93.

Hand, K. S., V. H. Baird, W. Van Paesschen, et al. 1997. Central benzodiazepine receptor autoradiography in hippocampal sclerosis. *British Journal of Pharmacology* 122: 358–64.

Heiss, W. D., J. Sobesky, U. Smekal, et al. 2004. Probability of cortical infarction predicted by flumazenil binding and diffusion-weighted imaging signal intensity: a comparative positron emission tomography/magnetic resonance imaging study in early ischemic stroke. *Stroke* 35(8): 1892–8.

Henry, T. R., K. A. Frey, J. C. Sackellares, et al. 1993. In vivo cerebral metabolism and central benzodiazepine-receptor binding in temporal lobe epilepsy. *Neurology* 43: 1998–2006.

Hoffman, E. J., S. C. Huang, and M. E. Phelps. 1979. Quantitation in positron emission computed tomography: 1. Effect of object size. *Journal of Computer Assisted Tomography* 3: 299–308.

Jalan, R., N. Turjanski, S. D. Taylor-Robinson, et al. 2000. Increased availability of central benzodiazepine receptors in patients with chronic hepatic encephalopathy and alcohol related cirrhosis. *Gut* 46(4): 546–52.

Johnson, E. W., N. C. de Lanerolle, J. H. Kim, et al. 1992. "Central" and "peripheral" benzodiazepine receptors: opposite changes in human epileptogenic tissue. *Neurology* 42: 811–5.

Juhász, C., F. Nagy, C. Watson, et al. 1999. Glucose and [¹¹C] flumazenil positron emission tomography abnormalities of thalamic nuclei in temporal lobe epilepsy. *Neurology* 53: 2037–45.

Juhász, C., D. C. Chugani, O. Muzik, et al. 2000. Electroclinical correlates of flumazenil and fluorodeoxyglucose PET abnormalities in lesional epilepsy. *Neurology* 55: 825–34.

Juhász, C., D. C. Chugani, O. Muzik, et al. 2001. Relationship of flumazenil and glucose PET abnormalities to neocortical epilepsy surgery outcome. *Neurology* 56: 1650–8.

Juhász, C., O. Muzik, D. C. Chugani, et al. 2001. Prolonged vigabatrin treatment modifies developmental changes of GABA_A-receptor binding in young children with epilepsy. *Epilepsia* 42(10): 1320–6.

Juhász, C., E. Asano, A. Shah, et al. 2009. Focal decreases of cortical GABAA receptor binding remote from the primary seizure focus: What do they indicate? *Epilepsia* 50(2): 240–50.

Koepp, M. J., M. P. Richardson, D. J. Brooks, et al. 1996. Cerebral benzodiazepine receptors in hippocampal sclerosis. An objective in vivo analysis. *Brain* 119: 1677–87.

Koepp, M. J., C. Labbé, M. P. Richardson, et al. 1997a. Regional hippocampal [^{11}C]flumazenil PET in temporal lobe epilepsy with unilateral and bilateral hippocampal sclerosis. *Brain* 120: 1865–76.

Koepp, M. J., M. P. Richardson, D. J. Brooks, et al. 1997b. Central benzodiazepine/gamma-aminobutyric acid A receptors in idiopathic generalized epilepsy: an [^{11}C] flumazenil positron emission tomography study. *Epilepsia* 38: 1089–97.

Koepp, M. J., M. P. Richardson, C. Labbé, et al. 1997c. ^{11}C -flumazenil PET, volumetric MRI, and quantitative pathology in mesial temporal lobe epilepsy. *Neurology* 49: 764–73.

Koepp, M. J., K. S. Hand, C. Labbé, et al. 1998a. In vivo [^{11}C] flumazenil-PET correlates with ex vivo [3H]flumazenil autoradiography in hippocampal sclerosis. *Annals of Neurology* 43: 618–26.

Koepp, M. J., M. P. Richardson, D. J. Brooks, et al. 1998b. Focal cortical release of endogenous opioids during reading-induced seizures. *Lancet* 352: 952–55.

Koepp, M. J., A. Hammers, C. Labbé, et al. 2000. ^{11}C -flumazenil PET in patients with refractory temporal lobe epilepsy and normal MRI. *Neurology* 54: 332–9.

Koepp, M. J., and J. S. Duncan. 2000. PET: Opiate neuroreceptor mapping. In T. R. Henry, J. S. Duncan, and S. F. Berkovic (Eds.), *Functional imaging in the epilepsies.* Vol. 83. Philadelphia: Lippincott Williams & Wilkins, 145–55.

Labbé, C., M. J. Koepp, J. Ashburner, et al. 1998. Absolute PET quantification with correction for partial volume effects within cerebral structures. In C. Carson, M. Daube-Witherspoon, and P. Herscovitch (Eds.), *Quantitative functional brain imaging with positron emission tomography.* San Diego: Academic Press, 59–66.

Lamusuo, S., A. Pitkänen, L. Jutila, et al. 2000. [^{11}C] Flumazenil binding in the medial temporal lobe in patients with temporal lobe epilepsy. Correlation with hippocampal MR volumetry, T2 relaxometry, and neuropathology. *Neurology* 54: 2252–60.

Levêque, P., S. Sanabria-Bohorquez, A. Bol, et al. 2003. Quantification of human brain benzodiazepine receptors using [^{18}F]fluoroethylflumazenil: a first report in volunteers and epileptic patients. *European Journal of Nuclear Medicine Molecular Imaging* 30(12): 1630–6.

Lingford-Hughes, A. R., S. J. Wilson, V. J. Cunningham, et al. 2005. GABA-benzodiazepine receptor function in alcohol dependence: a combined ^{11}C -flumazenil PET and pharmacodynamic study. *Psychopharmacology (Berlin)* 180(4): 595–606.

Meencke, H. J., and D. Janz. 1984. Neuropathological findings in primary generalised epilepsy: a study of eight cases. *Epilepsia* 5: 8–21.

Meltzer, C. C., J. P. Leal, H. S. Mayberg, et al. 1990. Correction of PET data for partial volume effects in human cerebral cortex by MR imaging. *Journal of Computer Assisted Tomography* 14: 561–70.

Meltzer, C. C., J. K. Zubieta, J. M. Links, et al. 1996. MR-based correction for brain PET measurements for heterogenous gray matter radioactivity distribution. *Journal of Cerebral Blood Flow Metabolism* 16: 650–8.

Millet, P., J. Delforge, F. Mauguiere, et al. 1995. Parameter and index images of benzodiazepine receptor concentration in the brain. *Journal of Nuclear Medicine* 36: 1462–71.

Mishina, M., M. Senda, Y. Kimura, et al. 2000. Intrasubject correlation between static scan and distribution volume images for [^{11}C]flumazenil PET. *Annals of Nuclear Medicine* 14: 193–8.

Muzik, O., E. A. da Silva, C. Juhasz, et al. 2000. Intracranial EEG versus flumazenil and glucose PET in children with extratemporal lobe epilepsy. *Neurology* 54: 171–9.

Niimura, K., O. Muzik, D. C. Chugani, et al. 1999. [^{11}C]flumazenil PET: activity images versus parametric images for the detection of neocortical epileptic foci. *Journal of Nuclear Medicine* 40: 1985–91.

Von Oertzen, J., H. Urbach, S. Jungbluth, et al. 2002. Standard magnetic resonance imaging is inadequate for patients with refractory focal epilepsy. *Journal of Neurology Neurosurgery Psychiatry* 73(6): 643–7.

Okazawa, H., H. Yamauchi, K. Sugimoto, et al. 2004. Effects of metabolite correction for arterial input function on quantitative receptor images with ^{11}C -flumazenil in clinical positron emission tomography studies. *Journal of Computer Assisted Tomography* 28: 428–35.

Olsen, R. W., R. T. McGabe, and J. K. Wamsley. 1990. GABAA receptor subtypes: autoradiographic comparison of GABA, benzodiazepine and convulsant binding sites in rat central nervous system. *Journal of Chemical Neuroanatomy* 3: 59–76.

Pearl, P. L., K. M. Gibson, Z. Quezado, et al. 2009. Decreased GABA-A binding on FMZ-PET in succinic semialdehyde dehydrogenase deficiency. *Neurology* 73: 423–29.

Prevett MC, Lammertsma AA, Brooks DJ, et al. 1995. Benzodiazepine- GABA, receptors in idiopathic generalised epilepsy measured with [11C]Flumazenil and positron emission tomography. *Epilepsia* 36: 113–21.

Richardson, M. P., M. J. Koepp, D. J. Brooks, et al. 1996. Benzodiazepine receptors in focal epilepsy with cortical dysgenesis: an ^{11}C-Flumazenil PET study. *Annals of Neurology* 40: 188–98.

Richardson, M. P., K. J. Friston, S. M. Sisodiya, et al. 1997. Cortical grey matter and benzodiazepine receptors in malformations of cortical development. A voxel-based comparison of structural and functional imaging data. *Brain* 120: 1961–73.

Richardson, M. P., M. J. Koepp, D. J. Brooks, et al. 1998. ^{11}C -flumazenil PET in neocortical epilepsy. *Neurology* 51: 485–92.

Rousset, O. G., Y. Ma, G. C. Léger, et al. 1993. Correction for partial volume effects in PET using MRI-based 3D simulations of individual human brain metabolism. In K. Uemura (Ed.), *Quantification of brain function, tracer kinetics and image analysis in brain PET.* New York: Elsevier Science, 113–25.

Ryvlin, P., S. Bouvard, D. Le Bars, et al. 1998. Clinical utility of flumazenil-PET versus [^{18}F]fluorodeoxyglucose-PET and MRI in refractory partial epilepsy. A prospective study in 100 patients. *Brain* 121: 2067–81.

Ryvlin, P., S. Bouvard, D. Le Bars, et al. 1999. Transient and falsely lateralizing flumazenil-PET asymmetries in temporal lobe epilepsy. *Neurology* 53: 1882–5.

Salmi, E., S. Aalto, J. Hirvonen, et al. 2008. Measurement of GABAA receptor binding in vivo with [¹¹C]flumazenil: a test-retest study in healthy subjects. *Neuroimage* 41(2): 260–9.

Savic, I., L. Widen, J. O. Thorell, et al. 1990. Cortical benzodiazepine receptor binding in patients with generalised and partial epilepsy. *Epilepsia* 31: 724–30.

Savic, I., L. Widen, and S. Stone-Elander. 1991. Feasibility of reversing benzodiazepine tolerance with flumazenil. *Lancet* 337: 133–7.

Savic, I., M. Ingvar, and S. Stone-Elander. 1993. Comparison of ¹¹C -flumazenil and ¹⁸F -FDG as PET markers of epileptic foci. *Journal of Neurology Neurosurgery & Psychiatry* 56: 615–21.

Savic, I., S. Pauli, J. O. Thorell, et al. 1994. In vivo demonstration of altered benzodiazepine receptor density in patients with generalised epilepsy. *Journal of Neurology Neurosurgery & Psychiatry* 57: 797–804.

Savic, I., J. O. Thorell, and P. Roland. 1995. [¹¹C]Flumazenil positron emission tomography visualises frontal epileptogenic regions. *Epilepsia* 36: 1225–32.

Savic, I., E. Svanborg, and J. O. Thorell. 1996. Cortical benzodiazepine receptor changes are related to frequency of partial seizures: a positron emission tomography study. *Epilepsia* 37: 236–44.

Szelies, B., G. Weber-Luxenburger, G. Pawlik, et al. 1996. MRI-guided Flumazenil- and FDG-PET in temporal lobe epilepsy. *Neuroimage* 3: 109–18.

Urbach, H., J. Hattingen, J. von Oertzen, et al. 2004. MR imaging in the presurgical workup of patients with drug-resistant epilepsy. *AJNR American Journal of Neuroradiology* 25: 919–26.

Vollmar, C., and S. Noachtar. 2004. Neuroimaging in epilepsy. *Turkish Journal of Neurology* 10: 185–200.

Wicks, P., M. R. Turner, S. Abrahams, et al. 2008. Neuronal loss associated with cognitive performance in amyotrophic lateral sclerosis: an (¹¹C)-flumazenil PET study. *Amyotrophic Lateral Sclerosis* 9(1): 43–9.

Woermann, F. G., S. L. Free, M. J. Koepp, et al. 1999. Abnormal cerebral structure in juvenile myoclonic epilepsy demonstrated with voxel-based analysis of MRI. *Brain* 122: 2101–8.

Chapter *12*

ALPHA-[¹¹C]METHYL-L-TRYPTOPHAN POSITRON EMISSION TOMOGRAPHY

Carlos E. A. Batista, Diane C. Chugani, and Harry T. Chugani

Alpha-[11C]Methyl-L-tryptophan (AMT) was developed initially as a tracer for positron emission tomography (PET) in order to measure brain serotonin synthesis (Diksic et al. 1990, 1991). This compound is an analog of the amino acid tryptophan, the precursor for serotonin synthesis. After validation studies in animal models, AMT PET was applied in normal adults and methods for estimating whole brain and regional values of "serotonin synthesis capacity" (rather than "absolute rates" of serotonin synthesis) were established (Chugani et al. 1998a; Chugani and Muzik 2000; Muzik et al. 1997).

Subsequently, AMT PET was applied in patients with drug-resistant epilepsy (Asano et al. 2000; Chugani et al. 1998b) based upon evidence suggesting that serotonin mechanisms might play a role in epilepsy. For example, in surgically resected brain tissue from human epileptic subjects, levels of 5-hydroxyindole acetic acid (5-HIAA, the breakdown product of serotonin) were found to be higher in actively spiking temporal cortex compared to non-spiking tissue (Louw et al. 1989; Pintor et al. 1990). Increased serotonin immunoreactivity has also been reported in human epileptic brain tissue (Trottier et al. 1996). Although these studies provided the rationale for applying AMT PET in studying epilepsy patients, subsequent findings indicated that AMT is a tracer not only for serotonin synthesis, but also for the metabolism of tryptophan via the kynurenine pathway, and it is perhaps the latter that is more relevant for epilepsy mechanisms (Chugani et al. 1998b).

This chapter will review important developments of AMT as a PET tracer that is capable of highlighting epileptogenic lesions in the interictal state, an important technical advance in neuroimaging of epilepsy. In the first section, we introduce the methodological aspects of this tracer. Subsequently, clinical applications and the current state of the art in the field will be discussed. Finally, possible new treatments for epilepsy based upon understanding of altered tryptophan metabolism in epilepsy will be discussed.

AMT PET METHODOLOGY

The molecule AMT is an analog of tryptophan with an incorporated methyl group, which is labeled with ¹¹C for PET studies. The properties of AMT make it a suitable tracer for PET studies because, unlike tryptophan, AMT is not incorporated into protein, and its metabolites are released into the blood circulation (Diksic 1990; Madras and Sourkes 1965). After administration of the tracer, AMT is converted into alpha-methyl-serotonin by a two-step enzymatic process. The presence of alpha-methyl-serotonin in serotonergic neurons has been confirmed by autoradiography and tryptophan-hydroxylase immunocytochemistry (Cohen et al. 1995). Furthermore, unlike serotonin, alpha-methyl-serotonin is not a substrate for monoamine oxidase (Missala and Sourkes 1988); hence, alpha-methyl-serotonin accumulates in nerve terminals equivalent to the rate of serotonin synthesis.

Kinetic modeling is applied for analysis of the AMT PET data. Animal studies conducted in the early 1990s (Diksic et al. 1990, 1991; Nagahiro et al. 1990) demonstrated that the distribution of the tracer AMT in brain can be explained by a three-compartment model using first-order rate constants (Fig. 12.1). The constants k1 and k2 represent respectively the inflow and outflow exchange rate between the vascular compartment and the cell cytoplasm, here representing the transport across the blood–brain barrier, the interstitial space, and the cell membrane. When the tracer is irreversibly trapped in the cell cytoplasm after conversion by enzymes, a third constant is then characterized (k3). All these three rate constants are combined to derive a factor called the K-complex, which is proportional to the unidirectional uptake of tracer into tissue. Since AMT utilizes the same transporters as the amino acid tryptophan to pass across the blood–brain barrier, this radioactive tracer is also subject to competition with large neutral amino acids (Lundquist et al. 2006). In addition, binding to albumin is a potential confounding factor, although the importance of the role of free versus total plasma tryptophan in the transport of tryptophan across the blood–brain barrier is still controversial due to evidence that tryptophan bound to albumin might become available as blood circulates through brain (Pardridge and Fierer 1990).

Since it is difficult to control all variables that determine the amount of plasma tryptophan available for extraction by brain tissue, PET study protocols usually require a period of fasting (4 to 6 hours) prior to scanning, and patients undergo study at around the same time of the day in order to avoid potential error from diurnal rhythms of serotonin synthesis. These standardized protocols improve the reliability of the measures of tryptophan kinetics, such as the K-complex. To estimate accurately the delivery of AMT to the brain during the scan, blood samples are drawn over predefined time intervals, generating a time–activity curve. This blood time–activity curve and the brain time–activity curve collected by dynamic PET imaging are then subjected to Patlak graphical analysis (Patlak et al. 1983) to determine the K-complex.

In the case of AMT, the value of the K-complex is thought to be proportional to tryptophan metabolism via the serotonin and kynurenine pathways when the blood–brain barrier is intact. However, circumstances that provoke breakdown of the blood–brain barrier may alter the K-complex due to increased permeability of the tracer; therefore, an estimate of the metabolic rate constant k3' and the volume of distribution (VD') of the tracer in the free precursor pool might be also calculated. The k3' parameter characterizes the enzymatic conversion of AMT, while the VD' parameter delineates the transport rate of AMT into the tissue. It has been demonstrated previously that the VD' value is increased when the blood–brain barrier is compromised (Juhász et al. 2006).

Originally, it was thought that AMT was a specific tracer for the absolute measurement of serotonin synthesis rates in brain. However, when AMT PET was applied to patient populations with epilepsy, it became clear that this tracer was less specific than previously thought. The original clinical study involved a child with intractable partial epilepsy and a left frontal epileptic focus on the EEG (Fig. 12.2). While the glucose metabolism PET scan showed left frontal hypometabolism, the AMT PET showed a focus of increased AMT uptake in the same area. Importantly, this increased AMT uptake was seen during the interictal state. This introduced the idea of applying AMT PET to patients with tuberous sclerosis who were being evaluated for epilepsy surgery in order to determine interictally the epileptogenic tuber, with the assumption that non-epileptogenic tubers would not show such an increase. Indeed, this proved to be the case (Chugani et al. 1998b). The applications of AMT PET in tuberous sclerosis subjects are reviewed below in greater detail.

Surprisingly, chemical analysis of the resected tubers showing increased AMT uptake on PET failed to show the expected high levels of serotonin. Instead, high levels of kynurenine pathway metabolites were found, suggesting that AMT PET might also trace tryptophan

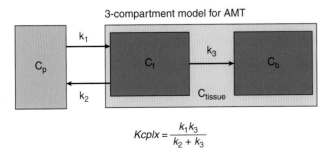

3-compartment model for AMT

$$Kcplx = \frac{k_1 k_3}{k_2 + k_3}$$

Figure 12.1 Three-compartment model for AMT kinetics.

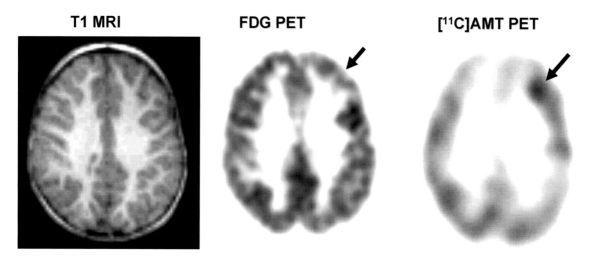

T1 MRI **FDG PET** **[¹¹C]AMT PET**

Figure 12.2 A 4-year-old girl with left frontal epileptic focus on the EEG. MRI was normal. Glucose metabolism PET showed left frontal hypometabolism (*arrow*), whereas AMT PET showed increased uptake interictally (*arrow*).

metabolism via the kynurenine pathway (Chugani et al. 1998c). Indeed, under certain circumstances, tryptophan may be preferentially metabolized by indoleamine 2,3-dioxygenase (IDO), the regulatory enzyme of the kynurenine pathway (Guillemin et al. 2005). Under normal conditions, kynurenine pathway metabolites are not expected to contribute to the accumulation of AMT in brain since the tryptophan metabolites of this pathway are between 100- and 1,000-fold lower than the concentration of tryptophan in the brain (Saito et al. 1993). In comparison, the sum of the concentrations of serotonin and its metabolite 5-HIAA is approximately one-fifth the concentration of tryptophan in brain (Hery et al. 1977). Therefore, when studying normal healthy individuals, AMT PET may provide reasonable estimates of serotonin synthesis capacity.

However, some pathologic states induce the kynurenine pathway by upregulation of IDO. For example, following ischemic brain injury or immune activation, induction of IDO can result in a 10-fold increase in quinolinic acid (a kynurenine pathway metabolite) in brain (Saito et al. 1993). Several metabolites of the kynurenine pathway, quinolinic acid, kynurenine, and 3-hydroxykynurenine, are convulsants through their action as agonists at N-methyl-D-aspartate (NMDA) receptors (Lapin et al. 1978, 1980, 1982; Perkins and Stone 1982, 1983; Vezzani et al. 1985). Quinolinic acid is a well-known excitotoxin whose effects are mediated via NMDA receptors. Its potential role in epileptogenesis has been intensively investigated and, in fact, it is used to induce seizures in animal models (Boeck et al. 2004; de Oliveira et al. 2004). More recent studies suggest that NMDA receptors may participate in quinolinate-induced seizures (Lehrmann et al. 2008; Tavares et al. 2008). On the other hand, kynurenic acid, which

is another metabolite in this pathway and is an NMDA *antagonist* (Perkins and Stone 1982), has been reported to suppress epileptiform activity in animal models of epilepsy (Sharfman and Ofer 1997). It has been postulated that metabolites of the kynurenine pathway might play a role in the initiation and maintenance of seizures in human seizure disorders (Feldblum et al. 1988; Heyes et al. 1990). While quinolinic acid concentrations were not increased in the seizure focus in adult temporal lobe epilepsy specimens (Heyes et al. 1990), our findings of five-fold higher concentrations of quinolinic acid in tubers showing elevated AMT accumulation (i.e., epileptogenic tubers) compared to tubers and brain tissue that do not show elevated AMT accumulation on PET (Chugani et al. 1998c) suggest that, in at least some patients with tuberous sclerosis, the mechanism of epileptogenesis may involve activation of the kynurenine pathway, leading to the production of endogenous convulsants.

CLINICAL APPLICATIONS

The unique capability of AMT to selectively highlight an epileptogenic lesion amidst a multitude of lesions without the necessity of capturing a seizure has led to several clinical applications of AMT PET, and these will now be reviewed.

Tuberous Sclerosis Complex

Tuberous sclerosis complex (TSC) is an autosomal dominant disorder characterized by multisystemic involvement, which includes the brain. TSC-related epilepsy is often refractory to medical treatment and, in infants and young children, may result in an epileptic encephalopathy. Mechanisms of epileptogenesis in TSC are not fully understood, but it is likely that the tuber and associated cortical dysplasia participates in the pathogenesis of seizures (Crino et al. 2004; Uhlmann et al. 2002). Identification of the epileptic tuber among numerous tubers that may be present in patients with TSC is often a challenge, and many patients with intractable epilepsy are denied surgical treatment because of insufficient localizing data. In some cases, bilateral intracranial electrodes are inserted for diagnostic purposes, but most epileptologists consider this approach too invasive. Therefore, a noninvasive neuroimaging method, such as AMT PET, capable of distinguishing epileptic from non-epileptic tubers (Fig. 12.3), was a welcome addition in the presurgical evaluation of TSC patients (Asano et al. 2000; Chugani et al. 1998b).

Following the initial report (Chugani et al. 1998b), the AMT PET approach to identify epileptogenic tubers was validated in several further studies. To determine the relationship between AMT uptake measured in tubers and epileptic activity on EEG, the AMT PET scans of 18 children with TSC and intractable epilepsy were analyzed after co-registration with the MRI (Asano et al. 2000). The AMT "uptake values" of 258 cortical tubers were measured using regions-of-interest delineated on co-registered MRI, and were divided by the value for normal-appearing cortex to obtain an AMT "uptake ratio." The measured tuber uptake ratios ranged from 0.6 to 2.0 (the majority of tubers appear as regions of *decreased* AMT uptake and, when compared to normal cortex, would have uptake ratios much lower than 1.0). Tuber uptake ratios in the epileptic lobes (as determined by ictal EEG) were found to be higher than those in non-epileptic lobes ($p < 0.0001$). All 15 patients with focal seizure activity showed at least one lesion with uptake ratio above 0.98

in the epileptic lobe. Receiver operating characteristics analysis demonstrated that a tuber uptake ratio of 0.98 resulted in a specificity of 0.91 for detection of the epileptic lobe. This study demonstrated that multi-modal imaging (AMT PET combined with FLAIR MRI) analysis of cortical tubers can select a subset of tubers that are epileptogenic based on ictal EEG recordings (Asano et al. 2000).

The usefulness of AMT PET in identifying epileptogenic tubers was confirmed by Fedi et al. (2003), who further reported a correlation between AMT uptake and interictal spike frequency. In their study, the K-complex was positively associated with the number of spikes per hour during the scan.

In a subsequent study (Kagawa et al. 2005), 87 patients with TSC and intractable seizures were evaluated with AMT PET. Seventeen of these children underwent epilepsy surgery, and 14 had intracranial EEG. Based on surgical outcome data, tubers showing increased AMT uptake (uptake ratio greater than 1.00) were classified into three categories: (1) epileptogenic (tubers within an EEG-defined epileptic focus whose resection resulted in seizure-free outcome), (2) non-epileptogenic (tubers that were not resected but the patient became seizure-free), or (3) uncertain (all other tubers). Increased AMT uptake was found in 30 tubers of 16 children, and 23 of these tubers (77%) were located in an EEG-defined epileptic focus. The tuber with the highest uptake was located in an ictal EEG onset region in each patient. Increased AMT uptake indicated an epileptic region not suspected by scalp EEG in four cases (Fig. 12.4). Twelve of the 17 children (71%) achieved seizure-free outcome. However, three of the five children who did not become seizure-free had a "planned incomplete resection" either because of eloquent cortex or because the homotopic cortex was severely hypometabolic on the glucose PET scan and, as a result, their

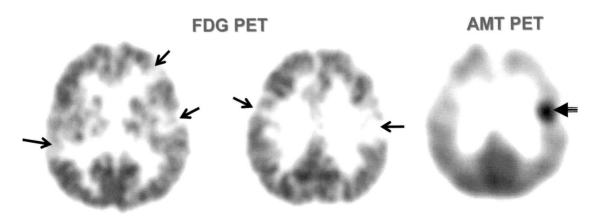

Figure 12.3 Patient with TSC whose FDG PET scan shows several tubers appearing as hypometabolic regions (*thin arrows*); the AMT scan shows increased uptake in the left central tuber (*thick arrow*).

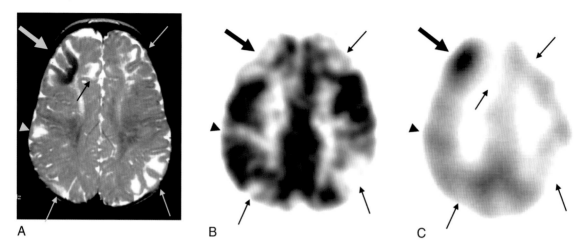

Figure 12.4 TSC patient with intractable epilepsy and non-lateralizing ictal EEG. Both the MRI (A) and FDG PET (B) showed multiple tubers (*thin arrows, arrowhead*) without indicating the epileptogenic one. The AMT PET (C) showed increased uptake in a right medial frontal tuber (*thick arrow*), the location of which accounted for the secondary bilateral synchrony on the EEG.

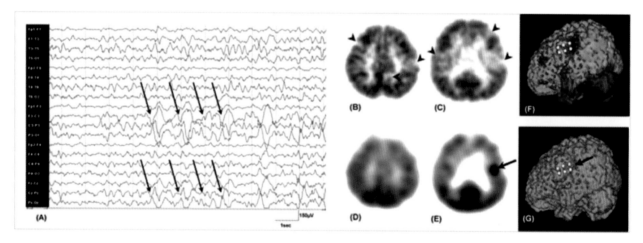

Figure 12.5 Confirmation of seizure onset on the intracranial EEG (A), co-registered with the MRI (F, G, white electrodes indicate seizure onset) in the region of increased AMT uptake (D, E, G, red indicates increased AMT) in a child with TSC. The FDG PET scan (B, C) showed multiple areas of cortical hypometabolism without indicating the epileptic lesion.

surgeries were considered palliative. Therefore, of the 14 patients who had a planned complete resection of the epileptogenic zone, 12 (86%) achieved seizure freedom.

Based on outcome criteria in this same study (Kagawa et al. 2005), 19 of 30 tubers (63%) with increased AMT uptake were epileptogenic, and these tubers had significantly higher AMT uptake than the non-epileptogenic ones ($p = 0.009$). Tubers with at least a 10% increase of AMT uptake (seen in nine patients) were all epileptogenic. Using a cutoff threshold of 1.02 for AMT uptake ratio provided an optimal accuracy of 83% for detecting tubers that needed to be resected to achieve a seizure-free outcome. The findings suggested that resection of tubers with

increased AMT uptake above a certain threshold is highly desirable to achieve a seizure-free surgical outcome in children with TSC and intractable epilepsy. AMT PET can provide independent complementary information regarding the localization of epileptogenic regions in TSC and enhance the confidence of patient selection for successful epilepsy surgery (Fig. 12.5). The disadvantages of AMT PET are that the AMT is labeled with [11]C (20-minute half-life), it is not widely available, and its sensitivity for detecting the epileptogenic tuber in intractable TSC patients is about 60% to 70%. Occasionally, more than one tuber with increased AMT uptake may be seen (Fig. 12.6) and, in such cases, usually the tuber with the highest AMT uptake ratio has the best correlation with the

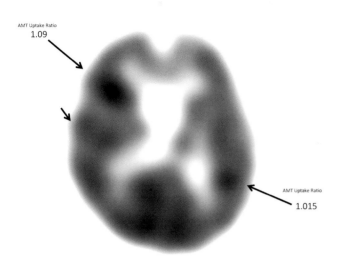

Figure 12.6 At least two tubers with increased AMT uptake (*long arrows*) in a child with TSC, intractable seizures, and a right frontal ictal focus on the scalp EEG. The left posterior temporal focus did not have an EEG accompaniment. A possible third suspicious tuber is seen in the right posterior frontal region (*short arrow*).

ictal EEG. It is possible that tubers with an intermediate AMT uptake ratio may evolve eventually into epileptogenic ones, but this remains to be shown.

Malformation of Cortical Development

Cerebral cortical development relies on three basic processes: cell proliferation, neuronal migration, and cortical organization. Errors in cortical development resulting in malformations of cortical development (MCD) may be focal or diffuse and are often associated with abnormal neuronal activity and seizures.

In most instances, areas of cortical malformation are readily identified on structural MRI. However, as reviewed in Chapter 3, structural MRI underestimates the extent of the MCD and may not even detect subtle areas of malformation.

In a recent large study, the sensitivity and specificity of AMT PET in identifying epileptic foci in children with and without MCDs were determined in 73 epileptic children classified into lesional and non-lesional groups (Wakamoto et al. 2008). The sensitivity and specificity of focally increased AMT uptake, using intracranial EEG localization of seizure onset as the standard, were compared between the two groups. While the specificity of AMT PET for detecting the seizure onset lobe was equally high in the lesional (97%) and non-lesional (100%) groups, the sensitivity was higher in the lesional than in the non-lesional group (47% vs. 29%; $p = 0.047$). The incidence of AMT uptake abnormality was higher in the lesional than the non-lesional group ($p < 0.01$). AMT PET localized and visualized epileptogenic regions in 25% of patients with non-localizing MRI and, in some cases, even non-localizing FDG PET (Fig. 12.7). Therefore, although the overall sensitivity of AMT PET in identifying neocortical epileptic foci is modest, the specificity is extremely high. When an AMT focus is detected, it likely represents the epileptic focus to be resected along with adjacent epileptogenic cortex as determined by intracranial EEG. This study found no distinctive pattern of AMT uptake among the types of MCD studied, which included focal cortical dysplasia (Fig. 12.8), subependymal heterotopia, polymicrogyria, and congenital perisylvian syndrome. Also, in contrast to the findings by Fedi et al. (2003), the authors of the Wakamoto et al. (2008) study did not find a relationship between frequency of spike activity and AMT uptake.

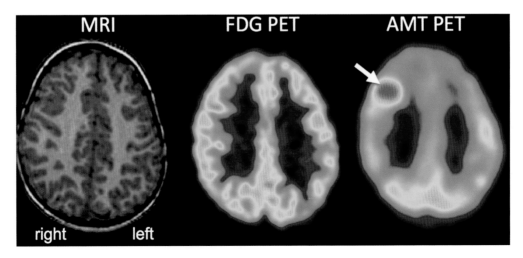

Figure 12.7 Increased AMT uptake (*arrow*) in epileptogenic cortex of a 3-year-old boy with right frontal lobe epilepsy. MRI and FDG PET were normal. EEG showed right frontal lobe seizure onset.

MRI AMT PET PATHOLOGY

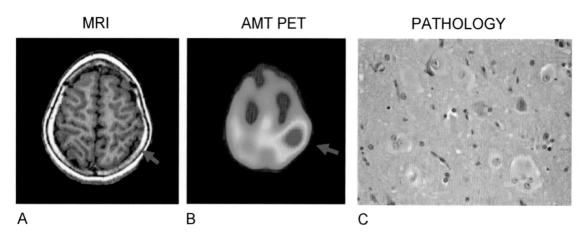

A B C

Figure 12.8 An 8-year-old girl with intractable focal epilepsy. (A) MRI showed subtle area of cortical dysplasia in left parietal cortex (*arrow*), (B) AMT PET showed increased uptake in the same region (*arrow*), and (C) pathology showed cortical dysplasia, type IIB with balloon cells. Intracranial EEG showed left central-parietal seizure onset.

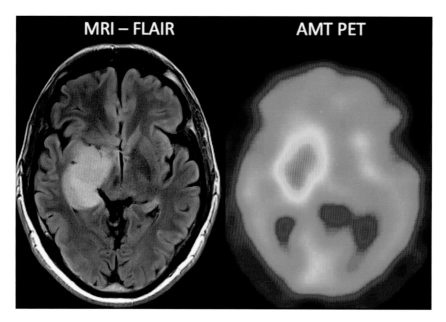

Figure 12.9 FLAIR MRI and AMT PET of a low-grade glioma located in the right medial temporal region, causing seizures. The tumor showed no contrast enhancement on gadolinium-enhanced MRI. Histology showed a grade II astrocytoma, a tumor type that often shows high metabolic rates of AMT, presumably due to activation of the kynurenine pathway of tryptophan metabolism. (Courtesy of Dr. Csaba Juhász.)

A different study performed on patients with periventricular nodular heterotopia and intractable seizures found a mismatch between the location of epileptic discharges and AMT uptake (i.e., high AMT uptake did not correspond to EEG epileptic focus), and the heterotopic nodules did not show any increase of AMT uptake (Natsume et al. 2008). However, there were major limitations in this study, such as the very low number of patients (n = 4) and no record of discharges coming from the nodules.

Tumors

Epilepsy is common in patients with brain tumors, reaching 30% or more depending on the tumor type (Hauser et al. 1993); in general, low-grade lesions (Figs. 12.9 and 12.10) have a higher seizure incidence than high-grade ones. Interestingly, human gliomas are capable of producing byproducts of the kynurenine pathway (Vezzani et al. 1990). In addition, low-grade tumor cells express the rate-limiting enzyme

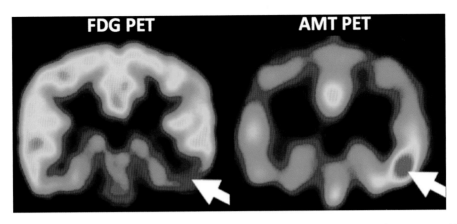

Figure 12.10 Increased AMT uptake in a left temporal epileptogenic glioneuronal tumor (dysembryoplastic neuroepithelial tumor). These low-grade tumors are typically hypometabolic on FDG PET. (Courtesy of Dr. Csaba Juhász.)

IDO more frequently than high-grade tumors (Batista et al. 2009). In one PET study, AMT uptake was measured in 40 patients with primary brain tumors using standard uptake values (Juhász et al. 2006). Tryptophan metabolism was further quantified in 23 patients using kinetic modeling. Grade II to IV gliomas and glioneuronal tumors showed increased AMT standard uptake values, including all recurrent/residual tumors. Gadolinium enhancement on MRI was associated with high VD' values, suggesting an impaired blood–brain barrier, while k3' values (associated with metabolism) were not related to contrast enhancement. In astrocytic tumors, low grade was associated with higher k3' and lower VD' in comparison to high-grade tumors, which showed the reverse pattern. Oligodendrogliomas showed high VD' values but lower k3' compared to normal cortex. Thus, increased AMT uptake in tumors is related to increased metabolism of tryptophan or transport depending on tumor type and grade, and it may be possible to predict tumor type based on AMT kinetics.

Nonlesional Epilepsy

Patients with intractable neocortical epilepsy and normal MRI (non-lesional epilepsy) are a challenging group of patients, generally with suboptimal surgical success unless there is strong *functional* neuroimaging localization of epileptogenic areas. Only a single paper has reported results of AMT PET on some patients with non-lesional temporal lobe epilepsy (Natsume et al. 2003). The authors compared FDG and AMT PET on 14 patients (7 with hippocampal sclerosis) against normal scans from 21 healthy subjects. The investigators did not report any diagnostic value of AMT PET on temporal lobe epilepsy, but the results were useful to help understand better the pathophysiology of the disease. Glucose metabolism of the lateral temporal lobe cortex ipsilateral to the seizure focus correlated negatively with AMT uptake in the ipsilateral hippocampus and positively with ipsilateral lenticular nucleus and cingulate cortex. The authors also reported that patients with normal hippocampal volume showed increased AMT uptake in the hippocampus ipsilateral to the seizure focus compared to uptake in sclerotic hippocampus, as well as compared to normal subjects.

In another study, the same group sought to determine the localizing value of AMT PET in intractable epilepsy of neocortical origin (Fedi et al. 2001). In 30% of cases where MRI did not show a detectable lesion, AMT PET uptake was increased in areas corresponding to localization from the ictal EEG. Several of these patients also underwent ictal SPECT and the results showed good concordance with the AMT PET findings.

In a study from our own group (Juhász et al. 2003), areas of increased AMT and decreased FDG uptake were marked objectively in 27 non-TSC children who underwent comprehensive evaluation for resective epilepsy surgery. The marked PET abnormalities were compared to the locations of scalp and subdural EEG epileptiform abnormalities, as well as histology and surgical outcome. Focal cortical increases of AMT uptake were found in 15 of the 27 patients. The lobar sensitivity (39.0%) of AMT PET for seizure onset was lower but its specificity (100%) was higher ($p < 0.0001$) than that of hypometabolism on FDG PET (sensitivity 73.2%, specificity 62.7%). AMT PET abnormalities were smaller than the corresponding FDG PET hypometabolic regions (p = 0.002), and increased AMT uptake occurred in two patients with non-localizing FDG PET (Fig. 12.7). Histologically verified MCDs were associated with increased AMT uptake ($p = 0.044$) (Fig. 12.8). Subdural electrodes adjacent to the area of increased AMT uptake were most often involved in seizure onset. Thus, AMT PET can assist in placement of subdural electrodes even when MRI and FDG PET fail to provide adequate localizing information. The authors also cautioned that cortical areas adjacent to increased AMT uptake should be carefully addressed by intracranial EEG because these regions often show a high degree of epileptogenicity.

Reoperation

When epilepsy surgery fails to provide substantial relief from seizures, reoperation may be considered in some cases. However, accurate identification of residual epileptogenic cortex becomes even more challenging following an initial resection. Interpretation of ictal scalp EEG is difficult due to alterations of the original brain anatomy as well as effects of skull and dural scarring. The current imaging modalities have serious limitations. MRI is not very helpful in cryptogenic epilepsy, and FDG PET typically reveals large areas of hypometabolism, most of which may be consequent to surgical tissue damage or deafferentation. Ictal SPECT and magnetic source imaging may be useful in some cases.

Since AMT PET may detect epileptogenic regions interictally, it was assessed as a potential tool to detect residual epileptogenic cortex in patients who had failed a previous neocortical resection (Juhász et al. 2004). Thirty-three patients (age 3 to 26 years; mean age 10.8 years) with intractable epilepsy of neocortical

origin and a previously failed cortical resection were studied. AMT PET scans were performed 6 days to 7 years after the first surgery. Cortical increases of AMT uptake were detected on the side of the previous resections in 12 of the 33 cases (Fig. 12.11). In two patients scanned shortly (within a week) after surgery, diffuse hemispheric increases were observed, without any further localization value. In contrast, in 10 (43%) of 23 patients scanned more than 2 months but within 2.3 years after surgery, focal cortical increases occurred, concordant with seizure onset on ictal EEG (Fig. 12.12). All patients with localizing AMT PET, who underwent reoperation, became seizure-free (n = 5) or showed a considerable reduction in seizure frequency (n = 2). Although the sensitivity is modest, this study showed that AMT PET can identify nonresected epileptic cortex in patients with a previously failed neocortical epilepsy surgery and can assist in planning reoperation.

Postoperative AMT PET scans have also provided some new insights into brain plasticity following cortical resection for epilepsy. Following removal of epileptic cortex, AMT uptake in the ipsilateral lentiform nucleus increased compared to the contralateral side (Fig. 12.13), suggesting functional reorganization of cortical-striatal projections associated with increased serotonin expression (Chugani et al. 2008). This phenomenon seems to be time-related, as it was more intense during early periods after surgery (Fig. 12.14). Interestingly, the AMT increase observed in the basal

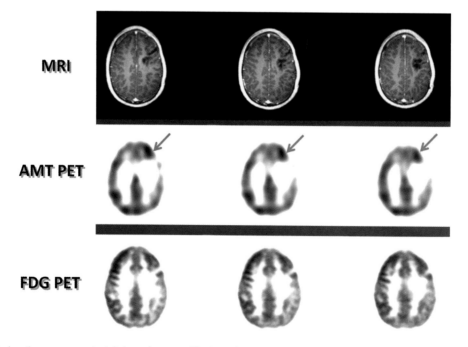

Figure 12.11 Failed epilepsy surgery in left frontal cortex. The MRI shows the extent of resection. While FDG PET shows a large area of hypometabolism, the AMT PET shows increased uptake anterior to the previous resection (*arrows*) corresponding to the intracranial EEG focus.

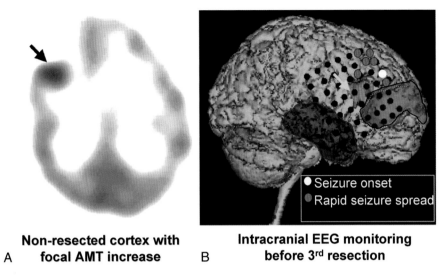

Non-resected cortex with
A   **focal AMT increase**   B

Intracranial EEG monitoring
before 3ʳᵈ resection

Figure 12.12 Two failed attempts of epilepsy surgery. FDG PET showed hemispheric hypometabolism of no localizing value, whereas AMT PET (A) showed increased uptake just posterior to the right frontal resection, concordant with the intracranial EEG (B).

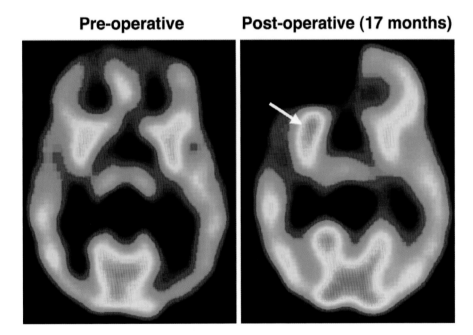

Figure 12.13 A 9-year-old boy with intractable right frontal lobe epilepsy before and after right frontal resection. Postoperative AMT PET scan at 17 months shows increased AMT uptake in the right striatum (*arrow*) compared to the left and compared to preoperative uptake in the striatum.

ganglia was apparently not driven by the extent of resection.

KYNURENINE PATHWAY AS A NEW PHARMACOLOGICAL TARGET FOR EPILEPSY

Several pharmacological approaches to treating epilepsy with agents aimed at the kynurenine pathway in animal models have been reported. Chiarugi et al. (1995) studied m-nitrobenzoylalanine (an inhibitor of kynurenine hydroxylase) and o-methoxybenzoylalanine (an inhibitor of kynureninase) in rats and found that both agents increased the concentration of kynurenic acid in hippocampal extracellular space. In addition, they showed that these agents protected against audiogenic seizures in DBA/2 mice. Nemeth et al. (2004) administered kynurenine with probenecid to rats with pentylentetrazol-induced seizures and

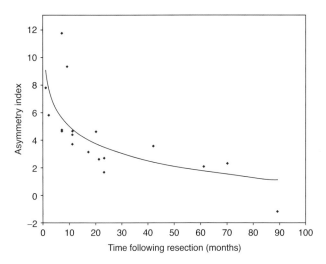

Figure 12.14 Striatal uptake of AMT expressed as asymmetry index (ipsilateral to resection/contralateral to resection) as a function of time after resection.

showed marked inhibition of electrophysiologic and behavioral seizure activity. Administration of 4-chloro-kynurenine, which is converted by astrocytes to the NMDA glycine-site antagonist 7-chloro-kynurenic acid, to rats with kainate-induced seizures delayed seizure onset, reduced total time in seizures, and prevented lesions in piriform cortex in the CA1 region of the hippocampus (Wu et al. 2002). In the chronic limbic epilepsy model, administration of 4-chloro-kynurenine resulted in decreased amplitude and number of population spikes in response to electrical stimulation, but showed no effect on the evoked response in control animals (Zhang et al. 2005). The same group reported enhanced formation of 7-chloro-kynurenic acid from administered 4-chloro-kynurenine in the pilocarpine seizure model (Wu et al. 2005). They hypothesized that the enhanced conversion was related to astrocytosis induced by pilocarpine treatment. These pharmacological agents, as well as others under development for treating tumors, are potential agents for the treatment of epilepsy. Importantly, selection of patients could be facilitated by the use of AMT PET as a biomarker to identify epileptic patients with increased tryptophan metabolism.

SUMMARY

AMT PET is a relatively recently developed imaging modality that has already demonstrated promising results, especially in situations where the seizures arise from one of multiple lesions in the brain, such as tuberous sclerosis and multifocal cortical dysplasia. It has shown an impressive specificity, but modest sensitivity, in identifying the epileptic focus. In addition,

AMT PET may also enhance our understanding of the basic mechanisms of epilepsy, and suggest new therapeutic approaches for epilepsy. The restricted number of sites available worldwide that are currently performing AMT PET is perhaps the biggest limitation that this technique encounters today, but this is expected to grow.

REFERENCES

Asano, E., D. C. Chugani, O. Muzik, et al. 2000. Multimodality imaging for improved detection of epileptogenic foci in tuberous sclerosis complex. *Neurology* 54: 1976–84.

Batista, C. E., C. Juhász, O. Muzik, et al. 2009. Imaging correlates of differential expression of indoleamine 2,3-dioxygenase in human brain tumors. *Molecular Imaging Biology* 11: 460–6.

Boeck, C. R., M. Ganzella, A. Lottermann, et al. 2004. NMDA preconditioning protects against seizures and hippocampal neurotoxicity induced by quinolinic acid in mice. *Epilepsia* 45: 745–50.

Chiarugi, A., R. Carpenedo, M. T. Molina, et al. 1995. Comparison of the neurochemical and behavioral effects resulting from the inhibition of kynurenine hydroxylase and/or kynureninase. *Journal of Neurochemistry* 65: 1176–1183.

Chugani DC, Muzik O. 2000. [C–11]Methyl-L-tryptophan PET maps brain serotonin synthesis and kynurenine pathway metabolism. *Journal of Cerebral Blood Flow Metabolism* 20: 2–9.

Chugani, D. C., H. T. Chugani, O. Muzik, et al. 1998b. Imaging epileptogenic tubers in children with tuberous sclerosis complex using alpha-[11C]methyl-L-tryptophan positron emission tomography. *Annals of Neurology* 44: 858–66.

Chugani, D. C., M. P. Heyes, D. M. Kuhn, et al. 1998c. Evidence that [C–11]methyl-L-tryptophan PET traces tryptophan metabolism via the kynurenine pathway in tuberous sclerosis complex. *Society of Neuroscience Abstracts* 24: 1757.

Chugani, D. C., O. Muzik, P. K. Chakraborty, et al. 1998a. Human brain serotonin synthesis capacity measured in vivo with alpha-[C–11]methyl-L-tryptophan. *Synapse* 28: 33–43.

Chugani, H. T., C. Juhász, D. C. Chugani, et al. 2008. Increased striatal serotonin synthesis following cortical resection in children with intractable epilepsy. *Epilepsy Research* 78: 124–30.

Cohen, Z., K. Tsuiki, A. Takada, et al. 1995. In vivo synthesis of radioactively labeled alpha-methyl-serotonin as a selective tracer for visualization of brain serotonin neurons. *Synapse* 21: 21–8.

Crino, P. B. 2004. Molecular pathogenesis of tuber formation in tuberous sclerosis complex. *Journal of Child Neurology* 19: 716–25.

De Oliveira, D. L. J. F. Horn, J. M. Rodrigues, et al. 2004. Quinolinic acid promotes seizures and decreases glutamate uptake in young rats: reversal by orally administered guanosine. *Brain Research* 1018: 48–54.

Diksic, M., S. Nagahiro, T. L. Sourkes, et al. 1990. A new method to measure brain serotonin synthesis in vivo. I. Theory and basic data for a biological model. *Journal of Cerebral Blood Flow Metabolism* 10: 1–12.

Diksic, M., S. Nagahiro, T. Chaly, et al. 1991. Serotonin synthesis rate measured in living dog brain by positron emission tomography. *Journal of Neurochemistry* 56: 153–62.

Fedi, M., D. Reutens, H. Okazawa, et al. 2001. Localizing value of alpha-methyl-L-tryptophan PET in intractable epilepsy of neocortical origin. *Neurology* 57: 1629–36.

Fedi, M., D. C. Reutens, F. Andermann, et al. 2003. Alpha-[11C]-Methyl-L-tryptophan PET identifies the epileptogenic tuber and correlates with interictal spike frequency. *Epilepsy Research* 52: 203–13.

Feldblum, S., A. Rougier, H. Loiseau, et al. 1988. Quinolinic acid phosphoribosyl transferase activity is decreased in epileptic human brain tissue. *Epilepsia* 29: 523–9.

Guillemin, G. J., G. Smythe, O. Takikawa, et al. 2005. Expression of indoleamine 2,3-dioxygenase and production of quinolinic acid by human microglia, astrocytes, and neurons. *Glia* 49: 15–23.

Hauser, W. A., J. F. Annegers, and L. T. Kurland. 1993. Incidence of epilepsy and unprovoked seizures in Rochester, Minnesota: 1935–1984. *Epilepsia* 34: 453–68.

Hery, F., G. Chouvet, J. P. Kan, et al. 1977. Daily variations of various parameters of serotonin metabolism in the rat brain. II. Circadian variations in serum and cerebral tryptophan levels: lack of correlations with 5-HT turnover. *Brain Research* 123: 137–45.

Heyes, M. P., A. R. Wyler, O. Devinsky, et al. 1990. Quinolinic acid concentrations in brain and cerebrospinal fluid of patients with intractable complex partial seizures. *Epilepsia* 31: 172–7.

Juhász, C., D. C. Chugani, O. Muzik, et al. 2003. Alpha-methyl-L-tryptophan PET detects epileptogenic cortex in children with intractable epilepsy. *Neurology* 60: 960–8.

Juhász, C., D. C. Chugani, U. N. Padhye, et al. 2004. Evaluation with alpha-[^{11}C]methyl-L-tryptophan positron emission tomography for reoperation after failed epilepsy surgery. *Epilepsia* 45: 124–30.

Juhász, C., D. C. Chugani, O. Muzik, et al. 2006. In vivo uptake and metabolism of alpha-[^{11}C]methyl-L-tryptophan in human brain tumors. *Journal of Cerebral Blood Flow Metabolism* 26: 345–57.

Kagawa, K., D. C. Chugani, E. Asano E, et al. 2005. Epilepsy surgery outcome in children with tuberous sclerosis complex evaluated with alpha-[11C]methyl-L-tryptophan positron emission tomography (PET). *Journal of Child Neurology* 20: 429–38.

Lapin, I. P. 1978. Stimulant and convulsant effects of kynurenines injected into brain ventricles in mice. *Journal of Neural Transmission* 32: 37–43.

Lapin, I. P. 1980. Effect of kynurenine and quinolinic acid on the actions of convulsants in mice. *Pharmacology Biochemistry Behavior* 13: 17–20.

Lapin, I. P. 1982. Convulsant action of intracerebroventricularly administered L-kynurenine sulphate, quinolinic acid and of derivatives of succinic acid, and effects of amino acids, structure-activity relationships. *Neuropharmacology* 21: 1227–33.

Lehrmann, E., P. Guidetti P, A. Löve, et al. 2008. Glial activation precedes seizures and hippocampal neurodegeneration in measles virus-infected mice. *Epilepsia* 49 (Suppl 2): 13–23.

Louw, D., G. B. Sutherland, G. B. Glavin, et al. 1989. A study of monoamine metabolism in human epilepsy. *Canadian Journal of Neurological Sciences* 16: 394–7.

Lundquist, P., P. Hartvig, G. Blomquist, et al. 2007. 5-Hydroxy-L-[beta–11C]tryptophan versus alpha-[11C] methyl-L-tryptophan for positron emission tomography imaging of serotonin synthesis capacity in the rhesus monkey brain. *Journal of Cerebral Blood Flow Metabolism* 27: 821–30.

Madras, B.K., and T. L. Sourkes. 1965. Metabolism of alpha-methyltryptophan. *Biochemistry Pharmacology* 14: 1499–506.

Missala, K., and T. L. Sourkes. 1988. Functional cerebral activity of an analogue of serotonin formed in situ. *Neurochemistry International* 12: 209–14.

Muzik, O., D. C. Chugani, P. Chakraborty, et al. 1997. Analysis of [C–11]alpha-methyl-tryptophan kinetics for the estimation of serotonin synthesis rate in vivo. *Journal of Cerebral Blood Flow Metabolism* 17: 659–69.

Nagahiro, S., A. Takada, M. Diksic, et al. 1990. A new method to measure brain serotonin synthesis in vivo. II. A practical autoradiographic method tested in normal and lithium-treated rats. *Journal of Cerebral Blood Flow Metabolism* 10: 13–21.

Natsume, J., Y. Kumakura, N. Bernasconi, et al. 2003. Alpha-[11C] methyl-L-tryptophan and glucose metabolism in patients with temporal lobe epilepsy. *Neurology* 60: 756–61.

Natsume, J., N. Bernasconi, Y. Aghakhani, et al. 2008. Alpha-[11C]methyl-L-tryptophan uptake in patients with periventricular nodular heterotopia and epilepsy. *Epilepsia* 49: 826–31.

Nemeth, H., H. Robotka, Z. Kis, et al. 2004. Kynurenine administered together with probenecid markedly inhibits pentylenetetrazol-induced seizures. An electrophysiological and behavioural study. *Neuropharmacology* 47: 916–925.

Pardridge, W. M., and G. Fierer. 1990. Transport of tryptophan into brain from the circulating, albumin-bound pool in rats and in rabbits. *Journal of Neurochemistry* 54: 971–6.

Patlak, C. S., R. G. Blasberg, and J. D. Fenstermacher. 1983. Graphical evaluation of blood-to-brain transfer constants from multiple-time uptake data. *Journal of Cerebral Blood Flow Metabolism* 3: 1–7.

Perkins, M. N., and T. W. Stone. 1982. An iontophoretic investigation of the actions of convulsant kynurenines and their interaction with endogenous excitant quinolinic acid. *Brain Research* 247: 183–7.

Perkins, M. N., and T. W. Stone. 1983. Pharmacology and regional variation of quinolinic acid-evoked excitations in rat central nervous system. *Journal of Pharmacology & Experimental Therapeutics* 226: 551–7.

Pintor, M., I. N. Mefford, I. Hutter, et al. 1990. The levels of biogenic amines, their metabolites and tyrosine hydroxylase in the human epileptic temporal cortex. *Synapse* 5: 152–6.

Saito, K., T. S. Nowak Jr., and K. Suyama. 1993. Kynurenine pathway enzymes in brain: Responses to ischemic brain injury versus systemic immune activation. *Journal of Neurochemistry* 61: 2061–70.

Scharfman, H. E., and A. Ofer. 1997. Pretreatment with L-kynurenine, the precursor to the excitatory amino acid antagonist kynurenic acid, suppresses epileptiform activity in combined entorhina/hippocampal slices. *Neurosci Letters* 224: 115–8.

Tavares, R. G., A. P. Schmidt, C. I. Tasca, et al. 2008. Quinolinic acid-induced seizures stimulate glutamate uptake into synaptic vesicles from rat brain: effects prevented by guanine-based purines. *Neurochemistry Research* 33: 97–102.

Trottier, S., B. Evrard, J. P. Vignal, et al. 1996. The serotonergic innervation of the cerebral cortex in man and its changes in focal cortical dysplasia. *Epilepsy Research* 25: 79–106.

Uhlmann, E. J., M. Wong, R. L. Baldwin, et al. 2002. Astrocyte-specific TSC1 conditional knockout mice exhibit abnormal neuronal organization and seizures. *Annals of Neurology* 52: 285–96.

Vezzani, A., J. B. Gramsbergen, P. Versari, et al. 1990. Kynurenic acid synthesis by human glioma. *Journal of Neurologi Science* 99: 51–7.

Wakamoto, H., D. C. Chugani, C. Juhász, et al. 2008. Alpha-methyl-l-tryptophan positron emission tomography in epilepsy with cortical developmental malformations. *Pediatric Neurology* 39: 181–8.

Wu, H. Q., S-C. Lee, H. E. Scharfman, et al. 2002. L-4-chlorokynurenine attenuates kainate-induced seizures and lesions in the rat. *Experimental Neurology* 177: 222–32.

Wu, H. Q., A. Rassoulpour, J. H. Goodman, et al. 2005. Kynurenate and 7-chlorokynurenate formation in chronically epileptic rats. *Epilepsia* 47: 1010–6.

Zhang, D. X., J. M. Williamson, H. Q. Wu, et al. 2005. In situ-produced 7-chlorokynurenate has different effects on evoked responses in rats with limbic epilepsy in comparison to naive controls. *Epilepsia* 46: 1708–15.

Chapter *13*

OTHER PET LIGANDS USED IN EPILEPSY

William H. Theodore

In addition to 2-deoxy-2(^{18}F)-fluoro-D-glucose (FDG; see Chapters 8, 9, 10), ^{11}C-flumazenil (see Chapter 11), and ^{11}C-alpha-methyl-L-tryptophan (AMT; see Chapter 12), a number of other PET ligands have been used to investigate the role of opiate, serotonin, dopamine, and several other neurotransmitter-receptor systems in epilepsy. This chapter will review the findings from such studies, which at present are much more important for understanding basic mechanisms of epilepsy than for application in clinical care—although, as illustrated in Chapters 11 and 12, clinical applications appear to be expanding for some ligands.

OPIATE RECEPTORS

Mu-opiate receptors were studied with ^{11}C-carfentanil and a PET scanner with 8 mm of spatial resolution in 13 patients with temporal lobe epilepsy (TLE). There was 9% to 15% increased binding in temporal neocortex ipsilateral to temporal seizure foci compared to the non-focus side, but no significant asymmetry was detected in the amygdala or hippocampus. These findings were interpreted as probably due to an increase in affinity or the number of unoccupied receptors in temporal neocortex (Frost et al. 1988). In contrast, the cerebral metabolic rate for glucose

(CMRglc) measured by FDG PET was decreased in both mesial and lateral temporal regions in these same patients. There was a significant inverse relation between ^{11}C-carfentanil binding and hypometabolism on FDG PET. Increased opiate receptor binding in temporal neocortex might be related to an endogenous antiepileptic response to seizure activity, but interpretation of these data raised issues faced by subsequent epilepsy PET receptor studies as well. Does increased binding imply increased receptor number (B_{max}), a conformational change leading to increased binding affinity (K_d), or reduction in the intrasynaptic availability of an endogenous ligand? Interestingly, one patient who had a seizure preceding the scan had relatively increased ^{11}C-carfentanil binding ipsilateral to the epileptic focus similar to the group as a whole, suggesting that ictal endogenous opiate release does not occur at a level high enough to affect binding (Frost et al. 1988). Although radiation dosimetry limits would make it difficult to perform the PET studies using multiple doses for Scatchard analysis and thus make the distinction, altered receptor availability is more likely than a change in affinity to account for increased binding.

A subsequent study of 11 patients with TLE from the same investigators compared ^{11}C-carfentanil to ^{11}C-diprenorphine (a ligand with comparable affinity for mu, delta, and kappa receptors), as well as to FDG

PET scans (Mayberg et al. 1991). ^{11}C-Carfentanil binding was increased in temporal neocortex and decreased in amygdala ipsilateral to the epileptic focus. In contrast, ^{11}C-diprenorphine binding was not significantly different between temporal regions ipsilateral and contralateral to the focus. CMRglc was decreased in mesial and lateral temporal lobe ipsilateral to the epileptogenic focus. This study suggested that an increase in mu-receptor binding might be offset by a decrease in delta and/or kappa receptor binding (Mayberg et al. 1991). The contrasting ^{11}C-carfentanil binding results in amygdala between the two studies from the same laboratory underlines the difficulty in drawing firm conclusions when studies consist of small numbers of subjects.

A third study, which included 10 patients, compared ^{11}C-carfentanil binding to the delta-receptor-selective antagonist ^{11}C-methylnaltrindole (^{11}C-MeNTI). Increased ^{11}C-MeNTI binding was present in mid-inferior and anterior aspects of the middle and superior temporal cortex ipsilateral to the seizure focus, while mu receptors were increased only in middle inferior temporal cortex (Madar et al. 1997). There was a nonsignificant trend for delta-receptor binding to be higher in ipsilateral amygdala, while mu-receptor binding was again significantly lower ipsilateral than contralateral to the epileptic focus.

Eleven patients were studied with ^{18}F-cyclofoxy, a potent opiate antagonist with affinity for mu and kappa receptors. Individual patients appeared to have higher binding in temporal lobe ipsilateral to the EEG focus compared to the non-focus side, but there was no asymmetry for the patients as a group (Theodore et al. 1992). There was a significant reduction of relative binding in frontal cortex, a region that normally shows low binding, that is difficult to explain. Nevertheless, at least for temporal lobe, this study suggested that kappa-receptor downregulation might offset mu-receptor upregulation.

In a very small study, two patients with TLE had PET scans using FDG and ^{11}C-diprenorphine before and 5 months after selective amygdalo-hippocampectomy; both became seizure-free. Before surgery CMRglc was decreased in mesial and lateral temporal lobe ipsilateral to the EEG focus. ^{11}C-diprenorphine binding was reduced in the same regions (but within 2 SD of the normal range). Postoperatively, there was a greater reduction of CMRglc in the ipsilateral lateral temporal cortex in one patient and somewhat less in the other; however, both patients had a greater reduction of ^{11}C-diprenorphine binding compared to the preoperative scans. Since mu, kappa, and delta receptors are all imaged by this ligand, the results are difficult to interpret but might reflect downregulation of mu receptors after successful surgery, thus reversing the epilepsy-induced upregulation that had been present preoperatively (Bartenstein et al. 1994).

The effect of naloxone on cerebral blood flow (CBF) measured with ^{15}O-water and CMRglc measured with ^{18}F-FDG was studied in 15 patients with complex partial seizures (Theodore et al. 1993). Following infusion of 1 mg/kg naloxone, there was no effect on glucose metabolism, but blood flow was reduced by 7% to 12% between 45 and 60 minutes after infusion, as was the degree of lateral temporal CBF asymmetry in patients with more than 10% baseline hypoperfusion. This study suggested that elevated opiate levels might be related to CBF abnormalities in TLE.

Unfortunately, none of the studies discussed above was performed with MRI-based partial volume correction, a technique that has become important for interpretation of receptor-binding studies. This is particularly important in TLE, since tissue loss could lead to artifactual reductions in receptor binding. However, increased binding cannot be explained purely on the basis of mesial and lateral temporal lobe atrophy.

Patients with generalized epilepsy syndromes have also been studied using PET ligands of opiate receptors. In one such study of eight subjects with childhood and juvenile absence epilepsy, there was no difference in ^{11}C-diprenorphine V_d between patients and controls in either cortex or thalamus, structures implicated in the pathogenesis of absence seizures (Prevett et al. 1994). These scans were performed in the interictal state with spike-wave activity ranging from 0% to 1.5% of the time on EEG recorded during the scans. In a study of the effect of absence seizures on opiate-receptor binding, hyperventilation for 10 minutes was started 30 to 40 minutes after ^{11}C-diprenorphine injection (Bartenstein et al. 1993). Generalized spike-wave discharges on the EEG occupied 10% to 51% of the time during hyperventilation. There was increased elimination of ^{11}C-diprenorphine from association cortex, but not from the thalamus, basal ganglia, or cerebellum, suggesting that endogenous opioids may be released, leading to increased receptor occupancy during serial absences.

Several opiate receptor studies using PET have been performed in the ictal state. In one such study, five patients with reading epilepsy had ^{11}C-diprenorphine scans while reading a string of symbols (baseline) or a scientific paper (activation) (Koepp et al. 1998). The patients with reading epilepsy had 7% to 11% lower ^{11}C-diprenorphine binding while reading the paper than during the control task. In comparison, six healthy volunteers had 10% to 12% increased binding while reading the paper. The difference was significant in the left parieto-temporo-occipital cortex (Brodmann area 37) when compared to the six controls. Three of the patients had seizures during the activated scan. The investigators suggested that an endogenous opioid-like substance might be released during reading-induced seizures to account for the decreased ictal binding (Koepp et al. 1998). Since this study included patients who were having seizures during the tracer uptake, it does not conflict with the report of the one TLE patient who had had a seizure about an hour before a ^{11}C-carfentanil scan; this subject had an ipsilateral increase in mu-receptor binding comparable to the patient group as a whole (Frost et al. 1988).

To examine postictal effects on opiate-receptor binding, nine patients were scanned with ^{11}C-diprenorphine PET within hours of spontaneous temporal lobe seizures (Hammers et al. 2007). Opiate-receptor availability increased in the temporal pole and fusiform gyrus ipsilateral to the seizure focus following seizures, showing an inverse correlation with time since last seizure, suggesting an early postictal increase of opiate-receptor availability and gradual return to baseline. This postictal increase in binding, combined with the previous reports of decreased binding when scans were performed acutely during absence and reading-induced seizures, suggests early peri-ictal endogenous opioid release, causing decreased binding site availability for the exogenous PET tracer (Hammers et al. 2007) (Fig. 13.1). Subsequently, a gradual fall in endogenous ligand receptor occupancy leads to an overshoot to below basal levels, shown by increased receptor availability for the exogenous tracer up to 8 hours after seizures.

The development of microPET has facilitated ligand studies in animal models. One recent study in rats used ^{18}F-MK-9470 and a microPET system to evaluate the effects of the anticonvulsants valproate (VPA) and levetiracetam (LEV) on the type 1 cannabinoid receptor (CB1R), which may be involved in epilepsy (Goffin et al. 2008). There was a significant increase in global cerebral ^{18}F-MK-9470 binding after chronic VPA but not LEV administration compared to sham-treated animals. Since VPA does not show high affinity for CB1R, the increased binding is most likely due to an indirect effect on the endocannabinoid system (Goffin et al. 2008).

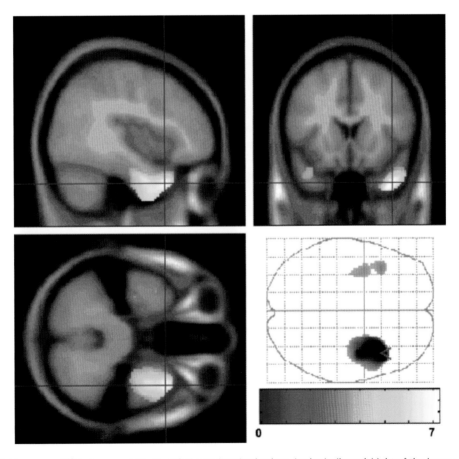

Figure 13.1 Postictal increase of ^{11}C-diprenorphine V_d, relative to interictal values, in the ipsilateral (right of the image, crosshairs) anterior temporal lobe. Thresholded *t* map overlaid onto MNI/ICBM152 average. Maximum intensity projection showing nonsignificant contralateral increases and absence of changes elsewhere. Color bar: *t* scores. (Reprinted from A. Hammers, M. C. Asselin, R. Hinz, et al. 2007. Upregulation of opioid receptor binding following spontaneous epileptic seizures. *Brain* 130(Pt 4): 1009–16.)

MONOAMINE OXIDASE RECEPTOR IMAGING

Deprenyl is an irreversible monoamine oxidase type B inhibitor (MAO-B) with a very high enzyme affinity. In brain, MAO-B has high levels in astrocytes, and increased binding to MAO-B in sclerotic hippocampi has been shown in vitro (Kumlien et al. 1992). In a PET study to examine MAO-B involvement in TLE, nine patients (seven with unilateral foci) were evaluated with both ^{18}F-FDG and ^{11}C-deuterium-deprenyl (Kumlien et al. 1995). There was significantly increased ^{11}C-deuterium-deprenyl uptake in the temporal lobe ipsilateral to the EEG focus in the patients overall, and in six of seven patients with unilateral seizure onset individually; however, there was no asymmetry in the two patients with bilateral seizure onset. There was good correlation between in vivo and in vitro binding data, regardless of whether metabolite corrected plasma or modified cerebellar uptake values were used as input function, with lower initial distribution and higher late tracer accumulation ipsilateral to the epileptic focus (Bergstrom et al. 1998).

In a subsequent study from the same group of investigators, 14 patients with mesial TLE, 9 with extratemporal neocortical epilepsy, and 6 healthy control subjects were reported (Kumlien et al. 2001). In the TLE group, initial tracer distribution volume was significantly lower in temporal lobe ipsilateral to the seizure focus compared to the contralateral side, probably reflecting reduced CBF. Although individual patients had increased accumulation, there was no significant difference between temporal lobes, in contrast to the earlier results. No asymmetries were found in either extratemporal lobe epilepsy patients or controls.

In a study using single photon emission computed tomography (SPECT) with the radiotracer [^{123}I]Ro 43-0463, an MAO-B inhibitor, nine patients with TLE had increased uptake in the mesial temporal lobe and putamen ipsilateral to the seizure focus (Buck et al. 1998). The increased uptake in ipsilateral putamen was unexpected. Overall, these data from PET and SPECT are consistent with the prominent gliosis found in mesial TLE and may be relevant to the increasing interest concerning the role of inflammation in the pathophysiology of mesial TLE (Vezzani and Granata, 2005).

SEROTONIN RECEPTORS

Serotonin (5HT) is an important neurotransmitter that influences a wide range of neurophysiologic processes and behavioral functions. 5HT$_{1A}$ receptors have recently received increasing attention in PET studies of epilepsy. Three receptor ligands, ^{18}F-FCWAY100635 (Giovacchini et al. 2005; Toczek et al. 2003), ^{11}C-WAY100635 (Savic et al. 2004), and ^{18}F-MPPF (Merlet et al. 2004a, 2004b) have been used. The ^{18}F ligands have the advantage of higher signal-to-noise ratio, but FCWAY has a fluorinated metabolite that can accumulate in bone, leading to partial volume effects that need to be corrected. MPPF has lower specific activity and is sensitive to endogenous 5HT levels but can be studied with a reference region approach. In general, however, all three ligands have shown similar results in patients with TLE. There was reduced binding in mesial temporal regions, including hippocampus, amygdala, and parahippocampal and fusiform gyrus ipsilateral to the epileptic focus, with lesser degrees of reduction in contralateral mesial temporal structures. The abnormalities were present in patients with normal MRI and could still be detected in patients with mesial temporal sclerosis after partial volume correction (Giovacchini et al. 2005) (Fig. 13.2). Correlation between findings from ^{18}F-MPPF PET and subdural electrodes showed that the magnitude of reduced binding was greater in the seizure onset zone than in regions of seizure spread or only interictal spiking (Merlet et al. 2004a). Although reduced binding potential was significantly influenced by MRI lesions, it was still correlated with seizure activity in regions with normal MRI. In 7 patients studied with ^{18}F-MPPF, those without hippocampal atrophy had reduced 5HT$_{1A}$ binding restricted to the temporal pole, without hippocampal reduction (Merlet et al. 2004b).

These findings suggest that PET scanning of 5HT$_{1A}$ receptors might have a role in presurgical evaluation for intractable epilepsy, particularly when MRI is normal. In a recent larger study, 42 patients with TLE had ^{18}F-MPPF PET using a simplified reference tissue model (Didelot et al. 2008); 38 of the 42 patients had focal areas of decreased binding potential on visual analysis. A specific pattern was encountered in the mesial TLE subgroup, consisting of decreased binding potential involving hippocampus, amygdala, and temporal pole altogether. Decreased binding potential corresponded to the epileptogenic zone in 40% of patients with mesial TLE and 33% with other TLE subtypes, but about 80% had decreases in the ipsilateral epileptogenic lobe. Statistical parametric mapping (SPM) analysis had lower sensitivity (67%) to detect decreases of binding potential in the epileptogenic temporal lobe and revealed areas of *increased* binding potential outside the epileptogenic zone as well as bitemporal decreases in binding potential of undetermined clinical significance in 29%.

A series of MRI-negative TLE patients studied with ^{18}F-FCWAY PET and ^{18}F-FDG PET had the location of their epileptic focus confirmed either by surgery or subdural electrode recording (Liew et al. 2009).

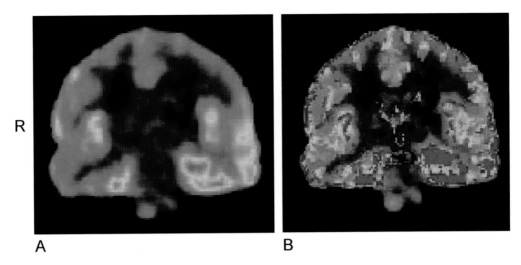

Figure 13.2 ^{18}F-FCWAY images before (A) and after (B) partial volume correction to account for the effect of mesial temporal sclerosis both show reduced binding in mesial temporal cortex in a patient with a right temporal lobe EEG focus. About 20% of the reduction in ipsilateral activity is accounted for by reduced hippocampal volume.

In this study, after partial volume correction for brain atrophy, side-to-side asymmetry indices (AIs) were computed to assess relative reduction in FCWAY V_d and CMRglc in the epileptic focus, and ^{18}F-FCWAY PET and ^{18}F-FDG PET results were compared with scalp video-EEG, intracranial EEG, and surgical outcome. Confirming previous results, mean ^{18}F-FCWAY free fraction-corrected volume of distribution (V/f1), compared with normal controls, was decreased significantly in fusiform gyrus, hippocampus, and parahippocampus ipsilateral to epileptic foci, and AIs were significantly greater in hippocampus, parahippocampus, fusiform gyrus, amygdala, and inferior temporal regions. Eleven patients had clearly lateralized epileptogenic zones. Nine had congruent, and two non-lateralized, ^{18}F-FCWAY PET. One patient with bitemporal seizure onset had non-lateralized ^{18}F-FCWAY PET. The ^{18}F-FDG PET showed congruent hypometabolism in 7 of 11 EEG-lateralized patients, bilateral hypometabolic regions in one, contralateral hypometabolism in one, as well as lateralized hypometabolism in the patient with bitemporal subdural seizure onset.

Finally, in a study of patients with juvenile myoclonic epilepsy, a generalized epilepsy syndrome, ^{11}C-WAY binding was reported to be reduced in bilateral dorsolateral prefrontal cortex, raphe nuclei, and hippocampus (Meshaks et al. 2005).

DEPRESSION, EPILEPSY, AND 5HT$_{1A}$ RECEPTOR BINDING

Depression is a major complication of epilepsy. However, it is uncertain whether people with epilepsy are depressed due to their suffering a chronic and unpredictable illness that leads to social stigma as well as economic problems, or whether there is an underlying biological mechanism that might be shared with major depressive disorders, such as altered serotonergic transmission (Drevets et al. 1999; Sargent et al. 2000).

Several studies have used WAY100635 to investigate the link between 5HT$_{1A}$ receptors and depression in epilepsy. In one study, reduced ^{11}C-WAY binding potential in anterior cingulate was found to have a significant correlation with the Montgomery-Asberg mood rating scale (Savic et al. 2004). Another study, which used ^{18}F-FCWAY, reported a significant correlation between hippocampal binding ipsilateral to the epileptic focus and the Beck Depression Inventory (Theodore et al. 2007) (Fig. 13.3). Both of these measures reflect the patient's state rather than an underlying depressive condition.

In a relatively large study on 37 patients with TLE and diagnosis of major depressive disorder based on the Structured Clinical Interview for DSM IV, greater reductions in FCWAY binding were found in the patients than in controls or patients with epilepsy alone; affected areas included limbic regions and cingulate gyrus (Hasler et al. 2007). Age, gender, age of seizure onset, or duration of epilepsy as covariates to the primary analysis had little effect on the results. Focus side and the presence of mesial temporal sclerosis were not associated with the presence of comorbid depression and did not affect 5HT$_{1A}$ results.

In a more recent study, 24 patients with TLE evaluated with ^{18}F-MPPF PET had Beck Depression Inventory (BDI-2) scores from 0 to 34, with 9 patients having a score above 11 (Lothe et al. 2008). Total BDI score, as well as symptoms of psychomotor anhedonia and

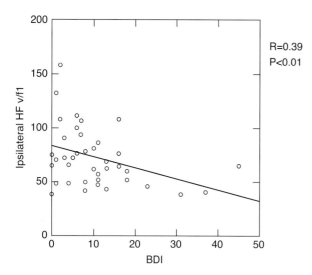

Figure 13.3 Relation of the Beck Depression Inventory (BDI) to hippocampal ^{18}F-FCWAY volume of distribution ipsilateral to the epileptic focus. (Reprinted from W. H. Theodore, G. Hasler, G. Giovacchini, et al. 2007. Reduced hippocampal 5HT1A PET receptor binding and depression in temporal lobe epilepsy. *Epilepsia* 48: 1526–30.)

negative cognition, correlated positively with ^{18}F-MPPF binding potential in raphe and insula contralateral to seizure onset. Somatic symptoms correlated positively with binding potential in hippocampal/parahippocampal region ipsilateral to seizure onset. The difference between this study and previous results using ^{18}F-FCWAY or ^{11}C-WAY probably can be explained by the high sensitivity of the ^{18}F-MPPF to synaptic 5HT levels. The K_d of ^{18}F-MPPF is 3.3 nM, and that of 5HT is 4.2 nM, while the K_d of FCWAY is 1.0 nM (Zimmer et al. 2002). Thus, low levels of endogenous serotonin, expected in depression, would lead to relatively increased binding in depressed compared with nondepressed epilepsy patients. This process would not affect FCWAY, consistent with findings of decreased binding in patients with epilepsy, as well as major depressive disorders (Hasler et al. 2007; Savic et al. 2004; Theodore et al. 2007). Patients with major depressive disorders have reductions of $5HT_{1A}$ receptor binding in limbic regions and cingulate cortex (Drevets et al. 1999; Sargent et al. 2000).

The effect of antiepileptic drugs (AEDs), including carbamazepine, oxcarbazepine, phenytoin, lamotrigine, valproic acid, levetiracetam, and phenytoin, on $5HT_{1A}$ receptor binding has been investigated using ^{18}F-FCWAY (Theodore et al. 2006). After correction for tracer plasma free fraction, which could be affected due to protein binding interactions, no AED effects were found. Similar results have been reported for patients on selective serotonin reuptake

inhibitors (SSRIs), probably due to the much lower $5HT_{1A}$ receptor K_d for ^{18}F-FCWAY than for serotonin itself (Drevets et al. 2007; Sargent et al. 2000).

One study of $5HT_{1A}$ receptor binding in sleep may be of interest, although not directly related to epilepsy. This study exploited the sensitivity of ^{18}F-MPPF to synaptic serotonin levels (Derry et al. 2006) and was based on animal studies suggesting that serotonin release promotes wakefulness and suppresses REM sleep. Fourteen subjects with narcolepsy/cataplexy underwent ^{18}F-MPPF PET scans in wakefulness and in sleep. There was a significant increase in ^{18}F-MPPF binding in sleep compared to wakefulness in whole brain, temporal cortex, mesial temporal region, and cingulate cortex. These findings are consistent with the animal studies in that higher $5HT_{1A}$ receptor binding in sleep might be due to lower endogenous serotonin receptor occupancy.

5HT transport has been studied extensively in patients with mood disorders. Studies with PET have suggested that limbic 5HT transport may be decreased in unipolar major depressive disorder and increased in bipolar disorders (Cannon et al. 2006; Parsey et al. 2006). In a preliminary study, there was significantly reduced binding of the 5HT transporter ligand ^{11}C-DASB in the amygdala, thalamus, and midbrain (the site of 5HT presynaptic autoreceptors) in patients with TLE (Lim et al. 2008). These data support the notion that $5HT_{1A}$ receptor reductions form a link between major depressive disorders and epilepsy (Fig. 13.4).

DOPAMINE RECEPTORS

Several studies of dopamine receptors using PET have been performed in patients with epilepsy. For example, in patients with epilepsy and ring chromosome 20, a severe inherited syndrome, ^{18}F-fluoro-L-DOPA uptake was significantly decreased bilaterally in the putamen and in the caudate nucleus (Biraben et al. 2004). The investigators suggested that the PET findings might reflect impaired striatal function related to the patients' prolonged seizures. Using a region-of-interest analysis to calculate the ^{18}F-fluoro-L-DOPA uptake constant, patients with generalized epilepsy and TLE showed striatal uptake reductions (Bouilleret et al. 2005). In patients with TLE, SPM but not region-of-interest analysis showed decreased striatal uptake ipsilateral to the seizure focus, and in bilateral substantia nigra (Fig. 13.5). The investigators suggested that some of their findings could be due to differences in seizure frequency as well as the epilepsy syndromes themselves (Bouilleret et al 2005).

In another study, seven patients with TLE (all with mesial temporal sclerosis) and nine age-matched

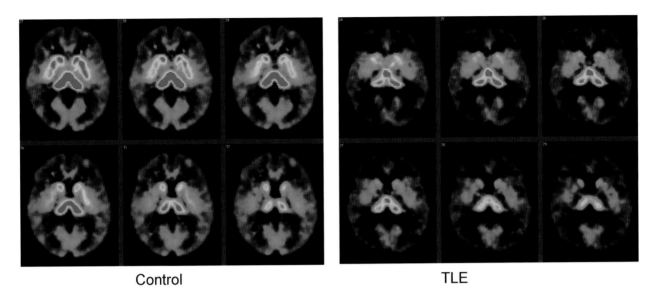

Control   TLE

Figure 13.4 Ratio of decrease of ^{18}F-fluoro-L-DOPA uptake in the three groups of patients with SPM analysis. Decrease of ^{18}F-fluoro-L-DOPA uptake occurs mainly in substantia nigrabut also in putamen. This decrease is bilateral in groups 1 and 2 ($P < 0.001$) and ipsilateral to hippocampal sclerosis in group 3 at a less conservative statistical level ($P <\_0.005$). (Reprinted from V. Bouilleret, F. Semah, A. Biraben, et al. 2005. Involvement of the basal ganglia in refractory epilepsy: an ^{18}F-fluoro-L-DOPA PET study using 2 methods of analysis. *Journal of Nuclear Medicine* 46: 540–47.)

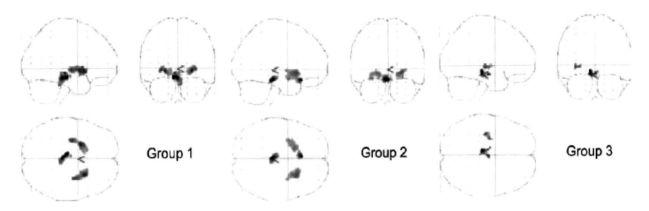

Group 1   Group 2   Group 3

Figure 13.5 Comparison of ^{11}C-DASB PET in a control subject (left) and TLE patient (right). The patient has reduced activity in amygdala and thalamus.

controls underwent PET scanning with both FDG and the high-affinity dopamine D2/D3-receptor ligand ^{18}F-fallypride (^{18}F-FP) suitable for imaging extrastriatal binding (Werhahn et al. 2006). Binding potential for ^{18}F-FP was calculated with a simplified reference tissue model. Compared with controls, ^{18}F-FP binding potential was significantly decreased in the epileptogenic temporal lobe in all patients, including temporo-polar and lateral temporal regions surrounding the seizure-onset zone. Reduced D2/D3 binding did not correlate with hippocampal atrophy.

It has been suggested that increased striatal dopamine release may be caused by increased acetylcholine sensitivity in patients with autosomal dominant nocturnal frontal lobe epilepsy (ADNFLE), which is associated with the alpha4-Ser248Phe mutation (Fedi et al. 2008). To test this hypothesis, 12 patients with ADNFLE and 19 controls were studied with PET and the D_1 receptor ligand ^{11}C-SCH23390 and a simplified reference region method. There was a small but significant reduction (about 4%) of D_1 receptor binding in the right putamen of ADNFLE patients. This could be due either to increased extracellular dopamine levels or to receptor downregulation. The investigators suggested this might be a potential mechanism for the paroxysmal nocturnal motor activity seen in ADNFLE.

EXCITATORY AMINO ACIDS, NICOTINIC AND HISTAMINE RECEPTORS

As illustrated thus far in this chapter, a number of studies have been performed to illustrate the wide potential applications of PET in evaluating epilepsy. Potentially the most interesting of these is the use of excitatory amino acid ligands. Several recent studies in primates and human have used mGlur5 ligands to evaluate the role of excitatory amino acid mechanisms in epilepsy (Brown et al. 2008; Sanchez-Pernaute et al. 2008).

In one such study, [11]C-(S)-[N-methyl]ketamine was used to image N-methyl-D-aspartate receptors in patients with TLE. Reduced tracer activity was found ipsilateral to the side of seizure onset, congruent with FDG PET hypometabolism (Kumlien et al. 1999). However, it was uncertain whether this was due to focal atrophy, since partial volume correction was not performed. Since excitotoxic mechanisms are thought to play an important role in epileptogenesis and epileptic brain injury, future PET studies of excitatory amino acid receptors have great potential in elucidating pathophysiologic processes in epilepsy.

As briefly mentioned above, ADNFLE is a familial form of frontal lobe epilepsy associated with mutations in subunits of nicotinic acetylcholine receptors (nAChRs). The PET ligand ^{18}F-F-A-85380, which is a high-affinity agonist at alpha4beta2 nAChRs, was applied to patients with ADNFLE. These studies showed increased binding in midbrain, pons, and cerebellum and decreased binding in dorsolateral prefrontal cortex (Picard et al. 2006). The investigators suggested that the increased mesencephalic nAChR binding might reflect altered ascending cholinergic arousal mechanisms.

Brain histamine receptors have been imaged with PET and ^{11}C-doxepin, an antidepressant with high affinity for histamine H_1 receptors. In the brain, histamine is involved in termination of seizures and may function as an endogenous anticonvulsant. Nine patients with complex partial seizures and temporal or frontal seizure foci were studied by PET using both FDG and ^{11}C-doxepin. H_1 receptor binding was 10% to 50% higher in temporal neocortex ipsilateral to the seizure focus. CMRglc was inversely correlated with binding of ^{11}C-doxepin in the focus. This study suggests that increased H_1 receptor binding may represent a defensive mechanism counteracting the spread of epileptic discharges.

IMAGING INFLAMMATION

There is increasing evidence for the role of inflammation in epilepsy. Several PET studies have been performed with ^{11}C-PK11195, a ligand for the "peripheral benzodiazepine receptor" that actually has nothing to do with benzodiazepines, but is found on astrocyte mitochondrial membranes and activated microglia (Sauvageau et al. 2002).

Compared with four healthy controls, patients with Rasmussen encephalitis showed diffusely increased ^{11}C-PK11195 specific binding in the affected hemisphere (Banati et al. 1999). Patients with TLE and mesial temporal sclerosis, who were not considered to be surgery candidates due to low seizure frequency, showed no differences in ^{11}C-PK11195 binding from controls. In hippocampal CA_1 subfields, patients with TLE and mesial temporal sclerosis had increased ^{3}H-PK11195 binding sites, immunoreactivity, and mRNA expression compared to TLE patients without mesial temporal sclerosis and postmortem controls without epilepsy (Sauvageau et al. 2002).

Several cases of ^{11}C-PK11195 PET have been reported in epilepsy that may have been due to encephalitis of unknown origin. In a 30-year-old woman with a 12-year history of simple partial seizures, right-sided homonymous hemianopia, severely impaired verbal memory, dyscalculia, and finger agnosia, the binding potential for ^{11}C-PK11195 in the occipito-temporal cortex was increased compared with healthy controls (Goerres et al. 2001). Occipital biopsy showed chronic vasculitis with perivascular mononuclear accumulations, and activated microglia. Azathioprine and prednisone led to clinical improvement. Another case report involved a 5-year-old boy with intractable epilepsy due to encephalitis of unknown etiology (Kumar et al. 2008). PET with ^{11}C-PK11195 revealed an area of increased uptake in the left temporal-occipital cortex, whereas FDG PET had shown diffuse bilateral hypometabolism. Seizures improved dramatically following cortical resection of the area showing increased binding, guided also by intraoperative electrocorticography. Immunostaining of the resected tissue with CD-68 showed microglial activation.

These studies suggest that pathophysiologic alterations can be imaged with specific ligands in certain epileptic syndromes that have clinical features suggestive of inflammatory processes. It is uncertain whether the findings can be applied to more common forms of epilepsy such as TLE with mesial temporal sclerosis. However, recent data suggest that at least some patients with TLE may have evidence for persistent viral infection (Theodore et al. 2008). Furthermore, limbic encephalitis of various etiologies may be a precursor of TLE (Bien et al. 2007). The application of PET with ^{11}C-PK11195 in other epileptic disorders will prove interesting.

p-GLYCOPROTEIN

Development of resistance to AEDs in patients whose seizures had responded initially is a common clinical problem in the treatment of epilepsy. The mechanism for this phenomenon is uncertain, but one possibility is enhanced transport of AEDs out of epileptogenic regions by the p-glycoprotein transporter that has been implicated in chemotherapy resistance in patients with cancer. A study with PET and ^{11}C-verapamil, a p-glycoprotein substrate, showed some increases in tracer influx and efflux rate constants but no statistically significant differences compared with contralateral non-epileptogenic regions; this was a preliminary study that included only a small number of subjects (Langer et al. 2007) (Fig. 13.6).

WHAT ARE THE USES OF RECEPTOR PET IN EPILEPSY?

In general, the clinical role of FDG PET in people with epilepsy is limited to presurgical evaluation. If structural MRI shows a clear lesion that correlates with ictal onset on video-EEG, there is apparently a lesser role for PET, but the argument is made that the structural abnormality is often not entirely visualized on MRI.

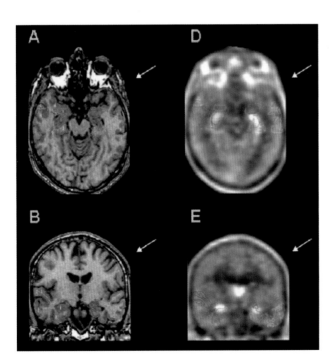

Figure 13.6 T1-weighted MR images (voxel size 0.9 × 0.9 × 4 mm) showing voxels of interest (A, B) and PET summation images (20 frames) (D, E) showing distribution of radioactivity after intravenous injection of *R*-[^{11}C]verapamil in a patient with TLE. The side of the seizure focus (left hemisphere) is indicated by an *arrow*. In the PET images, dark shades of gray represent low and light shades of gray high radioactivity concentrations. (Reprinted from O. Langer, B. Bauer, A. Hammers, et al. 2007. Pharmacoresistance in epilepsy: a pilot PET study with the p-glycoprotein substrate *R*-[^{11}C]verapamil. *Epilepsia* 48: 1774–84.)

There will be only a few patients for whom MRI and FDG PET fail to provide adequate clinical imaging data. In such cases, some studies (reviewed in Chapters 11 and 12) suggest a role for ^{11}C-flumazenil and AMT PET in preoperative evaluation. Encouraging preliminary data also exist for 5HT$_{1A}$ receptor imaging, and "peripheral benzodiazepine receptor" ligands may be of value in patients suspected of having inflammation as part of the pathophysiologic process underlying their seizure disorder. Indeed, many of the PET ligands reviewed in this chapter have not been adequately evaluated for their potential roles in the localization of epileptic foci, and many more studies could be performed with currently available ligands for clinical translation.

PET receptor imaging is particularly suited to forging links between clinical and preclinical investigations, and with the use of microPET scanners, receptor imaging studies also have great potential in advancing our knowledge of the basic mechanisms of epilepsy. Finally, a major role of receptor imaging is to help elucidate mechanisms of comorbidities, such as depression, in epileptic patients.

REFERENCES

Banati, R. B., G. W. Goerres; R. Myers, et al. 1999. [11C] (R)-PK11195 positron emission tomography imaging of activated microglia in vivo in Rasmussen's encephalitis. *Neurology* 53: 2199–203.

Bartenstein, P. A., J. S. Duncan, M. C. Prevett, et al. 1993. Investigation of the opioid system in absence seizures with positron emission tomography. *Journal of Neurology Neurosurgery & Psychiatry* 56(12): 1295–302.

Bartenstein, P. A., M. C. Prevett, J. S. Duncan, et al. 1994. Quantification of opiate receptors in two patients with mesiobasal temporal lobe epilepsy, before and after selective amygdalohippocampectomy, using positron emission tomography. *Epilepsy Research* 18: 119–25.

Bergström, M., E. Kumlien, A. Lilja, et al. 1998. Temporal lobe epilepsy visualized with PET with 11C-L-deuterium-deprenyl—analysis of kinetic data. *Acta Neurologica Scandinavica* 98: 224–31.

Bien, C. G., H. Urbach, J. Schramm, et al. 2007. Limbic encephalitis as a precipitating event in adult-onset temporal lobe epilepsy. *Neurology* 69(12): 1236–44.

Biraben, A., F. Semah, M. J. Ribeiro. 2004. PET evidence for a role of the basal ganglia in patients with ring chromosome 20 epilepsy. *Neurology* 63: 73–7.

Bouilleret, V., F. Semah, A. Biraben, et al. 2005. Involvement of the basal ganglia in refractory epilepsy: an 18F-fluoro-L-DOPA PET study using 2 methods of analysis. *Journal of Nuclear Medicine* 46: 540–7.

Brown, A. K., Y. Kimura Y, S. S. Zoghbi, et al. 2008. Metabotropic glutamate subtype 5 receptors are quantified in the human brain with a novel radioligand for PET. *Journal of Nuclear Medicine* 49(12): 2042–8.

Buck, A., L. D. Frey, P. Bläuenstein, et al. 1998. Monoamine oxidase B single-photon emission tomography with [123I]Ro 43-0463: imaging in volunteers and patients with temporal lobe epilepsy. *European Journal of Nuclear Medicine* 25(5): 464–70.

Derry, C., C. Benjamin, P. Bladin, et al. 2006. Increased serotonin receptor availability in human sleep: evidence from an [18F]MPPF PET study in narcolepsy. *Neuroimage* 30(2): 341–8.

Didelot, A., P. Ryvlin, A. Lothe, et al. 2008. PET imaging of brain 5-HT1A receptors in the preoperative evaluation of temporal lobe epilepsy. *Brain* 131(Pt 10): 2751–64.

Drevets, W. C., E. Frank, J. C. Price, et al. 1999. PET imaging of serotonin 1A receptor binding in depression. *Biological Psychiatry* 46: 1375–87.

Drevets, W. C., M. E. Thase, E. L. Moses-Kolko, et al. 2007. Serotonin-1A receptor imaging in recurrent depression: replication and literature review. *Nuclear Medicine Biology* 34: 865–77.

Fedi, M., S. F. Berkovic, I. E. Scheffer, et al. 2008. Reduced striatal D1 receptor binding in autosomal dominant nocturnal frontal lobe epilepsy. *Neurology* 71(11): 795–8.

Friston, K. J., C. D. Frith, P. F. Liddle, et al. 1991. Comparing functional (PET) images: the assessment of significant change. *Journal of Cerebral Blood Flow Metabolism* 11: 690–9.

Frost, J. J., H. S. Mayberg, R. S. Fisher, et al. 1988. Mu-opiate receptors measured by positron emission tomography are increased in temporal lobe epilepsy. *Annals of Neurology* 23: 231–7.

Goerres, G. W., T. Revesz, J. Duncan, et al. 2001. Imaging cerebral vasculitis in refractory epilepsy using [11C](R)-PK11195 positron emission tomography. *AJR Am J Roentgenol* 176: 1016–8.

Giovacchini, G., M. T. Toczek, R. Bonwetsch, et al. 2005. 5-HT 1A receptors are reduced in temporal lobe epilepsy after partial-volume correction. *Journal of Nuclear Medicine* 46: 1128–35.

Goffin, K., G. Bormans, C. Casteels, et al. 2008. An in vivo [18F]MK-9470 microPET study of type 1 cannabinoid receptor binding in Wistar rats after chronic administration of valproate and levetiracetam. *Neuropharmacology* 54(7): 1103–6.

Hammers, A., M. C. Asselin, R. Hinz, et al. 2007. Upregulation of opioid receptor binding following spontaneous epileptic seizures. *Brain* 130(Pt 4): 1009–16.

Hasler, G., R. Bonwetsch, G. Giovacchini, et al. 2007. 5-HT1A receptor binding in temporal lobe epilepsy patients with and without major depression. *Biological Psychiatry* 62: 1258–64.

Iinuma, K., H. Yokoyama, T. Otsuki, et al. 1993. Histamine H1 receptors in complex partial seizures. *Lancet* 341: 238.

Koepp, M. J., M. P. Richardson, D. J. Brooks, et al. 1998. Focal cortical release of endogenous opioids during reading-induced seizures. *Lancet* 352: 952–5.

Kumar, A., H. T. Chugani, A. Luat, et al. 2008. Epilepsy surgery in a case of encephalitis: use of 11C-PK11195 positron emission tomography. *Pediatric Neurology* 38(6): 439–42.

Kumlien, E., P. Hilton-Brown, B. Spännare, et al. 1992. In vitro quantitative autoradiography of (3H)-L-deprenyl and (3H)-PK 11195 binding sites in human epileptic hippocampus. *Epilepsia* 1992;33: 610–17.

Kumlien, E., M. Bergström, A. Lilja, et al. 1995. Positron emission tomography with [11C]deuterium-deprenyl in temporal lobe epilepsy. *Epilepsia* 36: 712–21.

Kumlien, E., P. Hartvig, S. Valind, et al. 1999. NMDA-receptor activity visualized with (S)-[N-methyl-11C]ketamine and positron emission tomography in patients with medial temporal lobe epilepsy. *Epilepsia* 40(1): 30–7.

Kumlien, E., A. Nilsson, G. Hagberg, et al. 2001. PET with 11C-deuterium-deprenyl and 18F-FDG in focal epilepsy. *Acta Neurologica Scandinavica* 103(6): 360–6.

Langer, O., B. Bauer, A. Hammers, et al. 2007. Pharmacoresistance in epilepsy: a pilot PET study with the p-glycoprotein substrate R-[11C]verapamil. *Epilepsia* 48: 1774–84.

Liew, C. J., Y. M. Lim, R. Bonwetsch, et al. 2009. 18F-FCWAY and 18F-FDG PET in MRI-negative temporal lobe epilepsy. *Epilepsia* 50(2): 234–9.

Lothe, A., A. Didelot, A. Hammers, et al. 2008. Comorbidity between temporal lobe epilepsy and depression: a [18F]MPPF PET study. *Brain* 131(Pt 10): 2765–82.

Madar, I., R. P. Lesser, G. Krauss, et al. 1997. Imaging of delta- and mu-opioid receptors in temporal lobe epilepsy by positron emission tomography. *Annals of Neurology* 41: 358–67.

Mayberg, H. S., B. Sadzot, C. C. Meltzer, et al. 1991. Quantification of mu and non-mu opiate receptors in temporal lobe epilepsy using positron emission tomography. *Annals of Neurology* 30: 3–11.

Merlet, I., K. Ostrowsky, N. Costes, et al. 2004a. 5-HT1A receptor binding and intracerebral activity in temporal lobe epilepsy: an [18F]MPPF-PET study. *Brain* 127: 900–13.

Merlet, I., P. Ryvlin, N. Costes, et al. 2004b. Statistical parametric mapping of 5-HT1A receptor binding in temporal lobe epilepsy with hippocampal ictal onset on intracranial EEG. *Neuroimage* 22(2): 886–96.

Meschaks, A., P. Lindstrom, C. Halldin, et al. 2005. Regional reductions in serotonin 1A receptor binding in juvenile myoclonic epilepsy. *Archives of Neurology* 62: 946–50.

Muller-Gartner, H. W., J. M. Links, J. L. Prince, et al. 1992. Measurement of radiotracer concentration in brain gray matter using positron emission tomography: MRI-based correction for partial volume effects. *Journal of Cerebral Blood Flow Metabolism* 12: 571–83.

Picard, F., D. Bruel, D. Servent, et al. 2006. Alteration of the in vivo nicotinic receptor density in ADNFLE patients: a PET study. *Brain* 129: 2047–60.

Prevett, M. C., V. J. Cunningham, D. J. Brooks, et al. 1994. Opiate receptors in idiopathic generalised epilepsy measured with [11C]diprenorphine and positron emission tomography. *Epilepsy Research* 19: 71–7.

Sanchez-Pernaute, R., J. Q. Wang, D. Kuruppu, et al. 2008. Enhanced binding of metabotropic glutamate receptor type 5 (mGluR5) PET tracers in the brain of parkinsonian primates. *Neuroimage* 42(1): 248–51.

Sargent, P. A., K. H. Kjaer, C. J. Bench, et al. 2000. Brain serotonin1A receptor binding measured by positron emission tomography with [11C]WAY-100635: effects of depression and antidepressant treatment. *Archives of General Psychiatry* 57: 174–180.

Sauvageau, Anny, Paul Desjardins, Violina Lozeva, et al. 2002. Increased expression of "peripheral-type" benzodiazepine receptors in human temporal lobe epilepsy: implications for PET imaging of hippocampal sclerosis. *Metabolic Brain Disease* 17(1): 3–11.

Savic, I., P. Lindstrom, B. Gulyas, et al. 2004. Limbic reductions of 5-HT1A receptor binding in human temporal lobe epilepsy. *Neurology* 62: 1343–51.

Theodore, W. H., R. E. Carson, P. Andreasen, et al. 1992. PET imaging of opiate receptor binding in human epilepsy using [18F]cyclofoxy. *Epilepsy Research* 13: 129–39.

Theodore, W. H., D. Leiderman, W. D. Gaillard, et al. 1993. The effect of naloxone on cerebral blood flow and glucose metabolism in patients with complex partial seizures. *Epilepsy Research* 16(5): 1–54.

Theodore, W. H., G. Giovacchini, R. Bonwetsch, et al. 2006. The effect of antiepileptic drugs on 5-HT1A receptor binding measured by positron emission tomography. *Epilepsia* 47: 499–503.

Theodore, W. H., G. Hasler, G. Giovacchini, et al. 2007. Reduced hippocampal 5HT1A PET receptor binding and depression in temporal lobe epilepsy. *Epilepsia* 48: 1526–30.

Theodore, W. H., L. Epstein, W. D. Gaillard, et al. 2008. Human herpes virus 6B: a possible role in epilepsy? *Epilepsia* 49(11): 1828–37.

Toczek, M. T., R. E. Carson, L. Lang, et al. 2003. PET imaging of 5-HT1A receptor binding in patients with temporal lobe epilepsy. *Neurology* 60: 749–56.

Vezzani, A., and T. Granata. 2005. Brain inflammation in epilepsy: experimental and clinical evidence. *Epilepsia* 46(11): 1724–43.

Werhahn, K. J., C. Landvogt, S. Klimpe, et al. 2006. Decreased dopamine D2/D3-receptor binding in temporal lobe epilepsy: an [18F]fallypride PET study. *Epilepsia* 47(8): 1392–6.

Zimmer, L., G. Mauger, D. Le Bars, et al. 2002. Effect of endogenous serotonin on the binding of the 5-hT1A PET ligand 18F-MPPF in the rat hippocampus: kinetic beta measurements combined with microdialysis. *Journal of Neurochemistry* 80: 278–86.

Chapter 14

SPECT SCANNING FOR EPILEPTIC SEIZURES

R. Edward Hogan, Elson L. So, and Terence J. O'Brien

There are numerous useful electrophysiologic and imaging tests that localize the area of seizure onset (epileptogenic zone) in patients with refractory partial epilepsy. Traditionally, scalp and invasive electroencephalography (EEG) were the standard for localization of the epileptogenic zone. However, recent advances in neuroimaging have enabled measurement of brain function during the ictal state. Notably, ictal single photon emission computed tomography (SPECT) allows measurement of brain perfusion patterns during seizures, which is useful for localizing regional blood flow changes in the epileptogenic zone in patients with partial epilepsy (Norden and Blumenfeld 2002; Rowe et al. 1991a).

HISTORY OF CEREBRAL BLOOD FLOW AND SEIZURES

There is a long history of the association of increased cerebral blood flow during epileptic seizures. Sir Victor Horsley first reported that partial seizures were associated with a focal, transient increase in blood flow in the region of the seizure focus (Horsley 1892). Throughout his career, Wilder Penfield had an interest in cerebral blood flow changes during seizures (Penfield 1933, 1971). Early in his career he attempted to improve seizure control by effecting cerebrovascular regulation changes through cervical or dorsal sympathectomy (Penfield 1933). In his later work, he noted striking vascular changes during observation of the exposed cerebral cortex during neurosurgical procedures, which he summarized in three stages: (1) dilation of the capillary bed, (2) cortical anemia, and (3) spasmodic closure of large arteries (Penfield 1933). Correlating observed operative blood flow changes with intraoperative electrocorticographic recordings, he commented: "Visible pulsation of the cortex disappears at the onset of a seizure. Careful observation makes this almost as reliable an evidence of fit onset as the electrocorticogram. This means, I suppose, . . . (there is) immediate increase in blood flow. This increase occurred in the area of cortex where epileptogenic discharge was taking place, not in the cortex at a distance. As the discharge spreads, the blood flow acceleration spreads with it" (Penfield 1971). Subsequent investigators have confirmed the close association of increased cerebral blood flow associated with epileptic seizures, both in humans and animal models (Dymond and Crandall 1976; Gibbs et al. 1934; Plum et al. 1968; Schridde et al. 2008).

RADIOPHARMACEUTICALS FOR SPECT SCANNING IN EPILEPSY

While there is a long history of the association of localized blood flow changes during epileptic seizures, the recent development of modern SPECT techniques to measure cerebral perfusion changes during seizures has enabled measurement of ictal cerebral blood flow changes in a clinical setting. Important in the application of SPECT imaging for seizures was the development of radiopharmaceuticals for SPECT scans that could be administered during the peri-ictal state.

The ideal agent for brain ictal SPECT imaging would have the following characteristics:

1. Stability for hours in vitro so that it can be stored near the patient for immediate intravenous injection as soon as it is recognized that the patient is having a seizure
2. A rapid brain uptake across the blood–brain barrier that is linearly proportional to blood flow at all physiologic and pathologic blood flow rates, and minimal back-diffusion after uptake, ensuring that the relative concentration of radiopharmaceutical will closely reflect the relative regional cerebral blood flow
3. Minimal extracerebral uptake and a rapid blood clearance, to maximize brain to background contrast (O'Brien 2000)

While no available radiopharmaceutical fulfills all the above criteria, modern radiopharmaceuticals are suitable for ictal SPECT studies. Earlier agents, such as Xenon 133 and ^{123}I-based radiopharmaceuticals, are not typically used due to issues with preparation or administration of the agents. The commonly used agents for clinical ictal SPECT are ^{99m}Tc-hexamethylpropylene amine oxime (Tc-HMPAO) and ^{99m}Tc-bicisate (Tc-ECD) (O'Brien 2000). Comparison of these agents shows that Tc-HMPAO and Tc-ECD share similar pharmacokinetic profiles for brain uptake, with the major pharmacokinetic difference between the agents being a proportionally greater amount of extracerebral uptake with Tc-HMPAO.

For Tc-HMPAO, the majority of brain uptake (3.6% to 7% of the injected dose) occurs within 1 minute of the injection (O'Brien 2000), with final, stable maximal uptake occurring at 2 minutes (Leveille et al. 1992). Tc-ECD displays similar pharmacokinetic profiles for brain uptake after intravenous injection (Leveille et al. 1992). Both Tc-HMPAO and Tc-ECD are irreversibly converted from lipophilic to hydrophilic compounds after they cross the blood–brain barrier, allowing very little back-diffusion after initial brain uptake of the agents (O'Brien 2000). Both radiopharmaceuticals show a net brain washout of less than 5% during the first 20 minutes after drug administration. However, during the same initial 20-minute period, 99mTc-ECD images of the head show significantly less background facial uptake and retention than 99mTc-HMPAO images (Leveille et al. 1992). Quantitative region-of-interest analysis of SPECT

images confirms that cortical-to-extracerebral uptake ratios are better with Tc-ECD (O'Brien et al. 1999a). Despite some relative differences in pharmacokinetic profiles of Tc-HMPAO and Tc-ECD, comparative studies using either Tc-HMPAO or Tc-ECD for ictal SPECT studies show no significant differences between the radiotracer groups in the sensitivity or specificity of seizure localization when studies are matched for time of injection in relationship to the associated ictal (or postictal) state (O'Brien et al. 1999a).

Important in conceptual understanding of the pharmacokinetic profiles of the radiopharmaceutical agents is the temporal uptake of the agents in the brain relative to blood flow changes induced by seizures. The time resolution of ictal perfusion SPECT uptake, which as outlined above roughly gives an average "snapshot" of brain perfusion changes over approximately 1 minute, is relatively long compared to seizure onset, propagation, and evolution. Electrographic onset and propagation of epileptic seizures often occurs over seconds, thus evolving over a shorter time period than measured by radiopharmaceutical uptake for ictal SPECT, and therefore some ictal SPECT studies will show patterns of seizure propagation (Kaiboriboon et al. 2002; Van Paesschen et al. 2007). Overall, ictal SPECT is very useful in localization of the epileptogenic zone in partial epileptic seizures. However, due to the relatively long uptake of radiopharmaceutical uptake, careful attention to the association of administration of the radiopharmaceutical agent in respect to seizure onset, propagation, and duration is very important in final interpretation of ictal SPECT results (Hogan et al. 1999; Spanaki et al. 1999; Stefan et al. 1990).

SPECT IN TEMPORAL LOBE EPILEPSY

Early in the course of the investigation of temporal lobe epilepsy (TLE) with SPECT, investigators reported false lateralization of interictal SPECT (Newton et al. 1995; Rowe et al. 1991a, 1991b) (Table 14.1). In addition, interictal SPECT localization is more difficult in patients with extratemporal epilepsy (Ho et al. 1994; Marks et al. 1992; Newton et al. 1995). Therefore, the current

Table 14.1 SPECT Lateralization

	Interictal (n = 119)	*Postictal* (n = 77)	*Ictal* (n = 51)
Correct	48	71	97
Inconclusive	42	25	3
Incorrect	10	4	0

From M. R. Newton, S. F. Berkovic, M. C. Austin, et al. 1995. SPECT in the localisation of extratemporal and temporal seizure foci. *Journal of Neurology Neurosurgery & Psychiatry* 59: 26–30.

role of interictal SPECT is primarily for comparison with ictal SPECT studies.

Important early studies in patients with TLE showed the usefulness of ictal SPECT in localization of epileptic seizures (Rowe et al. 1989). Ictal SPECT perfusion patterns during temporal lobe seizures, when compared with ictal EEG onset of seizures, show good correlation with lateralization of seizure onset. Typical patterns of perfusion show hyperperfusion in the entire anterior temporal lobe during ictal SPECT injections. The image of cerebral blood flow after temporal lobe seizures shows two distinct components: ongoing hyperperfusion in the anteromesial temporal lobe, and hypoperfusion in the lateral cortex, both on the side of the ictal EEG onset of seizures. Postictal perfusion changes evolve relatively rapidly after seizures, with hyperperfusion of the anteromesial temporal region typically resolving within the first few postictal minutes, while hypoperfusion of adjacent lateral cortex may persist for up to 10 to 20 minutes (Rowe et al. 1991a). Figure 14.1 shows the typical evolution of patterns in peri-ictal blood flow in TLE (Rowe et al. 1991a). Because of relatively rapid changes in cerebral blood flow in the postictal state,

localization of temporal lobe seizures is enhanced by earlier ictal injection of the radiopharmaceutical agent, as suggested by early investigation of ictal SPECT studies (Rowe et al. 1991a) and confirmed by subsequent quantitative SPECT studies (Newton et al. 1995; O'Brien et al. 1999b). Table 14.1 shows percentage lateralization accuracy of epileptic foci using interictal, postictal, and ictal SPECT in 119 cases of unilateral TLE (Newton et al. 1995).

The co-registration of ictal SPECT studies with MRI can help in their interpretation. The images in Figure 14.2 show typical perfusion changes in the posterior, mid-portion, and anterior temporal lobe.

DIFFERENTIAL SPECT PERFUSION PATTERNS IN TLE

Ictal SPECT shows distinct patterns of cerebral perfusion in subtypes of TLE (Ho et al. 1996). Patients with mesial temporal foci show ipsilateral hyperperfusion involving predominantly the mesial and lateral temporal regions. In subjects with lateral temporal foci, hyperperfusion is frequently bilateral in the temporal lobes, with predominant changes in the region of the lesion.

Ictal SPECT in patients with normal temporal lobe pathology and a good surgical outcome shows a pattern of hyperperfusion largely restricted to the ipsilateral anteromesial temporal region. Neuroanatomical connections of the temporal lobe may help explain these SPECT findings. The mesial temporal structures project to all major divisions of the ipsilateral temporal neocortex, with the most prominent projections ending in the cortex of the temporal pole and the rostral superior temporal gyrus, explaining the medial temporal perfusion pattern. The amygdala receives anterior commissural fibers from the contralateral temporal neocortex, although not from the contralateral amygdala; therefore, anterior commissure may be a potential major seizure-propagation pathway that can explain the bilateral temporal lobe hyperperfusion changes seen in seizures of lateral temporal origin (Ho et al. 1996).

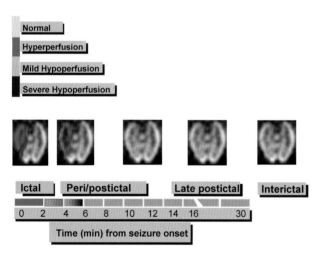

Figure 14.1 Typical perfusion changes during temporal lobe seizures. Changes are projected over the right temporal region. During the ictal state, there is temporal hyperperfusion, with surrounding severe hypoperfusion. In the peri-ictal/postictal state, there is a "postictal switch" during which there is severe hypoperfusion throughout the temporal lobe, with the exception of persistent hyperperfusion in the mesial temporal region. As the postictal state progresses, there is gradual progression to more mild hypoperfusion, which is more diffuse in the temporal lobe in the later postictal period. These changes eventually evolve to the typical interictal pattern of hypoperfusion in the anterior temporal lobe. (Adapted from C. C. Rowe, S. F. Berkovic, M. C. Austin, et al. 1991a. Patterns of postictal cerebral blood flow in temporal lobe epilepsy: qualitative and quantitative analysis. *Neurology* 41: 1096–103.)

SPECT IN EXTRATEMPORAL LOBE EPILEPSY

Successful epilepsy surgery is more elusive in extratemporal lobe epilepsy (ETLE) than in TLE. The surgical epileptogenic zone is often more difficult to localize precisely, particularly in the absence of an associated structural brain abnormality. Overall, the outcome after ETLE surgery is significantly poorer than after TLE surgery. Approximately two thirds of patients are

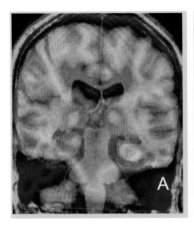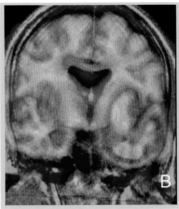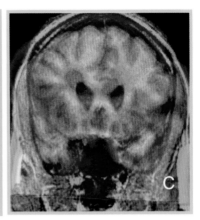

Figure 14.2 Images of a single ictal SPECT scan, obtained during a left mesial temporal seizure, co-registered to the patient's MRI. The "rainbow" color scale shows regions of "cooler" colors (purple and blue) representing areas of relative hypoperfusion, with "warmer" colors showing regions of relative hyperperfusion. The white regions show the areas of greatest hyperperfusion. (A) Coronal section through the posterior temporal lobe, with associated hyperperfusion in the left mesial temporal region and bilateral thalami. (B) Coronal section through the amygdalo-hippocampal complex with hyperperfusion throughout the temporal lobe and basal ganglia. (C) Section through the temporal tip, showing hyperperfusion in the most anterior temporal region.

free of disabling seizures after surgery for TLE, with 11% to 15% of subjects showing no change in seizure frequency. By contrast, in selected well-localized ETLE, 50% of subjects will be rendered free of disabling seizures after surgery, while 21% will show no improvement in seizure frequency (Engel Jr. et al. 2003). Application of ictal SPECT in ETLE plays an important role in localizing seizures for epilepsy surgery. Accurate methods are required to identify the site and the extent of the surgical epileptogenic zone in ETLE to optimize surgical outcome.

Extratemporal seizures are often brief, hypermotor, and nocturnal, making ictal injection more difficult. Often, ictal or interictal scalp EEG findings are poorly localizing, and the ictal EEG discharge tends to spread quickly (Quesney 1991), which results in a less focal and sustained increase in regional cerebral blood flow. However, studies show that ictal SPECT plays a useful role in the evaluation of ETLE.

Initial studies of ictal SPECT showed that subjects with ETLE, as would be predicted by the shorter duration and rapid propagation of ETLE seizures, require earlier ictal injection for seizure localization as compared to TLE seizures. In past comparisons of subjects with similar delays in radiopharmaceutical injection, the diagnostic yield of SPECT in patients with ETLE was much lower than in TLE subjects (Newton et al. 1995). This suggests that postictal perfusion patterns in temporal lobe seizures and in seizures of extratemporal origin evolve at different rates. Therefore, it is likely that the sequence of ictal to postictal changes in regional cortical perfusion, referred to as the "postictal switch" of perfusion, in ETLE seizures evolves over a much shorter time frame than in temporal lobe

seizures (Avery et al. 1999; O'Brien et al. 1999b). In addition, comparison of ictal SPECT studies shows that the topography of cortical blood flow distribution after ETLE seizures seemed to differ from that of temporal lobe seizures. The examples of postictal hypoperfusion shown by SPECT in ETLE seizures were restricted to the immediate region of the seizure focus. In comparison, temporal lobe seizures are usually followed by the characteristic widespread ipsilateral cortical depression of blood flow, often sparing the mesial temporal region. These early observations about temporal and extratemporal ictal perfusion patterns, which likely reflect variations in the underlying physiology of regional cortical blood flow that accompany seizures arising from different sites, have important implications for the use of SPECT and the underlying pathophysiology of global brain changes and consciousness during epileptic seizures (Blumenfeld and Taylor 2003). In a study of 89 patients with neocortical epilepsy and normal MRI, Lee et al. (2005) demonstrated localization of 41.1% with ictal SPECT. However, in a subset of 56 patients with seizure-free outcome after epilepsy surgery, the association of localized ictal SPECT with seizure freedom postoperatively was not statistically significant (Lee et al. 2005). While other studies, especially those that apply subtraction SPECT techniques (O'Brien et al. 2000), show that ictal SPECT can be useful in ETLE, the lower yield of diagnostic information from late injection or postictal SPECT in suspected ETLE seizures stresses the importance of injecting the radiopharmaceutical as soon as possible during the seizure to facilitate the interpretation of ictal hyperperfusion.

SUBTRACTION ICTAL SPECT

Initial methods of ictal–interictal SPECT comparison included visual evaluation of perfusion changes between ictal and interictal scans to determine the region of ictal hyperperfusion. However, visual interpretation is complicated by lack of normalization of ictal and interictal studies, differences in quantities of injected radiopharmaceutical, inability to accurately compare concordant matched slices, and the relatively poor spatial resolution of SPECT (Zubal et al. 1995). Also, due to the underlying epileptogenic process or an associated structural lesion (which is commonly associated with chronic epileptic seizures [Jack Jr. 1993]), there is often associated hypoperfusion on interictal SPECT scans, which further confounds the interpretation of perfusion differences between ictal and interictal SPECT scans. Occasionally, ictal SPECT studies may show "normalization," where a region of the brain that shows interictal hyperperfusion appears to show symmetrical perfusion during the ictal state. Figure 14.3 illustrates ictal and interictal SPECT studies in a patient with right TLE. In the interictal image there is right temporal hyperperfusion. In the ictal image there is relatively symmetrical perfusion within the temporal lobes, with associated cerebellar diaschisis. Interpretation of the ictal SPECT study alone would be difficult.

While initial studies using ictal SPECT showed good lateralization of TLE seizures, most of those studies investigated cases with TLE foci that were well localized using interictal scalp EEG, ictal video-EEG, or MRI (O'Brien et al. 1998b). For techniques such as ictal SPECT to have an important role in the evaluation of partial epilepsy patients, it should provide localizing information beyond what is provided by more standard tests. This is particularly important in patients with ETLE, or with poorly localized seizures, where localization of epileptic seizures is inadequate to proceed with surgery. Computer-aided subtraction of the interictal from the ictal SPECT images addresses the difficulties of visual interpretation of ictal and interictal SPECT scans, allows more definitive localization of localized regions of hyperperfusion during epileptic seizures, and assists in localization of seizures in subjects where other tests do not show definitive localization (O'Brien et al. 1998b).

Zubal et al. published the first series of ictal–interictal subtraction SPECT studies in epilepsy (1995) and outlined one of the initial techniques for performing ictal–interictal subtraction. Many subsequent studies have described different techniques of computer-aided ictal–interictal SPECT subtraction (Barber et al. 1995; Brinkmann et al. 1999; Chang et al. 2002; Lee et al. 2000; McNally et al. 2005) and co-registration of SPECT to MRI (Hogan et al. 1996; Turkington et al. 1993). O'Brien et al. (1998a) described SPECT-to-SPECT co-registration using brain surface matching and validated the accuracy of this technique in a phantom model and in partial epilepsy patients. The SPECT-to-SPECT co-registration was shown to produce accurate and reliable results, with the worst errors being considerably less than one voxel diameter and the resolution of the imaging system (O'Brien et al. 1998a).

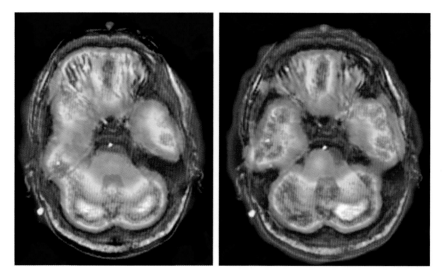

Figure 14.3 Example of ictal "normalization" of a region of hypoperfusion in the right temporal lobe. The SPECT images are co-registered to the MRI, with color scale as described in Figure 14.2. (Left) Interictal study with right temporal hypoperfusion. (Right) Ictal study acquired during a right temporal seizure. On the ictal SPECT study, there is apparent symmetrical perfusion of the temporal regions. However, there is also associated cerebellar diaschisis, with hyperperfusion of the contralateral (left) cerebellum, during the ictal SPECT study.

The method of subtraction ictal SPECT co-registered to MRI (SISCOM) (O'Brien et al. 1998a) has been extensively evaluated, comparing results of visual inspection of ictal and interictal studies. In a study of 51 consecutive intractable partial epilepsy patients who had interictal and ictal scans, SPECT studies were blindly reviewed and classified as either localizing to 1 of 16 sites in the brain or as non-localizing. SISCOM images were localizing in 45 of 51 (88.2%) compared with 20 of 51 (39.2%) for traditional visual inspection of ictal and interictal SPECT images ($p < 0.0001$). Inter-rater agreement for two independent reviewers was better for SISCOM. Concordance of seizure localization with the more established tests for localizing epileptic seizures was also higher for SISCOM (O'Brien et al. 1998b). Figure 14.4 shows ictal and interictal SPECT studies, with an associated SISCOM image. The use of quantitative methods such as SISCOM has enabled more precise investigation of perfusion changes in relationship to the time of radiotracer injection in respect to seizure onset, surgical outcomes after epilepsy surgery, and timing of postictal hypoperfusion changes after epileptic seizures.

SUBTRACTION ICTAL SPECT IN ETLE

SISCOM has advantages of improving surgical localization in ETLE patients with complex and intractable epilepsy, particularly if the methods are used with stereotactic image-guided surgical techniques (O'Brien et al. 2000). In a SISCOM study of 36 extratemporal lobe epilepsy patients, O'Brien et al. (2000) showed 24 patients (66.7%) had localizing SISCOM, including 13 (76.5%) of those without a focal MRI lesion. Subjects with localizing SISCOM concordant with the surgical site, compared with non-localizing or non-concordant SISCOM, had a statistically significant improvement in excellent outcome. SISCOM findings were predictive of postsurgical outcome, independently of MRI or scalp ictal EEG findings. The extent of resection of the cortical region of the SISCOM focus was significantly associated with the rate of excellent outcome (100% with complete resection, 60% with partial resection, and 20% with nonresection).

A study by Knowlton et al. (2008) using logistical regression analysis to control for similar covariates of MRI and scalp EEG classification of epilepsy localization showed a statistically significant ratio for prediction of Engel stage 1 surgical outcome with subtraction ictal SPECT, similar to the results of O'Brien et al. (2000) Sensitivity of SISCOM in their study was 62%, compared with 31% for magnetic source imaging and 54% for PET. Specificity was 86% for either SISCOM or PET, and 79% for magnetic source imaging.

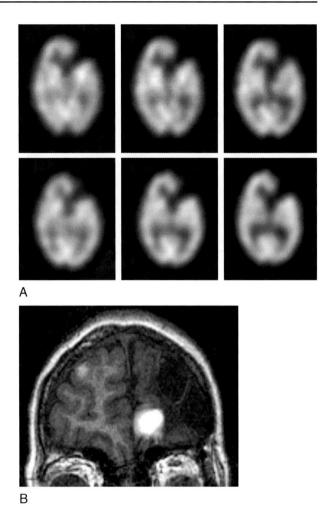

Figure 14.4 (A) Interictal (top row) and ictal (bottom row) SPECT studies in a patient with frontal lobe epilepsy. (B) SISCOM image with a region of hyperperfusion in the left basal frontal region. This example illustrates the difficulty of interpreting perfusion changes using visual comparison of ictal and interictal images, especially when there is a structural lesion affecting perfusion and the region of hyperperfusion is at the margin of the structural lesion.

EARLY INJECTION OF RADIOTRACER

The importance of prompt injection of SPECT radiopharmaceuticals after seizure onset cannot be overemphasized. As has been discussed, late radiotracer injection increases the probability of non-localizing or falsely localizing results (O'Brien et al. 1998b). Also, postictal radiotracer injection is more likely to be associated with the finding of regional hypoperfusion changes, which are usually more widespread than hyperperfusion changes (O'Brien et al. 1999b). Several strategies can be used to enhance the opportunity of early ictal SPECT injection. Patients, families, and caregivers should be counseled on being vigilant for symptoms or signs of seizure onset and should be aware of the importance of early ictal injection of the radiotracer. Patients should be situated in rooms closest to the station where staff responsible for the injection is located. The path between the station and the patient's room should be clear, and nonessential traffic in the area should be restricted. The seizure alarm triggered by patient and family should include a flashing light by the door of the room.

Staff should be experienced in recognizing early clinical and EEG seizure activity. They should preferably be gloved and ready to grab the radiopharmaceutical as soon as seizure activity is detected. Intravenous access of the patient should be ensured by frequent scheduled checks of its patency. It also helps to postpone the injection until a sufficient number of seizures have been recorded to familiarize staff with the features of seizure onset in the particular patient, and also to increase the likelihood that more seizures are soon to follow. When seizures are very frequent or are likely to occur at a particular time in the day or night, staff could wait by the patient's bed to conduct radiotracer injection very soon after seizure onset. If patient's habitual seizures typically occur during sleep, sleep could be limited at night and encouraged in the daytime, when more staff is available to conduct the radiotracer injection and subsequent imaging.

Automated injection systems triggered by EEG seizure activity, or by patient or staff, have been described (Feichtinger et al. 2007; Sepkuty et al. 1998), but they need further evaluation to determine the degree of safety to the patient and persons in the room. Injection with the use of these systems should also be triggered by several indicators, rather than a single indicator, of seizure activity. It should also have the capability of being overridden, in order to reduce the chance of injection following false alarms.

SISCOM IN THE POSTICTAL STATE

As discussed previously, early investigators commented on conversion of hyperperfusion to hypoperfusion after temporal lobe seizures, and on patterns of postictal switch of perfusion as measured by SPECT (Newton et al. 1995; Rowe et al. 1991a). SISCOM studies can show regions of significant hypoperfusion as well as hyperperfusion, and thus can define trends of postictal perfusion changes. To determine patterns of hyperperfusion and hypoperfusion after seizures, 35 subjects with intractable partial epileptic seizures who had postictal SPECT injections were assessed using SISCOM (O'Brien et al. 1999b). Whereas the time of radiopharmaceutical injection in patients with hyperperfusion-dominant SISCOM images was earlier than that in patients with hypoperfusion-dominant images, the difference did not reach statistical significance. Importantly, the plot of the timing of postictal radiopharmaceutical

injection showed a wide overlap between the hypoperfusion and hyperperfusion patterns. Hyperperfusion-dominant images were obtained with injections as late as 159 seconds after seizures ended; conversely, hypoperfusion-dominant images occurred even as soon as 2 seconds after radiotracer injection. Normalization of injection timing to the seizure length, therefore taking into account effects of the length of seizures, did not show a significant difference between the two patterns of perfusion. These data strongly suggest that the timing of the postictal switch varies greatly in individual patients.

Due to the variability of perfusion changes among patients, evaluation of both hyperperfusion and hypoperfusion patterns for either ictal or postictal SPECT injection is helpful. Concordance with other modalities of seizure localization is higher for the combined hyperperfusion and hypoperfusion SISCOM evaluation than for either the hyperperfusion or the hypoperfusion SISCOM images alone. This is especially true for postictal SPECT injection, which is associated with focal hyperperfusion changes, rather than hypoperfusion changes, in a third of the patients (O'Brien et al. 1999b). Moreover, ictal SPECT injection occasionally results in focal hypoperfusion changes and not the expected hyperperfusion changes.

FALSE LOCALIZATION AND NON-LOCALIZATION SISCOM

While subtraction ictal SPECT studies often provide additional, useful information for localization of seizures, there are limitations to SPECT studies that make interpretation in the context of other studies extremely important. Whereas localization of seizures is improved with computerized subtraction of images, there is still an important proportion (Kaiboriboon et al. 2002; O'Brien et al. 1998b) (approximately 15% to 25%) of patients who show non-localizing subtraction ictal SPECT findings. Perhaps more importantly, some patients will show false localization with SISCOM; this occurred in 3 of 38 patients in one series (Kaiboriboon et al. 2002).

An important, well-established factor for falsely localizing or non-localizing SISCOM is late (more than 45 seconds postictal) injection of the radiopharmaceutical (O'Brien et al. 1999b). However, occasional subjects with "early" radiopharmaceutical injections may also have falsely localizing or lateralizing findings. This could be related to a number of factors. Because propagation of ictal discharges occurs within seconds in some epileptic seizures, some ictal SPECT studies will show increased perfusion in areas of ictal propagation rather than the primary ictal onset zone (epileptogenic zone) (Van Paesschen et al. 2007). As discussed previously, persistence of postictal hyperperfusion varies greatly between individuals. Conceptually, given the uptake time of radiopharmaceutical agents, which occurs predominantly over 1 minute and continues for over 2 minutes, a proportion of the agent will be taken up by the brain in the postictal period in most seizures. Therefore, rapid resolution of hyperperfusion after a seizure in an individual subject would likely cause variability in the overall SPECT perfusion pattern, and possibly lead to falsely localizing or non-localizing studies. The variability of findings in interictal SPECT studies, which show falsely lateralizing hypoperfusion in approximately 10% of cases (Newton et al. 1995), may also play a role in falsely localizing SISCOM. Findings of occasional false localization with SISCOM stress the need to correlate SISCOM results with other tests for localization of epileptic seizures.

The ictal SPECT study shown in Figure 14.5 is from a 30-year-old patient who presented with a history of complex partial seizures since childhood. His MRI showed significant left hippocampal volume loss, and he had associated ictal events that were stereotypical, with arrested activity, staring, and postictal confusion. He underwent an ictal SPECT study, with an injection occurring 25 seconds after seizure onset. The seizure semiology consisted of passive head turning to the left and right upper extremity dystonic posturing during the ictal SPECT study. Scalp ictal

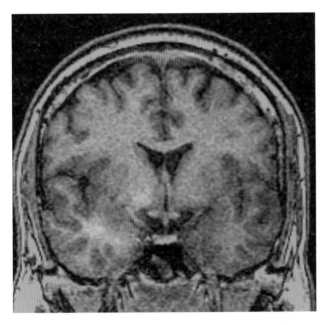

Figure 14.5 SPECT study from a patient with otherwise well-localized seizures to the left temporal lobe, but with right temporal hyperperfusion on SISCOM. SISCOM can be falsely lateralizing and should always be interpreted in the context of other diagnostic tests for localization of seizures.

EEG recording showed left temporal onset of the seizure. He later underwent epilepsy surgery, with a standard left amygdalo-hippocampectomy and anterior temporal lobectomy, with subsequent seizure freedom. Despite this history, the patient showed clear lateralized hyperperfusion of the right temporal lobe with SISCOM. This case represents false lateralization with SISCOM.

RELATIONSHIP OF CEREBRAL BLOOD FLOW AND THE EPILEPTOGENIC ZONE IN PARTIAL EPILEPSY WITH SECONDARILY GENERALIZED TONIC-CLONIC SEIZURES

The underlying pathophysiology of the relationship of region of seizure onset, or epileptogenic zone, and secondarily generalized tonic-clonic seizures is an important issue for many aspects of epileptology. Because some patients will have associated secondarily generalized tonic-clonic seizures during ictal SPECT studies, the relationship of ongoing involvement, and associated perfusion changes, of the epileptogenic region during secondarily generalized tonic seizures is particularly important.

Studies evaluating the localization of subtraction SPECT show that while late injection of the radiopharmaceutical (more than 45 seconds) was associated with false localization or non-localization, secondarily generalized tonic-clonic seizures was not (O'Brien et al. 1999b). This finding suggests that despite secondary generalization of partial seizures, the epileptogenic zone continues to show focal increased perfusion.

To study the patterns of SPECT imaging perfusion changes in secondarily generalized tonic clonic seizures, Blumenfeld et al. (2000a, 2000b) used SPECT imaging in patients with secondarily generalized tonic-clonic seizures induced by electroconvulsive therapy (ECT). During treatment with ECT, subjects underwent either bilateral fronto-temporal stimulation or right unilateral fronto-temporal stimulation for induction of secondarily generalized tonic-clonic seizures. After bilateral fronto-temporal ECT stimulation for seizure induction, subtraction SPECT studies showed hyperperfusion at symmetrical regions of presumed seizure onset in the anterior-inferior frontal and temporal cortex. In comparison, right unilateral ECT stimulation caused an asymmetrical pattern with more extensive hyperperfusion of the right prefrontal cortex and sparing of the left frontal and temporal cortex (Blumenfeld et al. 2003b). In comparing patients who had bifrontal ECT with patients who had bitemporal ECT, bifrontal ECT was found to cause hyperperfusion in prefrontal and anterior cingulate regions. Bitemporal ECT, however, caused hyperperfusion in the lateral frontal cortex and in the anterior temporal lobes (Blumenfeld et al. 2003a). These findings are consistent with the notion that the epileptogenic zone continues to show focal hyperperfusion during secondarily generalized tonic-clonic seizures.

In addition to the finding of hyperperfusion at brain regions near ECT stimulation, there are regions of frontal and parietal association cortex that showed relative hyperperfusion. There are also asymmetries of remote perfusion patterns in subjects with different sites of ECT stimulation for induction of seizures. These findings have important implications, both in the underlying pathophysiology of secondarily generalized tonic-clonic seizures as well as in the interpretation of ictal SPECT findings for localization of seizures. They suggest that certain neuronal networks may be more important than others in secondarily generalized tonic-clonic seizures. The findings also support the concept that "generalization" of seizures is more complex than simple global, homogenous activation of all brain regions.

EVALUATING THE NEED FOR REPEAT EPILEPSY SURGERY

The probability of excellent seizure control following repeat epilepsy surgery is generally more modest than first surgeries (Salanova et al. 2005; Siegel et al. 2004). Moreover, repeat surgeries often require intracranial EEG recordings to delineate the extent of resection to improve seizure outcome and reduce postoperative deficits. Ictal subtraction SPECT has been used to localize seizures that recurred following initial epilepsy surgery. In a study of 58 patients with previous temporal or extratemporal epilepsy surgeries, SISCOM was positive in nearly 80% (Wetjen et al. 2006). Most SISCOM localization (72%) was adjacent or in close proximity to the location of prior resection. Although concordance of SISCOM localization with ictal scalp EEG onset was good (70%), its concordance with intracranial onset was poor (47%). Nonetheless, many non-concordant SISCOM localizations were still close to the intracranial EEG seizure focus. Therefore, SISCOM localization should be used in conjunction with other evidence of seizure localization. It can also serve as a guide for the location and extent of intracranial electrode implantation.

PARAMETRIC MAPPING OF ICTAL SPECT

As outlined previously, past investigators have described ictal hyperperfusion patterns in TLE. Using visual interpretation of large numbers of ictal studies, Rowe et al. (1991a) described hyperperfusion throughout the anterior and mesial temporal region. However, as studies with ictal SPECT progressed with higher-resolution images and broader experience with larger groups of patients, subsequent investigators showed variability in perfusion patterns in some patients with TLE. Investigators described variability with multiple patterns of hyperperfusion changes in the temporal lobe during complex partial seizures of mesial temporal onset (Ho et al. 1996; Wichert-Ana et al. 2001). Such patterns included hyperperfusion throughout the anterior and mesial temporal region (Rowe et al. 1991b) and a predominant lateral as well as posterolateral rather than mesial temporal hyperperfusion (Ho et al. 1997). Furthermore, ictal hyperperfusion of other structures, such as the insular cortex (Shin et al. 2002) and the basal ganglia (Shin et al. 2001; Sojkova et al. 2003), were frequently observed in mesial TLE.

Parametric mapping of groups of subjects with localized epileptic seizures offers the advantage of evaluating common perfusion patterns among subjects with seizures originating from the same region in the brain. There are multiple techniques to statistically average subtraction ictal SPECT images for groups of subjects (Blumenfeld et al. 2004a; Hogan et al. 2004; Tae et al. 2005; Van Paesschen et al. 2003). While the techniques for parametric mapping vary, the general principles of all techniques involve non-linear registration of subtraction SPECT brain images to a common space. After non-linear co-registration to a common space, probabilities and covariance of perfusion changes occurring in specific brain regions can be calculated for the group as a whole. Past techniques have involved comparisons of groups of ictal–interictal subtraction SPECT studies (Hogan et al. 2004), as well as comparing groups of subjects with ictal and interictal SPECT studies with normal control subjects (Tae et al. 2005). These images can provide information for both hyperperfusion and hyperperfusion patterns to objectively define regional perfusion changes in defined epilepsy syndromes.

Using parametric mapping techniques in groups of patients with well-defined mesial TLE due to mesial temporal sclerosis, Van Paesschen et al. (2003) reported ictal hyperperfusion of the temporal lobe ipsilateral to the seizure focus, the border of the ipsilateral middle frontal and precentral gyrus, both occipital lobes, and two small regions in the contralateral postcentral gyrus. There was ictal hypoperfusion in the frontal lobes, contralateral posterior cerebellum, and ipsilateral precuneus. They also found a statistical association between ipsilateral temporal lobe hyperperfusion and ipsilateral frontal lobe hypoperfusion. Because of the significant regions of common hyperperfusion and hypoperfusion, they concluded that the involved structures make up a neuronal network of perfusion changes during complex partial seizures due to mesial temporal sclerosis.

Analyzing a group of subjects with TLE who received postictal SPECT injections, Blumenfeld et al. (2004a) performed parametric analysis of interictal and postictal studies. In patients with complex partial temporal lobe seizures, there was hyperperfusion in the temporal lobe, followed by increases in bilateral midline subcortical structures. They also found marked bilateral hypoperfusion in the frontal and parietal association cortex. In contrast, in subjects with simple partial temporal lobe seizures, there were no associated widespread cerebral blood flow changes in higher-order association cortex. Comparing subjects with complex partial seizures who had 60- to 90-second postictal injections versus those with greater-than-90-second postictal injections also showed differences in perfusion patterns. The maximal region of hyperperfusion in the 60- to 90-second group was the ipsilateral hippocampus, while the greater-than-90-second group showed maximal hyperperfusion in the bilateral hypothalamus. The maximal region of hypoperfusion in the 60- to 90-second group was the contralateral orbitofrontal and ipsilateral precuneus, while the greater-than-90-second group showed maximal hypoperfusion in the contralateral insula.

Using a parametric mapping technique to perform group analysis of SISCOM studies ("composite SISCOM"), Kaiboriboon et al. (2005) analyzed groups of subjects who underwent ictal radiopharmaceutical injection. Composite SISCOM studies in patients with well-localized mesial TLE most commonly showed a region of hyperperfusion in the anterior temporal region, which often also involved the basal ganglia and insula, likely representing the primary regions of seizure propagation. The authors concluded that identifying this pattern of hyperperfusion as typical for mesial temporal onset seizures would assist in clinical interpretation and localization of ictal SPECT studies. Images also showed other regions of hyperperfusion distant from the ipsilateral temporal lobe. These more distant perfusion changes included the orbitofrontal regions and contralateral temporal lobe. Because ictal SPECT studies reflect the location of ictal discharge as measured by simultaneous intracranial EEG (Spanaki et al. 1999), and the orbitofrontal and contralateral temporal lobe are common regions for propagation of mesial temporal lobe seizures (Spencer et al. 1990), it is likely these changes represented patterns of seizure propagation. Figure 14.6 shows a composite

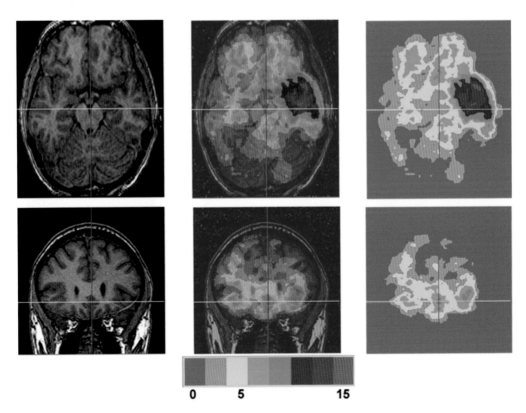

Figure 14.6 Composite SISCOM images were derived from 15 subjects with left mesial TLE. The color scale represents regions of hyperperfusion greater than one standard deviation from all subjects. Using parametric analysis to determine regions of significance (Kaiboriboon et al. 2005), regions colored yellow are the borderline of significant hyperperfusion. In this image the most significant hyperperfusion is in the anterior temporal lobe. However, less commonly hyperperfused but still significant regions of hyperperfusion include the bilateral basal frontal regions, as well as the contralateral temporal lobe, which are common sites of propagation pathways for temporal lobe seizures.

SISCOM combining a group of 15 subjects with left mesial TLE, illustrating temporal hyperperfusion as well as hyperperfusion in the bilateral orbitofrontal regions and contralateral temporal lobe.

Tae et al. (2005) examined cerebral perfusion changes in mesial TLE using statistical parametric mapping of brain SPECT in 38 TLE patients and 19 normal controls. Ictal and interictal SPECT studies were independently compared with control SPECT studies, and ictal–interictal SPECT studies were directly compared as well. The left TLE group showed interictal hypoperfusion in the ipsilateral hippocampus, bilateral thalami, and paracentral lobules. The right TLE group showed interictal hypoperfusion in bilateral hippocampi, contralateral insula, bilateral thalami, and paracentral lobules. Both right and left TLE groups showed ictal hyperperfusion in bilateral temporal lobes with ipsilateral predominance, as well as in the anterior frontal white matter bilaterally. Using statistical comparison, ictal hyperperfusion was found in the ipsilateral temporal lobe, hippocampus, thalamus, putamen, insula, and bilateral precentral gyri, whereas ictal hypoperfusion was found in bilateral frontal poles and middle frontal gyri. The authors propose that their findings indicate ictal activation of a cortico-thalamo-hippocampal-insular network with associated ictal hypoperfusion of the anterior frontal cortex.

In the initial studies using parametric mapping to assess patterns of TLE, to assist with statistical analysis the right temporal scans were rotated so the entire group would show changes on the left side (Blumenfeld et al. 2004a; Van Paesschen et al. 2003). Therefore, there were no conclusions about possible asymmetries between right and left temporal lobe seizures in these studies. Subsequently, comparison of right and left TLE perfusion patterns has shown asymmetries.

In groups of patient with right and left TLE, matched for clinical semiology of seizures, time of ictal SPECT radiopharmaceutical injection, and duration of seizures, Hogan et al. (2006) found similar regions of hyperperfusion change in the ipsilateral anteromedial temporal–corpus striatum–insula region in both groups. In the midbrain reticular formation, there was a significant difference in hyperperfusion between the left and right TLE groups, with the left TLE group showing an approximately 60-fold increased probability of hyperperfusion in the region of the midbrain reticular formation. In addition, the right, but not the left, TLE group showed contralateral hypoperfusion of the temporoparietal junction.

Tae et al. (2005) found, in groups matched for clinical semiology of seizures and timing of SPECT radiopharmaceutical injection, the following regions of ipsilateral hyperperfusion using parametric analysis to compare ictal and interictal SPECT scans. In left TLE seizures, the putamen, thalamus, mammillary body, hippocampus, insula, superior temporal gyrus, temporal white matter, precentral gyrus, and cuneus showed significant hyperperfusion. In right TLE, the anterior nucleus of the thalamus, amygdala, hippocampus, insula, middle temporal gyrus, temporal white matter, and precentral gyrus showed significant hyperperfusion. Tae et al. (2005) found significant ictal midbrain hyperperfusion in both right and left TLE subjects as compared to a group of controls, but not when comparing interictal to ictal scans.

With previous parametric mapping studies of patients with TLE, there are some commonalities and some differences in results. All studies have shown ictal hyperperfusion in the ipsilateral anterior temporal lobe, involving the temporal tip and anterior medial temporal structures. However, involvement of hyperperfusion of other structures has shown variability in different studies. For example, Van Paesschen et al. (2003) reported no associated basal ganglia hyperperfusion in their series of mesial TLE cases. However, Shin et al. (2001) demonstrated that associated ipsilateral basal ganglia hyperperfusion is common in TLE. Kaiboriboon et al. (2005) also found significant hyperperfusion of the ipsilateral basal ganglia during temporal lobe seizures. Regions of hypoperfusion also show similarities among studies, with all studies of TLE showing broad associated regions of hypoperfusion, which typically involve broad regions of the midline structures, as well as regions in the frontal and parietal lobes. However, there are also differences in reported patterns of hypoperfusion. Differences between studies are likely related to multiple factors, including duration of seizures, timing of SPECT injections (which in one study were postictal [Blumenfeld et al. 2004a]), and differences in post-image acquisition processing. However, commonalities of findings of perfusion changes, despite differences in study populations and techniques of parametric mapping, help to delineate patterns of ictal SPECT hyperperfusion and hypoperfusion in TLE, and aid in interpretation of ictal SPECT perfusion findings by establishing common regions of hyperperfusion.

To assess effects of seizure propagation on perfusion patterns in TLE, Kim et al. (2007) explored the relationship between ictal scalp EEG patterns and ictal hyperperfusion patterns in patients with unilateral hippocampal sclerosis-associated mesial TLE by using parametric SPECT analysis. In 39 consecutive subjects, ictal scalp EEG patterns were classified into two different lateralizing patterns: (1) a sustained regular 5- to 9-Hz rhythm with a restricted temporal or subtemporal distribution and (2) an irregular 2- to 5-Hz rhythm with a widespread distribution. Subjects with pattern 1 showed hyperperfusion mainly confined to the ipsilateral temporal lobe, whereas subjects with pattern

2 showed widespread hyperperfusion in the extratemporal structures such as ipsilateral basal ganglia, brain stem, and bilateral thalamus, in addition to the ipsilateral temporal lobe. Clinical characteristics, tracer-injection time, semiology, pathologic hippocampal sclerosis grade, and surgical outcome between two groups showed no significant differences. Among semiologic features, dystonic limb posturing was more frequently observed in subjects with EEG pattern 2. The investigators concluded that scalp ictal EEG patterns in TLE can be an important determining factor of ictal hyperperfusion patterns, and that the lack of difference in surgical outcome between the two groups implied that different hyperperfusion patterns reflect only preferential pathways of ictal propagation rather than the intrinsic epileptogenic region.

Other post-image acquisition techniques of ictal SPECT studies offer promise for further evaluation of ictal hyperperfusion patterns. Weder et al. (2006) studied mesial temporal lobe seizures in patients who showed oro-alimentary behavior within the first 20 seconds of clinical seizure manifestation. Comparing ictal and interictal SPECT images, as well as normal control subject images, they employed categorical comparisons with statistical parametric mapping and principal component analysis to assess functional connectivity. Principal component analysis supplemented the findings of the categorical analysis by decomposing the covariance matrix containing images of patients and healthy subjects into distinct component images of independent variance. Two principal components discriminated the subject groups: patients with right or left mesial temporal seizures and normal volunteers, indicating distinct neuronal networks implicated by the seizure. Because all subjects had early oro-alimentary signs, the authors proposed that the two principal components identify relay nodes related to oro-alimentary behavior: (1) right mesial temporal zone and ipsilateral anterior insula in right mesial temporal lobe seizures, and (2) temporal poles on both sides that are densely interconnected by the anterior commissure. Principal component analysis in ictal SPECT studies offers an interesting technique for measuring ictal functional connectivity between brain regions.

ICTAL SPECT AND PATHOPHYSIOLOGY OF EPILEPTIC SEIZURES

There is growing evidence that "partial" epilepsy involves not only a localized brain region but also interconnected structures in preferential patterns of neuronal networks (Nair et al. 2004; Spencer 2002). Within proposed models, there is a concept that the epileptogenic zone activates surrounding neuroanatomical structures (Nair et al. 2004) in what we will define for discussion as a "primary" neuronal network. Interpreting ictal SPECT findings in the context of neuronal network involvement, the region of the brain most commonly hyperperfused would represent the primary neuronal network activated in a defined epilepsy syndrome. In chronic TLE, for example, multiple investigatory studies have documented widespread interictal abnormalities in subjects with chronic TLE, including PET (Sperling 1993), SPECT (Rowe et al. 1991b), fMRI (Tasch et al. 1999), and structural MRI (Bonilha et al. 2004), implicating extensive effects of focal epileptic seizures and supporting the concept of neuronal network involvement of epilepsy. However, intracranial electrocorticographic recordings of preferential ictal propagation patterns are the traditional and best-documented work in defining ictal neuronal networks, so we review the documented involvement of the primary neuronal network in TLE in this context.

Wieser (1983, 1986) described neuroanatomical seizure propagation in TLE, the most common of which is a "mesio-basal limbic" pattern, which commonly propagates to the "temporo-polar" region. These findings correlate with findings of anteromedial temporal lobe hyperperfusion in parametric SPECT studies. More recently Isnard et al. (2000) performed depth electrode recordings of the insula in subjects with TLE and found insular cortex involvement in all of 81 recorded seizures, confirming the extremely common involvement of the insula in TLE. Intracranial EEG studies of the basal ganglia show no ictal discharge when TLE seizures remain localized to the seizure-onset zone, but do show changes dependent on seizure propagation (Rektor et al. 2002). Given the correlation of ictal SPECT hyperperfusion with ictal discharges (Spanaki et al. 1999), available intracranial electrographic studies support parametric SPECT findings of a primary neuronal network activation of the anterior temporal lobe, insula, and deep gray matter structures in TLE. Based on correlative analysis of global ictal brain perfusion changes, Blumenfeld et al. (2004a) have proposed neuronal networks involving the basal ganglia and temporal structures, and separate neuronal networks involving the thalamus, while Tae et al. (2005) propose an ictal activation of the cortico-thalamo-hippocampal-insular network. Interestingly, intracranial EEG data suggest that the centromedian thalamic nuclei participate little in the direct spread of complex partial seizures (Velasco et al. 1989), which would support the concept that the thalamus is not part of a primary neuronal network in TLE.

While regions of hyperperfusion represent regions of electrocortical ictal activation, regions of hypoperfusion may correlate with electrocortical inhibition, as represented by focal irregular slowing. Correlating intracranial EEG findings in patients with mesial TLE, Blumenfeld et al. (2004b) found prominent irregular slowing in bilateral frontal and ipsilateral parietal association cortex during and after temporal lobe seizures. They proposed that EEG slowing in the frontoparietal association cortex may signify physiologic impairment that contributes to widespread altered cerebral function during partial seizures. Regions of prominent irregular slowing may represent long-range neuronal network interactions during which there is decreased excitatory input or active inhibition of the frontal and parietal cortex. These regions correlate with regions of hypoperfusion seen in ictal SPECT studies during temporal lobe seizures (Blumenfeld et al. 2004b).

ICTAL SPECT AND CONSCIOUSNESS

Typical temporal lobe seizures cause alteration in consciousness, and therefore global changes of ictal perfusion may shed light on the pathophysiologic mechanisms of alterations of consciousness. Despite the longstanding interest in consciousness and epilepsy, definitions of consciousness and establishment of objective relationships between conscious states and epileptic seizures remain difficult (Blumenfeld and Taylor 2003; Hogan and Kaiboriboon 2003). In the 18th century, John Hughlings-Jackson proposed that deficits of consciousness during epileptic seizures occur due to both positive and negative symptoms, stating that epileptic seizures made consciousness "imperfect by deficit and imperfect by excess" (Hogan and Kaiboriboon 2003). He proposed a system of levels of consciousness and described positive or negative influences on different levels of consciousness during epileptic seizures. His concepts of positive and negative components of epileptic seizures provide an interesting background to contemporary findings during ictal SPECT studies, which show regions of hyperperfusion (representing "positive" phenomenon) and hypoperfusion (representing "negative" phenomenon).

Blumenfeld and Taylor (2003) have proposed the "network inhibition hypothesis" in TLE, which postulates that when a focal seizure involves the mesial temporal lobe unilaterally, there is subsequent propagation from the mesial temporal lobe to midline subcortical structures. Disruption of the normal activating functions of the midline subcortical structures, together with the resulting depressed activity in bilateral regions of the fronto-parietal association cortex, leads to loss of consciousness.

There is evidence from ictal SPECT studies to support global dysfunction and associated disruption of consciousness during temporal lobe seizures. Early investigators noted broad regions of SPECT hypoperfusion during temporal lobe seizures (Newton et al. 1995).

As discussed above in the section on parametric SPECT studies of TLE, several investigators have demonstrated widespread patterns of ictal hyperperfusion and hypoperfusion changes in TLE, during which subjects typically had associated deficits of consciousness.

Ictal SPECT studies in TLE aid in determining the involvement of different neuroanatomical structures responsible for the clinical semiology of seizures, such as ictal signs and symptoms that indicate lateralization of seizure onset. Ictal dystonia, which lateralizes the ictal onset zone to the hemisphere contralateral to the dystonia, is accompanied by hyperperfusion in the basal ganglia on the side of the ictal onset zone (Newton et al. 1992). Approximately 5% of all subjects with temporal lobe seizures have automatisms with preserved responsiveness. Such patients have relatively preserved consciousness and are able to respond to simple questions during their seizures, despite having other signs and symptoms of temporal lobe seizures, and show seizure onset from the non-language dominant temporal lobe (Ebner et al. 1995). Interestingly, past investigators have shown differences in ictal SPECT perfusion patterns in patients with right and left temporal lobe seizures (Hogan et al. 2006; Tae et al. 2005). In comparing SPECT studies in subjects with clinically comparable seizures, left temporal lobe seizures have an over 60-fold greater probability of hyperperfusion of the brain stem tegmentum compared to subjects with right temporal lobe seizures (Hogan et al. 2006). The differences in perfusion of the brain stem tegmentum correlate with the region of brain stem reticular formation, which plays a major role in regulation of consciousness, attentiveness, and awareness and exerts influences on autonomic functions. Therefore, the relative sparing of hyperperfusion of the brain stem reticular formation in right temporal lobe seizures may explain why right temporal lobe seizures cause a lesser degree of loss of consciousness in ictal automatisms with preserved responsiveness compared to left temporal lobe seizures.

Functional imaging will play an important role in correlation of peri-ictal semiologic changes with specific patterns of activation and deactivation in brain structures, which involves global brain regions in TLE. Whether positive symptoms in general, ranging from simple repetitive movements to complex motor automatisms, represent a direct activation of neuroanatomical structures from an epileptic discharge or are the result of a "release" phenomenon (during which an activating discharge allows manifestation of function in another brain region) remains an important question (Kotagal 2000). Adding further complexity to ictal semiology is the possibility that some symptoms are related to deactivation of some brain structures. This likely plays a major role in changes in consciousness, as discussed above in the "network inhibition hypothesis" (Norden and Blumenfeld 2002). There are further correlates of electrographic involvement of structures outside the temporal lobe during temporal lobe seizures. Depth electrode recordings of the insula in subjects with TLE document insular cortex involvement in recorded seizures, confirming the extremely common involvement of the insula in TLE (Hogan et al. 2006). Therefore, functional activation of the insula contributes to ictal TLE semiology. As the knowledge of the localization of neuronal networks involved in TLE grows, pathophysiologic definition of TLE syndromes will become more complete.

SUMMARY

There is a long history of the association of cerebral blood flow changes during epileptic seizures. The advent of radiopharmaceutical agents to measure cerebral perfusion during seizures has enabled a clinically feasible way to record ictal cerebral blood flow changes. Studies show that ictal SPECT findings, especially with the use of subtraction ictal SPECT techniques, correlate well with other measures of seizure onset and the epileptogenic zone. Ictal SPECT studies are also helpful in predicting outcome after epilepsy surgery. Applications of parametric mapping using ictal SPECT studies have helped to further define regions of perfusion changes in groups of patients with specific regions of seizure onset. The use of parametric mapping techniques in subjects with TLE has yielded interesting common patterns of ictal hyperperfusion and hypoperfusion. These studies help define expected patterns of ictal perfusion changes in TLE, as well as shed light on the associated pathophysiology of aspects of ictal semiology, such as ictal unilateral dystonia and the associated changes in consciousness during temporal lobe seizures.

REFERENCES

Avery, R. A., S. S. Spencer, M. V. Spanaki MV, et al. 1999. Effect of injection time on postictal SPET perfusion changes in medically refractory epilepsy. *European Journal of Nuclear Medicine* 26: 830–6.

Barber, D. C., W. B. Tindale, E. Hunt, et al. 1995. Automatic registration of SPECT images as an alternative to immobilization in neuroactivation studies. *Physics in Medicine & Biology* 40: 449–63.

Blumenfeld, H., K. A. McNally, R. B. Ostroff, et al. 2003a. Targeted prefrontal cortical activation with bifrontal ECT. *Psychiatry Research* 123: 165–70.

Blumenfeld, H., K. A. McNally, S. D. Vanderhill SD, et al. 2004a. Positive and negative network correlations in temporal lobe epilepsy. *Cerebral Cortex* 14: 892–902.

Blumenfeld, H., M. Rivera, K. A. McNally, et al. 2004b. Ictal neocortical slowing in temporal lobe epilepsy. *Neurology* 63: 1015–21.

Blumenfeld, H., and J. Taylor. 2003. Why do seizures cause loss of consciousness? *Neuroscientist* 9: 301–10.

Blumenfeld, H., M. Westerveld, R. B. Ostroff, et al. 2003b. Selective frontal, parietal, and temporal networks in generalized seizures. *Neuroimage* 19: 1556–66.

Bonilha, L., C. Rorden, G. Castellano, et al. 2004. Voxel-based morphometry reveals gray matter network atrophy in refractory medial temporal lobe epilepsy. *Archives of Neurology* 61: 1379–84.

Brinkmann, B. H., T. J. O'Brien, S. Aharon, et al. 1999. Quantitative and clinical analysis of SPECT image registration for epilepsy studies. *Journal of Nuclear Medicine* 40: 1098–105.

Chang, D. J., I. G. Zubal, C. Gottschalk, et al. 2002. Comparison of statistical parametric mapping and SPECT difference imaging in patients with temporal lobe epilepsy. *Epilepsia* 43: 68–74.

Dymond, A. M., and P. H. Crandall. 1976. Oxygen availability and blood flow in the temporal lobes during spontaneous epileptic seizures in man. *Brain Research* 102: 191–6.

Ebner, A., D. S. Dinner, S. Noachtar, et al. 1995. Automatisms with preserved responsiveness: a lateralizing sign in psychomotor seizures. *Neurology* 45: 61–4.

Engel, J., Jr., S. Wiebe, J. French, et al. 2003. Practice parameter: temporal lobe and localized neocortical resections for epilepsy: report of the Quality Standards Subcommittee of the American Academy of Neurology, in association with the American Epilepsy Society and the American Association of Neurological Surgeons. *Neurology* 60: 538–47.

Feichtinger, M., H. Eder, A. Holl, et al. 2007. Automatic and remote controlled ictal SPECT injection for seizure focus localization by use of a commercial contrast agent application pump. *Epilepsia* 48: 1409–13.

Gibbs, F. A., W. G. Lennox, and E. L. Gibbs. 1934. Cerebral blood flow preceding and acccompanying epileptic seizures in man. *Archives of Neurology and Psychiatry* 32: 257–72.

Ho, S. S., S. F. Berkovic, W. J. McKay, et al. 1996. Temporal lobe epilepsy subtypes: differential patterns of cerebral perfusion on ictal SPECT. *Epilepsia* 37: 788–95.

Ho, S. S., S. F. Berkovic, M. R. Newton, et al. 1994. Parietal lobe epilepsy: clinical features and seizure localization by ictal SPECT. *Neurology* 44: 2277–84.

Ho, S. S., M. R. Newton, A. M. McIntosh, et al. 1997. Perfusion patterns during temporal lobe seizures: relationship to surgical outcome. *Brain* 120: 1921–8.

Hogan, R. E., M. J. Cook, C. J. Kilpatrick, et al. 1996. Accuracy of coregistration of single-photon emission CT with MR via a brain surface matching technique. *AJNR American Journal of Neuroradiology* 17: 793–7.

Hogan, R. E., and K. Kaiboriboon. 2003. The "dreamy state": John Hughlings-Jackson's ideas of epilepsy and consciousness. *American Journal of Psychiatry* 160: 1740–7.

Hogan, R. E., K. Kaiboriboon, M. E. Bertrand, et al. 2006. Composite SISCOM perfusion patterns in right and left temporal seizures. *Archives of Neurology* 63: 1419–26.

Hogan, R. E., K. Kaiboriboon, and M. Osman. 2004. Composite SISCOM images in mesial temporal lobe epilepsy: technique and illustration of regions of hyperperfusion. *Nuclear Medicine Communication* 25: 539–45.

Hogan, R. E., V. J. Lowe, and R. D. Bucholz. 1999. Triple-technique (MR imaging, single-photon emission CT, and CT) coregistration for image-guided surgical evaluation of patients with intractable epilepsy. *AJNR American Journal of Neuroradiology* 20: 1054–8.

Horsley, V. 1892. An address on the origin and seat of the epileptic disturbance. *British Medical Journal* 1: 693–6.

Isnard, J., M. Guenot, K. Ostrowsky, et al. 2000. The role of the insular cortex in temporal lobe epilepsy. *Annals of Neurology* 48: 614–23.

Jack, C. R., Jr. 1993. Epilepsy: surgery and imaging. *Radiology* 189: 635–46.

Kaiboriboon, K., M. E. Bertrand, M. M. Osman, et al. 2005. Quantitative analysis of cerebral blood flow patterns in mesial temporal lobe epilepsy using composite SISCOM. *Journal of Nuclear Medicine* 46: 38–43.

Kaiboriboon, K., V. J. Lowe, S. I. Chantarujikapong, et al. 2002. The usefulness of subtraction ictal SPECT coregistered to MRI in single- and dual-headed SPECT cameras in partial epilepsy. *Epilepsia* 43: 408–14.

Kim, J. H., K. C. Im, J. S. Kim, et al. 2007. Ictal hyperperfusion patterns in relation to ictal scalp EEG patterns in patients with unilateral hippocampal sclerosis: a SPECT study. *Epilepsia* 48: 270–7.

Knowlton, R. C., R. A. Elgavish, A. Bartolucci, et al. 2008. Functional imaging: II. Prediction of epilepsy surgery outcome. *Annals of Neurology* 64: 35–41.

Kotagal, P. 2000. Automotor seizures. In H. O. Luders and S. Noachtar (Eds.), *Epileptic seizures, pathophysiology and clinical semiology*. New York: Churchill Livingstone: 449–57.

Lee, J. D., H. J. Kim, B. I. Lee, et al. 2000. Evaluation of ictal brain SPET using statistical parametric mapping in temporal lobe epilepsy. *European Journal of Nuclear Medicine* 27: 1658–65.

Lee, S. K., S. Y. Lee, K. K. Kim, et al. 2005. Surgical outcome and prognostic factors of cryptogenic neocortical epilepsy. *Annals of Neurology* 58: 525–32.

Leveille, J., G. Demonceau, and R. C. Walovitch. 1992. Intrasubject comparison between technetium–99m-ECD and technetium–99m-HMPAO in healthy human subjects. *Journal of Nuclear Medicine* 33: 480–4.

Marks, D. A., A. Katz, P. Hoffer, et al. 1992. Localization of extratemporal epileptic foci during ictal single photon emission computed tomography. *Annals of Neurology* 31: 250–5.

McNally, K. A., A. L. Paige, G. Varghese, et al. 2005. Localizing value of ictal-interictal SPECT analyzed by SPM (ISAS). *Epilepsia* 46: 1450–64.

Nair, D. R., A. Mohamed, R. Burgess, et al. 2004. A critical review of the different conceptual hypotheses framing human focal epilepsy. *Epileptic Disorders* 6: 77–83.

Newton, M. R., S. F. Berkovic, M. C. Austin, et al. 1992. Dystonia, clinical lateralization, and regional blood flow changes in temporal lobe seizures. *Neurology* 42: 371–7.

Newton, M. R., S. F. Berkovic, M. C. Austin, et al. 1995. SPECT in the localisation of extratemporal and temporal seizure foci. *Journal of Neurology Neurosurgery Psychiatry* 59: 26–30.

Norden, A. D., and H. Blumenfeld. 2002. The role of subcortical structures in human epilepsy. *Epilepsy & Behavior* 3: 219–31.

O'Brien, T. J. 2000. SPECT: methodology. *Advances in Neurology* 83: 11–32.

O'Brien, T. J., B. H. Brinkmann, B. P. Mullan, et al. 1999a. Comparative study of 99mTc-ECD and 99mTc-HMPAO for peri-ictal SPECT: qualitative and quantitative analysis. *Journal of Neurology Neurosurgery Psychiatry* 66: 331–9.

O'Brien, T. J., M. K. O'Connor, B. P. Mullan, et al. 1998a. Subtraction ictal SPET co-registered to MRI in partial epilepsy: description and technical validation of the method with phantom and patient studies. *Nuclear Medicine Communications* 19: 31–45.

O'Brien, T. J., E. L. So, B. P. Mullan, et al. 2000. Subtraction peri-ictal SPECT is predictive of extratemporal epilepsy surgery outcome. *Neurology* 55: 1668–77.

O'Brien, T. J., E. L. So, B. P. Mullan, et al. 1998b. Subtraction ictal SPECT co-registered to MRI improves clinical usefulness of SPECT in localizing the surgical seizure focus. *Neurology* 50: 445–54.

O'Brien, T. J., E. L. So, B. P. Mullan, et al. 1999b. Subtraction SPECT co-registered to MRI improves postictal SPECT localization of seizure foci. *Neurology* 52: 137–46.

Penfield, W. 1933. The evidence for a cerebral vascular mechanism in epilepsy. *Annals of Internal Medicine* 1933; 7: 303–10.

Penfield, W. 1971. Remarks on incomplete hypotheses for the control of cerebral circulation. *Journal of Neurosurgery* 1971; 35: 124–7.

Plum, F., J. B. Posner, and B. Troy. 1968. Cerebral metabolic and circulatory responses to induced convulsions in animals. *Archives of Neurology* 18: 1–13.

Quesney, L. F. 1991. Preoperative electroencephalographic investigation in frontal lobe epilepsy: electroencephalographic and electrocorticographic recordings. *Canadian Journal of the Neurological Sciences* 18: 559–63.

Rektor, I., R. Kuba, and M. Brazdil. 2002. Interictal and ictal EEG activity in the basal ganglia: an SEEG study in patients with temporal lobe epilepsy. *Epilepsia* 43: 253–62.

Rowe, C. C., S. F. Berkovic, M. C. Austin, et al. 1991a. Patterns of postictal cerebral blood flow in temporal lobe epilepsy: qualitative and quantitative analysis. *Neurology* 41: 1096–103.

Rowe, C. C., S. F. Berkovic, M. C. Austin, et al. 1991b. Visual and quantitative analysis of interictal SPECT with technetium–99m-HMPAO in temporal lobe epilepsy. *Journal of Nuclear Medicine* 32: 1688–94.

Rowe, C. C., S. F. Berkovic, S. T. Sia, et al. 1989. Localization of epileptic foci with postictal single photon emission computed tomography. *Annals of Neurology* 26: 660–8.

Salanova, V., O. Markand, and R. Worth. 2005. Temporal lobe epilepsy: analysis of failures and the role of reoperation. *Acta Neurologica Scandinavica* 111: 126–33.

Schridde, U., M. Khubchandani, J. E. Motelow, et al. 2008. Negative BOLD with large increases in neuronal activity. *Cerebral Cortex* 18: 1814–27.

Sepkuty, J. P., R. P. Lesser, C. A. Civelek, et al. 1998. An automated injection system (with patient selection) for

SPECT imaging in seizure localization. *Epilepsia* 39: 1350–6.

Shin, W. C., S. B. Hong, W. S. Tae, et al. 2002. Ictal hyperperfusion patterns according to the progression of temporal lobe seizures. *Neurology* 58: 373–80.

Shin, W. C., S. B. Hong, W. S. Tae, et al. 2001. Ictal hyperperfusion of cerebellum and basal ganglia in temporal lobe epilepsy: SPECT subtraction with MRI coregistration. *Journal of Nuclear Medicine* 42: 853–8.

Siegel, A. M., G. D. Cascino, F. B. Meyer, et al. 2004. Resective reoperation for failed epilepsy surgery: seizure outcome in 64 patients. *Neurology* 63: 2298–302.

Sojkova, J., P. J. Lewis, A. H. Siegel, et al. 2003. Does asymmetric basal ganglia or thalamic activation aid in seizure foci lateralization on ictal SPECT studies? *Journal of Nuclear Medicine* 44: 1379–86.

Spanaki, M. V., I. G. Zubal, J. MacMullan, et al. 1999. Periictal SPECT localization verified by simultaneous intracranial EEG. *Epilepsia* 40: 267–74.

Spencer, S. S. 2002. Neural networks in human epilepsy: evidence of and implications for treatment. *Epilepsia* 43: 219–27.

Spencer, S. S., D. D. Spencer, P. D. Williamson, et al. 1990. Combined depth and subdural electrode investigation in uncontrolled epilepsy. *Neurology* 40: 74–9.

Sperling, M. R. 1993. Neuroimaging in epilepsy: recent developments in MR imaging, positron-emission tomography, and single-photon emission tomography. *Neurologic Clinics* 11: 883–903.

Stefan, H., J. Bauer, H. Feistel, et al. 1990. Regional cerebral blood flow during focal seizures of temporal and frontocentral onset. *Annals of Neurology* 27: 162–6.

Tae, W. S., E. Y. Joo, J. H. Kim, et al. 2005. Cerebral perfusion changes in mesial temporal lobe epilepsy: SPM analysis of ictal and interictal SPECT. *Neuroimage* 24: 101–10.

Tasch, E., F. Cendes, L. M. Li, et al. 1999. Neuroimaging evidence of progressive neuronal loss and dysfunction in temporal lobe epilepsy. *Annals of Neurology* 45: 568–76.

Turkington, T. G., R. J. Jaszczak, C. A. Pelizzari, et al. 1993. Accuracy of registration of PET, SPECT and MR images of a brain phantom. *Journal of Nuclear Medicine* 34: 1587–94.

Van Paesschen, W., P. Dupont, S. Sunaert, et al. 2007. The use of SPECT and PET in routine clinical practice in epilepsy. *Current Opinion in Neurology* 20: 194–202.

Van Paesschen, W., P. Dupont, G. Van Driel, et al. 2003. SPECT perfusion changes during complex partial seizures in patients with hippocampal sclerosis. *Brain* 126: 1103–11.

Velasco, M., F. Velasco, A. L. Velasco, et al. 1989. Epileptiform EEG activities of the centromedian thalamic nuclei in patients with intractable partial motor, complex partial, and generalized seizures. *Epilepsia* 30: 295–306.

Weder, B. J., K. Schindler, T. J. Loher, et al. 2006. Brain areas involved in medial temporal lobe seizures: a principal component analysis of ictal SPECT data. *Human Brain Mapping* 27: 520–34.

Wetjen, N. M., G. D. Cascino, A. J. Fessler, et al. 2006. Subtraction ictal single-photon emission computed tomography coregistered to magnetic resonance imaging in evaluating the need for repeated epilepsy surgery. *Journal of Neurosurgery* 105: 71–6.

Wichert-Ana, L., T. R. Velasco, V. C. Terra-Bustamante, et al. 2001. Typical and atypical perfusion patterns in periictal SPECT of patients with unilateral temporal lobe epilepsy. *Epilepsia* 42: 660–6.

Wieser, H. G. 1983. Part 3, *Electroclinical Features of the Psychomotor Seizure*. London: Butterworths, 177–235.

Wieser, H. G. 1986. Psychomotor seizures of hippocampal-amygdalar origin. In T. A. Pedley (Ed.), *Recent advances in epilepsy*. Edinburgh: Churchill Livingstone: 57–79.

Zubal, I. G., S. S. Spencer, K. Imam, et al. 1995. Difference images calculated from ictal and interictal technetium–99m-HMPAO SPECT scans of epilepsy. *Journal of Nuclear Medicine* 36: 684–9.

Chapter 15

MULTIMODALITY NEUROIMAGING AND FUTURE DIRECTIONS

Otto Muzik and Harry T. Chugani

This volume has summarized the latest in application of various neuroimaging approaches to the evaluation of people with epilepsy. With ever-improving imaging technologies and boost in computational power, the medical imaging field has experienced a tremendous increase in the amount of collected information. In addition to the exponential increase in raw data acquisition, each modality also carries a qualitatively different information content associated with inherent strengths and limitations. For example, while T1-weighted magnetic resonance imaging (MRI) yields high-resolution anatomical images, the ability to absolutely quantify the obtained data is limited. In contrast, molecular imaging using a variety of positron emission tomography (PET) tracers provides accurate quantitative information, unfortunately with significantly less anatomical detail than MRI. In addition, electrophysiologic data provide excellent temporal resolution of brain currents, but employ a vastly different localization scheme than conventional imaging methods. Nevertheless, all these modalities provide invaluable clinical information to the epileptologist even when utilized qualitatively.

As is apparent from this volume, a large number of groups have successfully used data from PET, SPECT,

MRI, and EEG in the presurgical evaluation of epileptic children and have shown a significant improvement in seizure outcome, although still about one in three patients fails to become seizure-free following resective surgery. Further improvements in the localization of epileptogenic brain tissue can potentially be derived from the development of a unifying computational framework that is able to quantitatively describe relationships between many qualitatively diverse data sets. Once integrated within a rigorous computational framework, information entailed in one modality can be used to enhance, or even re-interpret, information derived from other complementing modalities. Thus, the information content inherent to such an approach is not simply additive, but likely to have an *amplifying* effect. Moreover, one important consequence of this approach is the ability to construct database structures that incorporate qualitatively different data sets within a common reference frame. As a result, meta-analyses of data patterns that are distributed over several modalities can be undertaken. Obviously, such analyses require, in addition to a formal mathematical structure, also well-developed visual interface tools that allow researchers to grasp the relationship between data patterns in an intuitive way and provide clinicians with important clues regarding the pathologic state of brain tissue under study.

THE PROBLEM OF BRAIN SURFACE PARCELLATION

The first step in the direction of a successful integrative computational framework for brain analysis is to achieve a mathematically consistent parcellation of the brain surface that yields homotopic cortical areas across patients, in order to relate diverse patient features to a group average. Unfortunately, a consistent parcellation of anatomical brain surface structures from medical images and their compact geometrical representation in a rigorous computational framework proves to be extremely challenging. The reason for this is that boundaries and extent of gyri are imprecise and major sulci show frequently variable branching patterns or may be absent, even in the normal population. To date, most studies have relied on the visual assessment of gross abnormalities in cortical gyration on 3D surface rendered MR images (Sisodya et al. 1996); however, quantitative analysis is not possible using this approach. Moreover, caveats typical of sampled data, such as sampling errors, spatial aliasing, and noise, further contribute to signal deterioration and often cause the boundaries of brain structures to appear indistinct and disconnected. Among various brain segmentation techniques, deformable models and level-set methods have been historically found to be successful since their introduction in the late 1980s. Terzopoulos et al. (1987) pioneered the theory of continuous (multi-dimensional) deformable models based on Lagrangian dynamics and formulated deformation energies for generalized splines with controlled continuity. Since then, an extensive body of literature emerged on deformable models in medical image analysis (for a review see Cootes and Taylor 2001). Fundamental work on level-set methods was pioneered by Osher and Sethian (1988) and this method has been widely applied to a variety of applications in the field of image processing (Caselles et al. 1997; Malladi et al. 1995; Whitaker 1998), with varying degrees of success.

TEMPLATE VERSUS SPACE ANALYSIS

In general, two brain segmentation strategies have been pursued in the neuroimaging field: a template-space and a native-space approach. The former strategy performs nonlinear spatial normalization of the brain to a predefined template with subsequent data analysis in template space, whereas the latter approach processes all data in the subject's own (native) space and subsequently matches the structure-specific results across individual subjects. In addition to their unquestionable strengths, both strategies pose limitations, and the choice of either strategy is dependent on the specific objectives of the study.

Voxel-based analyses, most prominent of which is the statistical parametric mapping (SPM) method (Friston et al. 1991), have proven to be powerful techniques for the comparison of functional imaging data sets among groups of patients or in individuals under different conditions. Their defining advantage is the very efficient processing of whole brain volumes in standard template space, without the bias of preselecting specific regions of interest. There is extensive literature describing the usefulness of SPM analysis in both adult (Kim et al. 2002; Richardson et al. 1998; Van Bogaert et al. 1998) and pediatric (Lee et al. 2005; Muzik et al. 2000) applications, including foci detection in mesial temporal lobe epilepsy (Juhasz et al. 2001), frontal lobe epilepsy (Bruggeman et al. 2004), and intrahemispheric language reorganization in complex partial epilepsy (Rosenberger et al. 2009). In general, there is consensus that voxel-based methods are more sensitive than region-of-interest–based approaches only in detecting abnormal functional regions in cortical areas that are normally asymmetrical. A serious limitation of voxel-based analyses methods is the conceptual problem of using individual image voxels as the unit of statistical analysis, as due to small-scale physiologic variation in brain structure among subjects it is impossible to assign identical anatomical locations to image voxels. As a consequence, the data must be heavily smoothed to increase the likelihood that image voxels correspond anatomically, resulting in suboptimal sensitivity and the necessity to exclude brains that significantly deviate from the chosen template. In contrast, methods that analyze brain image volumes in native space are highly sensitive to the specific characteristics of individual data sets; however, these techniques pose difficulties in terms of how to relate results obtained in different native spaces in a unified statistical framework. Nevertheless, the native-space approach appears to be better suited for multimodality data integration in clinical routine, as clinical management options are usually evaluated for a particular subject under very specific conditions.

MULTIMODALITY DATA INTEGRATION IN NATIVE SPACE

Owing to the limitations of template-space approaches to study patient data in a clinical setting, an increasing number of methods have focused on the analysis of brain image volumes in native space. Thompson et al. (1996), Lohman (1998), and Valiant et al. (1996) all used a manually labeled atlas brain, which was then warped to fit an individual subject's brain surface with subsequent transfer of labels onto the subject's cortical surface. More recently, conformal mapping techniques have gained a wider application in brain mapping (Drury 1999). For example, Hurdal and Stephenson (2004) proposed a discrete mapping approach that uses spherical packing in order to produce a "flattened" image of the cortical surface onto a sphere, resulting in maps that are quasi-conformal approximations of classical conformal maps. Gu et al. (2004) proposed optimization of the conformal parameterization method by composing an optimal Möbius transformation so that it minimizes the landmark mismatch energy. Finally, Wang et al. (2005a, 2005b) introduced the application of compound energy (harmonic and landmark matching energy) to optimize the brain conformal mapping.

Taking advantage of user-defined cortical landmarks, this approach was further improved by matching cortical landmarks that have been conformally mapped from native space into a spherical domain (Muzik 2007; Zou et al. 2006a, 2006b). The results showed that conformal mapping of the cortical surface to a sphere preserves angular relationships and is robust with respect to differences in data triangulation and resolution. Following skull removal, this method requires manual definition of cortical landmarks in native space (Fig. 15.1A), followed by parcellation of the cortical surface into patches. Next, these patches are conformally mapped to the surface of a unit sphere (Fig. 15.1B) and cortical landmarks are aligned to a template through minimization of the harmonic surface energy between individual and template landmarks. Once aligned, a recursive parcellation scheme is applied, resulting in the creation of finite surface elements on the spherical surface (Fig. 15.1C). These finite elements are subsequently reversely mapped into the subject's native space, where all data analysis takes place. Consequently, a regular surface parcellation in the spherical domain will transfer into an irregular, but homotopic, surface parcellation in native space of individual cortical surfaces (Fig. 15.1D), as each point in the spherical domain corresponds to homotopic points in native space of individual brains. The parcellation is realized by a regular recursive segmentation scheme, starting with the eight surface quadrants of the sphere followed by recursive division of each surface quadrant into four sub-elements. This approach yields a progression of 8 (level 0), 32, 128, 512, and 2,048 (level 4) finite surface elements covering the whole brain, with a surface area of ~1 cm^2 for the 512 (level 3) and ~0.3 cm^2 for the 2,048 (level 4) element parcellation.

Although the shape and location of the resulting finite elements differs between any two individual brains in native space, each finite grid element is characterized by the same spatial relationship to its own cortical landmarks. Consequently, finite surface elements characterized by the same index are homotopic across individuals. By extending these finite surface

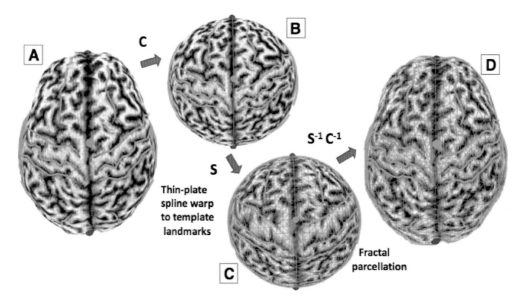

Figure 15.1 Sequence of steps to perform a landmark-constrained conformal mapping of the cortical surface. As the spatial relationship between cortical landmarks and finite cortical elements is identical, the resulting cortical finite elements are homotopic across individual subjects.

elements into the brain, standardized cortical volume elements are defined in native space of each subject. As the positions of cortical landmarks are affected by features of individual subjects, this method incorporates both physiologic variations as well as possible structural abnormalities into the mapping process. Thus, the set of cortical finite elements provides a basis for multimodality image data representation, information integration, and data mining, as well as statistical analysis across patient groups, that can be applied to the detection and characterization of cortical abnormalities in a large array of neurological disorders, including epilepsy.

In a sense, this method attempts to merge the advantages of both voxel-based and region-of-interest–based strategies, as the finite cortical elements can be compared to the "resolution elements" (RESELS) used in the context of SPM analysis. The major difference here is that instead of transferring image data into standard space where predefined regions are sampled, landmark-constrained conformal mapping is applied to transfer the parcellation scheme from the spherical domain into native space. Thus, the original data remain unchanged but are sampled in native space according to the conformally mapped parcellation. Although these two approaches are fairly similar if one considers only image intensities, the advantage of native space analysis becomes evident when non-scalar data sets are included, such as data from diffusion tensor imaging (DTI) or from EEG grid arrays. Not only is the non-linear spatial normalization of DTI vector fields conceptually problematic, but integration of multimodality data is also likely to be most accurate in native space where individual features of the data set can be used as additional information for integration. Moreover, the transfer of EEG electrode locations into template space is fraught with problems and not useful for epilepsy surgery in individual patients.

A similar method has been proposed also by Dale et al. (1999) and Fischl et al. (1999, 2002, 2004), although not in the context of epilepsy surgery data integration. These authors have developed the Freesurfer software environment that allows construction of a geometrically accurate and topologically correct model of the cortical sheet in canonical space. Using this method, the reconstructed surface of each individual subject is mapped onto a sphere using an isometric transformation. All surfaces are subsequently morphed into register with an average, canonical surface, guided by a combination of folding-alignment (sulcus/gyrus) and isometry-preserving forces. The difference between the Freesurfer software environment and the described conformal mapping approach is the physical location of analysis: the former performs data analysis in canonical space, whereas the finite element approach uses canonical space for the

definition of a surface coordinate system that is subsequently transformed back into native space for data analysis.

INTEGRATION OF MULTIMODALITY DATA SETS IN THE PRESURGICAL EVALUATION OF EPILEPSY PATIENTS

Although intracranial subdural EEG recordings still remain the gold standard for determination of the resection site in epilepsy surgery, the accuracy of foci localization using subdural electrodes depends greatly on the location of electrodes placed on the brain surface, and selection bias (i.e., area of cortex sampled) is a major limitation. In order to guide the placement of subdural electrodes, a combination of noninvasive imaging techniques (MR, PET) is used, yielding important clues to guide placement of subdural electrodes over epileptogenic brain regions based on the locations and extent of anatomical and functional abnormalities (Juhasz et al. 2000; So 2002). Furthermore, after the intracranial EEG grid electrodes are implanted, each electrode records a number of electrophysiologic parameters that need to be related to the imaging information to decide on the most effective course of surgical intervention.

Currently several groups worldwide are actively developing methods for integrative analysis of multimodality neuroimaging data in the context of epilepsy surgery. Among others, the goal of the University of Washington Brain Project is to develop software tools for processing, integrating, and visualizing multimodality language data obtained at the time of neurosurgery, both for surgical planning and for the study of language organization in the brain (Poliakov et al. 1999). In this model, data from a single patient consist of four MR-based image volumes: anatomy, veins, arteries, and fMRI activations. The data also include the location of sites that were electrically stimulated for the presence of language. The primary method of integration is the construction of a patient-specific model of the brain, obtained from structural MR scans. The three other MR image volumes (showing veins, arteries, and fMRI activation blobs) are then registered to the anatomical MR image volume; once aligned, the low-resolution cortical shell is used to mask non-cortical veins and arteries from the corresponding MR image volumes. Integration of the surgical stimulation data is based on a visualization-based approach: the cortical surface model is combined with the MR-based models of the cortical veins and arteries and rendered so as to visually match a photograph taken of the cortical surface exposed during neurosurgery. The veins and arteries provide landmarks that can be readily recognized on the photograph (Fig. 15.2A); an interactive

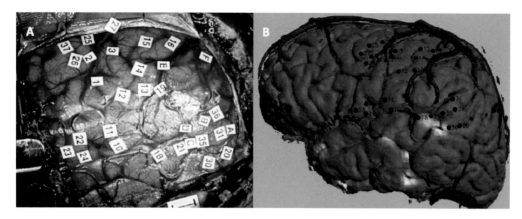

Figure 15.2 Visualization of five integrated sources of brain map data: cortex, arteries, veins, fMRI, and stimulation mapping sites. (A) Intra-operative photograph of the patient's cortical surface exposed during surgery. Numbered tags are the location of sites stimulated for mapping of language function. (B) Cortical surface rendering including venous vessels and the location of electrode transferred based on the photograph. Highlighted areas (in white) represent the fMRI activation sites that are close to the surface. (Reprinted from A. Poliakov, K. Hinshaw, C. Rosse, et al. 1999. Integration and visualization of multimodality brain data for language mapping. *Proceedings of AMIA Symposium* 349–53.)

tool is subsequently used to map the location of stimulation sites (as seen on the photograph) onto the reconstructed cortex (Fig. 15.2B). Given this integration, various forms of visualization and analysis techniques are applied to gain a better understanding of the relationships among the various data sources.

A similar approach, using interictal SPECT, T1-weighted FLAIR, and fMR images integrated with a subdural electrode grid display, has been developed at the University of Melbourne, Australia (Murphy et al. 2004). This integrative approach has since allowed several patients, previously considered ineligible for surgery, to undergo successful resection of their epileptogenic foci (Murphy et al. 2004). Alignment of the subdural electrode grid with the surface rendered T1-weighted MR image volume is accomplished using a spiral CT scan, acquired within 24 hours of implanting the intracranial electrodes. The high-attenuation electrode grid is initially segmented from CT images using in-house–developed software together with brain contours, which are subsequently co-registered to the previously obtained MR image volume. This procedure yields the position of the electrode grid on the rendered MR surface (Fig. 15.3) with a mean error of 3.4 mm (range 0.5–5.4 mm) (Morris et al. 2000).

INTEGRATION OF PET AND INTRACRANIAL EEG

Over the years, our group has made significant contributions to the multimodality integration of PET and intracranial EEG data in the context of presurgical evaluation of patients with epilepsy, particularly children. In applying PET imaging to the study of glucose

metabolism (2-deoxy-2-[^{18}F]fluoro-D-glucose, FDG) and GABA$_A$ receptor (^{11}C-flumazenil, FMZ) distribution in patients with epilepsy (Muzik et al. 2000; Juhász et al. 2001, 2009), it became increasingly clear that a better understanding of the underlying mechanisms can be achieved only by means of a computational framework that will allow a quantitative assessment of spatial relationships between PET imaging and intracranial EEG data. To provide a quantitative method for the assessment of the spatial relationship between image volumes and intracranial EEG electrodes, a method was developed that relies on the accurate alignment of a lateral planar X-ray image of the patient's head (with fiducial markers and intracranial EEG electrodes in place) with a 3D surface rendering of the T1-weighted MR image volume (Fig. 15.4) (Juhász et al. 2000; Thiel et al. 1998). Following insertion of an intracranial EEG grid, a lateral skull X-ray image is obtained at the patient's bedside using a portable X-ray machine. To encode orientation information into the skull X-ray image, three fiducial markers are placed at anatomically reproducible locations on the patient's head during the X-ray procedure. The X-ray film is then digitized and the three fiducial markers are identified. The T1-weighted volumetric MR image volume obtained prior to grid insertion is then surface rendered and three fiducial markers are then virtually defined at corresponding anatomical locations to those in the X-ray image (Fig. 15.4A). To reconstruct 3D brain surface views corresponding to the planar X-ray image, the digitized X-ray image is overlayed onto the image plane and an iterative algorithm is used to minimize the differences between the two sets of coordinate triplets (physical and virtual markers) by simultaneously adjusting the three euler-angles and the image

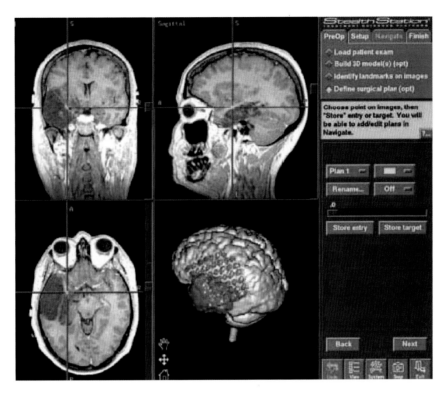

Figure 15.3 Coronal (upper left), sagittal (upper right), and axial (lower left) orthogonal slices and 3D volume-rendered image (lower right) of the head revealing the co-registration of segmented CT-derived subdural electrodes and 3D volumetric MR images. These images were obtained in a patient with longstanding refractory partial epilepsy associated with a dysembryoplastic neuroepithelial tumor in the left temporal lobe. In the volume-rendered image display (lower right) the electrodes are green and the tumor is red. (Reprinted from M. A. Murphy, T. J. O'Brien, K. Morris, et al. 2004. Multimodality image-guided surgery for the treatment of medically refractory epilepsy. *Journal of Neurosurgery* 100: 452–62.)

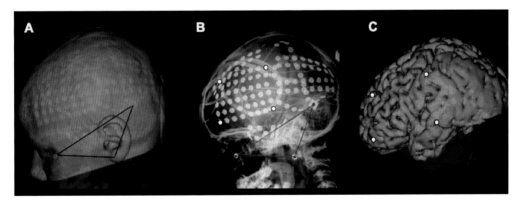

Figure 15.4 (A) Anatomical information is used to define virtual markers on the surface-rendered brain corresponding to (B) fiducial markers placed on the patient's head prior to X-ray imaging. (C) The result is a surface view where the location of the four corner electrodes of each of the EEG grids can be determined on the brain surface.

zoom (Fig. 15.4B). Upon completion of alignment, a surface view of the cortex is created that corresponds to the planar X-ray image and where the spatial coordinates of the four corner grid electrodes of each rectangular EEG grid can be determined on the brain surface (Fig. 15.4C). The accuracy of this method was previously reported as 1.24 ± 0.66 mm with a maximal misregistration of 2.7 mm (Thiel et al. 1998).

The accurate localization of EEG electrodes on the cortical surface is crucial to study the relationship between electrophysiology and anatomical as well as functional cortical abnormalities. The advantages of this method are that it does not require repeating an MRI scan after grid electrode placements and the skull X-ray is performed at the bedside. Our previous studies focused on the examination of the spatial proximity between functional abnormalities and epileptogenic cortex suggested that epileptogenic areas are frequently found *adjacent* to FDG PET abnormalities and only partially overlapping (Juhász et al. 2000b). This phenomenon is at present poorly understood, and possible mechanisms are discussed by Juhász et al. (2000b, 2001) and reviewed in Chapter 9 of this volume. Thus, although there exists a strong spatial relationship between epileptic cortex and functional abnormalities, both appear to be distinct, rendering a rigorous quantitative assessment of this relationship using a receiver operating characteristics (ROC) analysis problematic, as sensitivity and specificity measures are independent of the distance between the electrophysiologic and functional abnormalities. In contrast, the close proximity of the PET abnormality to the epileptogenic zone is of great practical value for the surgical treatment of epilepsy patients, as it initiates the insertion of a larger EEG grid that will include the border zone of the PET abnormality as well.

To assess this relationship quantitatively, we introduced the spatial proximity index (SPI), calculated based on the position of intracranial subdural EEG electrodes relative to PET abnormal cortical areas. The SPI is a continuous variable that equals zero for perfect overlap between seizure onset electrodes and PET-defined abnormal cortical elements and increases in proportion to the distance between EEG-defined onset electrodes and PET-defined abnormal cortical elements. To calculate the SPI, EEG electrodes are initially characterized either as EEG positive (E+) or negative (E-) for a particular electrophysiologic parameter (seizure onset or early spread). Moreover, a weighting factor w_i is used to account for the varying interictal spike frequencies at different electrode locations. When only seizure onset electrodes are considered,

the weighting factor is either 1 or 0, whereas when spike frequencies are considered the weighting factor is derived as the quotient between the spike frequency at a particular electrode location and the maximal spike frequency in the whole brain. Finally, electrodes located within the PET abnormality are designated as PET positive (P+) and those outside the PET abnormality are designated as PET negative (P-). Using these definitions, the (unitless) SPI is computed as the ratio of the penalized total weighted distance between EEG-positive and PET-positive electrodes and the total number of seizure onset electrodes:

$$SPI = \frac{\sum_{i=1}^{M} w_i d_i (E_i + | P_i +) + \sum_{i=1}^{K} P_i + (\neg E_i +)}{\sum_{i=1}^{M} E_i +} \qquad \text{Eq. (1)}$$

where M is the number of EEG-positive electrodes, K is the number of PET-positive electrodes, and w_i is the weighting factor. In the above equation, the first term in the numerator represents the total weighted distance between all EEG-positive electrodes and the nearest PET-positive electrode; the second term represents then the number of all false-positive PET electrodes (i.e., PET-positive electrodes that are not EEG-positive). Lastly, the denominator reflects the total number of EEG-positive electrodes.

To demonstrate the calculation of the SPI measure, Figure 15.5 shows a (5 × 4) electrode grid with seizure onset electrodes in red and electrodes that are not seizure onset electrodes coded in yellow. In Figure 15.5A the PET abnormality is adjacent to the seizure onset electrodes, resulting in a SPI(onset) value of 2.66, while in Figure 15.5B the PET abnormality is remote to the seizure onset electrodes, resulting in a higher

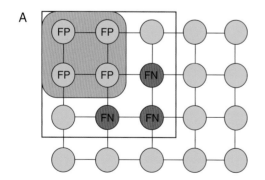
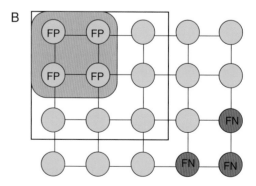

Figure 15.5 An intracranial EEG grid placed on the surface of the brain. Electrophysiologically normal electrodes are yellow, whereas electrodes determined as abnormal (either onset, spread, or frequent spiking) are shown in red. The area with abnormal PET tracer concentration is depicted in gray. Electrodes that are overlaying the PET abnormality but are electrophysiologically normal represent false-positive (FP) cases, whereas electrophysiologically abnormal electrodes not overlaying the PET abnormality represent false-negative (FN) cases. (A) PET abnormality in close spatial proximity to electrophysiologically abnormal electrodes prompts the insertion of an intracranial grid (*black square*) that will include the electrophysiologically abnormal area, whereas (B) a PET abnormality that is distant to the electrophysiologically abnormal area will trigger the insertion of intracranial grid electrodes likely to miss the electrophysiologically abnormal area.

SPI(onset) value of 5.66. In this example, the lower SPI represents a quantitative measure of the closer spatial proximity between PET abnormalities and EEG electrodes. Low SPI values are thus associated with situations in which PET imaging is successful in guiding the placement of an intracranial EEG grid (despite its partially or non-overlapping characteristics).

Subsequently, the PET tracer concentration in finite cortical elements is sampled and the extent and severity of PET abnormalities are objectively assessed in relationship to electrophysiologic information. Initially, the brain is extracted through removal of all extracerebral structures using well-established software tools in the field, such as MRIcro (Smith 2002) or BrainSuite (Shattuck 2001). Despite the best efforts, however, complete removal of all extracerebral structures is hard to achieve, especially in pediatric brains, where the dura mater is difficult to separate from cortex. As a result, the rendering quality of cortical sulci and gyri often varies widely among subjects, and in a large portion of pediatric patients only major cortical landmarks can be recognized. To improve visualization of minor cortical landmarks and achieve consistent rendering quality throughout the patient population, a computationally simple method was developed that takes advantage of the sharp transition between gray and white matter a short distance beneath the brain surface. Initially the brain surface is smoothed using alpha-shapes (Edelsbrunner and Mucke 1994) and a curvilinear shrink operation with 5-mm depth is performed on all surface voxels. This operation removes both the dura mater and the outer cortical layer, thus exposing the deep folding structure of the cortex (Fig. 15.6A). As a result, sharp border zones between white and gray matter are exposed and subsequently projected onto the original (non-shrinked) cortex, visualizing the location of major and minor cortical sulci. The normal surface vector is then calculated in each surface voxel and all normal vectors belonging to an individual finite element are averaged,

yielding one single normal direction for a particular finite element. Following triangulation of the brain surface, the PET tracer concentration in the co-registered PET image volume is then averaged along the inverse normal vector for each surface voxel (usually to a depth of 8 to 10 mm). As a result, 3D functional information derived from the cortical mantle is transferred and texture mapped onto the cortical surface, allowing the visual assessment of functional abnormalities relative to anatomical cortical landmarks (Fig. 15.6A). The functional data in individual finite cortical elements are then evaluated either using hemispheric asymmetry or by comparing each finite element against a normative scale. Hemispheric asymmetry is evaluated based on the asymmetry index (AI(%) = $(L - R)/(0.5(L + R)) \times 100\%$), where L and R is the PET tracer concentration in corresponding finite cortical elements in the left and right hemisphere. Normal asymmetry (mean ± 2 standard deviations [SD]) for five cortical areas (frontal, temporal, parietal, occipital, and central) (Fig. 15.6B) was previously obtained from a normal age-matched population. Figure 15.6C shows the extent of false-positive abnormalities in a normal subject, corresponding to a 5% error rate associated with the 2-SD threshold. (Figures 15.8, 15. 9, and 15.10 subsequently show application of this method in patients with epilepsy.)

The major limitation of hemispheric asymmetry for the definition of abnormal cortical areas is its reliance on the existence of unilateral abnormalities, as one hemisphere is a priori selected as normal. A second limitation is that definition of cortical abnormalities located in both the insular and mesial cortex is problematic. Although there is still no satisfactory solution to objectively define abnormal cortical areas in the insular region, we have extended our integrative approach to allow analysis of the mesial cortex. Objective assessment of the mesial cortex is accomplished by separating the brain into two hemispheres and then rendering each hemisphere separately,

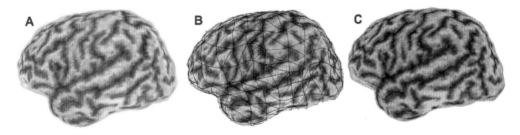

Figure 15.6 Integration of PET and MR images. (A) Inverse gradient fusion of co-registered PET and MR image volumes is used to color-code PET tracer concentration onto the cortical surface. Functional information can then be assessed with respect to anatomical cortical landmarks. (B) A set of finite elements is defined representing five bilateral cortical areas (frontal, temporal, parietal, occipital, and central). PET tracer concentration in these cortical areas is automatically sampled in normal subjects and used to define area-specific normal asymmetry. (C) Abnormal increases of PET tracer concentration (red areas) in a normal subject. Given 256 finite elements per hemisphere, about 12 elements are expected to be outside the normal range at the 5% level.

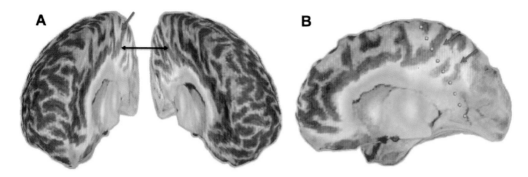

Figure 15.7 Assessment of PET abnormalities in the mesial cortex based on asymmetry. (A) To expose the mesial cortex, the brain is separated at the midplane and each hemisphere is rendered independently. Finite cortical elements are then defined in the mesial plane that spatially correspond between the two hemispheres (*black arrow*). The asymmetry index between PET tracer concentration in corresponding finite cortical elements is then calculated and used to objectively define PET abnormalities (*red arrow*). (B) Right mesial cortex in a representative patient showing decreased PET tracer uptake in the posterior cingulated region. Inserted electrodes showed early spread (yellow), which spatially corresponded with the PET abnormality.

thereby exposing the mesial cortical plane (Fig. 15.7). Finite cortical elements can be then defined on the mesial plane and used to calculate an asymmetry index between homotopic areas in the left and right mesial cortex.

Moreover, decisions about the presence of functional abnormalities at a given location can be also made based on a severity index that is independent from the condition of the contralateral (to the epileptic focus) hemisphere. The severity index is calculated as $(m_i - \mu_i)/\sigma_i$, where m_i is the average tracer concentration of a particular finite cortical element with index i, while μ_i and σ_i are the mean tracer concentration and SD derived from a control group for the same finite element. Values of the severity index within ±2 SD are then assumed to represent functionally normal cortex. Although conceptually preferable, the severity index analysis requires an age-matched database that carries for each finite cortical element the normative mean and SD values. In the absence of such a database and following a careful appraisal of the contralateral hemisphere, the asymmetry index technique is applicable, although the severity index method needs to be used for patient brains that are known to express bilateral abnormalities.

We have used the severity index methodology in the assessment of the clinical accuracy of FDG and ^{11}C-alpha-methyl-L-tryptophan (AMT) PET imaging to characterize epileptogenic tissue in young children (n = 11, ages 1 to 15 years) with intractable neocortical epilepsy (see also Chapter 12). Subdural EEG data were used to define the location of seizure onset and early spread electrodes. In addition, three distinct 10-minute segments of the continuous interictal subdural EEG recordings during the awake state were selected and quantitative interictal parameters (spike frequency and spike amplitude) for all electrode

channels were determined. Clinical performance of FDG and AMT PET imaging was then compared for both ictal (seizure onset and spread) and interictal (spike frequency and amplitude) EEG variables using the SPI (see Eq. (1)) measure (Fig. 15.8). Integrative analysis showed that AMT PET performed better than FDG PET for both seizure onset (SPI AMT 1.7 vs. SPI FDG 2.7) and spike amplitude (SPI AMT 0.8 vs. SPI FDG 4.8), while FDG PET was superior in detecting early seizure spread (SPI AMT 3.4 vs. SPI FDG 0.7). Moreover, there was no difference between AMT and FDG in detecting cortical areas with abnormal spike frequency (SPI AMT 1.7 vs. SPI FDG 1.8).

Integrative analysis of FDG PET and quantitative ictal/interictal subdural EEG data has been also applied to study the spatial relationship between hypometabolic cortical areas and electrophysiologic parameters (Asano et al. 2003; Luat et al. 2005; Fig. 15.9). Applying a similar analysis, Asano et al. (2000) assessed the spatial relationship between AMT PET and epileptic activity on EEG in patients with tuberous sclerosis. The results of this study showed that cortical tubers with AMT uptake greater than or equal to normal cortex are significantly related to epileptiform activity in that lobe and should be resected to achieve a seizure-free outcome, while AMT uptake lower than normal cortex indicated nonepileptic tubers (see also Chapter 12 for a more thorough discussion of AMT PET in tuberous sclerosis).

Finally, to quantitatively assess the spatial relationship among cortical areas of seizure onset, rapid seizure propagation, and hypometabolic cortical regions, we applied integrative PET/EEG analysis in a group of 14 children with refractory neocortical epilepsy (Alkonyi et al. 2009). Normative lobe-specific asymmetry index values (mean ± 2SD) were used as cutoff thresholds for the detection of abnormal glucose

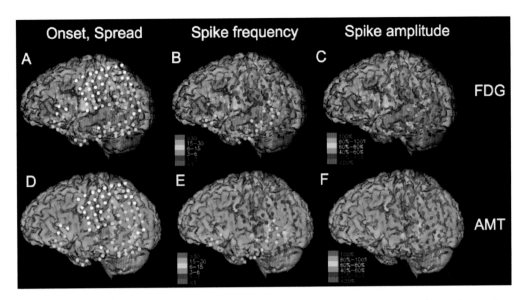

Figure 15.8 Spatial relationship between ictal (A, D) and quantitative interictal (BC, EF) subdural EEG variables and cortical areas of decreased FDG (upper row) and AMT (lower row) uptake in a 6-year-old girl. (Upper row) Multiple areas of glucose hypometabolism (highlighted in red) were objectively marked in the left hemisphere using the asymmetry index. (A) Seizure onset (red electrodes) occurred over a relatively large temporal region with a SPI of 2.7; early spread is indicated in yellow, SPI for spread is 0.7. (B) Electrodes with different interictal spike frequency (red: highest, purple: lowest) yielding a SPI of 1.8. (C) Amplitude of averaged spikes with SPI of 4.8. (Lower row) Areas of increased AMT uptake marked in red. (D) SPI for seizure onset (red electrodes) is considerably lower (1.7) than for FDG, but SPI for early spread (yellow electrodes) is higher (3.4). (E) Spike frequency; SPI = 1.7. (F) Amplitude of averaged spikes, SPI = 0.8.

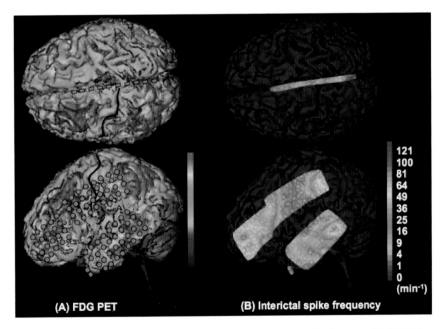

Figure 15.9 Integration of quantitative EEG data with PET to assess the spatial relationship between FDG PET abnormalities and interictal spike frequency. The figure shows data obtained from an 8-year-old boy with medically uncontrolled epilepsy associated with continuous spike-wave during slow-wave sleep. (A) Interictal FDG PET showed multifocal hypermetabolism in the left hemisphere. (B) Interictal spike frequency was tightly correlated with the severity of hypermetabolism. Surgical resection of the multiple lobes in the left hemisphere resulted in a seizure-free outcome (Luat et al. 2005).

metabolic areas in epilepsy patients (Fig. 15.10A,B). Results of this study suggest that cortical areas surrounding FDG PET-defined hypometabolic regions (2-cm border zone area, Fig. 15.10C,D) detect a similar proportion of seizure onset electrodes as do hypometabolic areas (46% vs. 41%) (Alkonyi et al. 2009). Thus, the predictive value of FDG PET is close to 90% if border zone areas are considered for seizure onset localization. These findings strongly support the notion that seizure onset areas often extend beyond

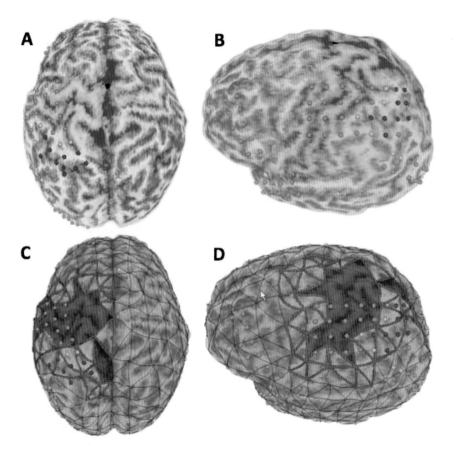

Figure 15.10 Integration of PET, MR, and EEG data to assess the spatial relationship between epileptogenic and hypometabolic cortex. (A) Inverse gradient fusion of co-registered PET data with the extracted cortical surface showing anatomical landmarks in a representative pediatric patient with refractory neocortical epilepsy. EEG grid electrodes are color-coded as red (seizure onset), yellow (early seizure propagation), and green (normal). (B) Following landmark-constrained cortical mapping, finite elements characterizing the frontal, temporal, occipital, parietal, and central cortical territory were automatically defined. Furthermore, location-specific asymmetry thresholds were applied to objectively determine hypometabolic cortical areas (blue). (C, D) Hypometabolic cortical areas (blue) together with the border zone area (finite elements highlighted in purple). It is apparent that seizure onset electrodes (red) are preferentially located in the normometabolic border zone as opposed to hypometabolic cortex.

the hypometabolic cortex to encompass adjacent normometabolic areas, while a large portion of the hypometabolic cortex is not involved in seizure onset or early seizure propagation. As a result, clinical utility of FDG PET in guiding subdural electrode placement is greatly enhanced if grid electrode coverage is extended to at least 2 cm beyond the FDG PET-defined hypometabolic areas (Fig. 15.10C,D).

There are several possible explanations for the observed complementary quality of hypometabolic and epileptogenic cortex. Animal studies have demonstrated that cortical epileptic foci and surrounding cortical zones display different electrophysiologic, metabolic, and neurochemical properties (Liang et al. 1997, 1998; Sherwin et al. 1984; Witte et al. 1994). Moreover, electrophysiologically hyperexcitable cortical regions may show normal metabolism in experimentally induced cortical dysplasia (Redecker et al. 1998). Taken together, it can be hypothesized that the

observed spatial relationship between electrophysiologic characteristics and functional abnormalities may protect cortical areas from ictal involvement and that severely hypometabolic cortex in the vicinity of epileptogenic brain tissue likely represents a functional disconnection from the seizure focus. Further insights into this mechanism are likely to come from the study of structural connectivity between involved brain regions.

STRUCTURAL CONNECTIVITY

Despite the fact that fiber tract anatomy and functional connectivity in brain have been widely studied in nonhuman primates through invasive procedures (Rye 1999), until recently it was not possible to assess fiber tract anatomy and structural connectivity in a living human. As discussed in detail in Chapter 6, with the advent of diffusion tensor imaging (DTI), it is now possible to study connectivity among cortical and subcortical brain areas in vivo. More importantly, quantitative assessment of connectivity between cortical areas appears to be an essential part in our understanding of the mechanisms underlying the origin and maturation of secondary epileptic foci. At present, the relevance of cortical hypometabolic areas observed by PET imaging that are located remotely to the primary seizure focus (and are shown to be electrophysiologically normal) is poorly understood. The fate of such remote functional abnormalities following resection of the primary epileptic focus remains uncertain. Cortical areas showing functional abnormalities on PET either can normalize following resection of the primary focus or may mature to become independent primary epileptic foci. Consequently, one of the goals of DTI in epilepsy is to predict whether a remote functional abnormality will likely become a future seizure onset area that needs to be resected, or whether this area will normalize and thus can be spared during surgery.

Although DTI provides directional information at the voxel level, it provides no explicit information about the link between neighboring voxels. The task to connect individual voxels according to their mathematical properties and to create a fiber tract that can be analyzed quantitatively remains problematic even today. In the past few years a number of different methods have been proposed to characterize fiber tracts in vivo based on DTI information. The most common fiber-tracking algorithms usually generate a fiber tract by following the direction corresponding to the largest eigenvalue of the diffusion tensor and at the same time observing certain consistency constraints (Conturo et al. 1999; Mori et al. 1999, 2002). These deterministic techniques allow only a very limited measure of connectivity, mostly based on the ratio between the number of fibers terminating in a target region normalized to those originating from a source region. Moreover, although deterministic models proved to be mathematically stable and computationally efficient, many, especially minor, pathways known to exist based on dissection and tract tracer studies could not be reproduced using deterministic fiber tracking. Other attempts have concentrated on probabilistic methods employing Monte Carlo simulations to determine the likelihood of a particle to diffuse in a particular direction based on the local values of the diffusion tensor components (Koch et al. 2002). More importantly, probabilistic methods have shown potential to detect minor fiber tracts, as they incorporate uncertainty stemming from both measurement noise as well as from the applied imperfect diffusion model into the calculation (Tuch et al. 2002). Apart from providing a quantitative method for describing regional connectivity in the brain based on probabilis-

tic measures, stochastic methods have also been shown to be computationally superior to deterministic methods in the presence of fiber crossings. Stochastic methods allow fibers to pass through low-anisotropy areas (which is impossible for deterministic methods) as well as to penetrate deeper into gray matter areas where the fibers start and end (Behrens et al. 2003). Due to their superior performance, probabilistic methods appear to be well suited for quantitative connectivity studies in the epileptic brain, where the relationship among cortical territories, white matter fiber bundles, functional PET abnormalities, and electrophysiologic measures is largely unclear. Consequently, there is a need to extend integrative techniques so that they allow quantitative evaluation of the relationship between the proximity of primary to remote PET abnormalities with respect to the location of major fiber bundles.

Recently, Friman et al. (2006) proposed a Bayesian approach in which the local probability density function in each voxel is based on the angular distribution of the primary eigenvectors in all 18-connect neighboring voxels. This probability distribution is then multiplied with a prior distribution giving preference for continuation in the previous-step direction and evaluated at a large number of predefined unit length vectors obtained by a fourfold tessalation of an icosahedron. To calculate a fiber path originating from a predefined seed point, random samples are drawn from the probability distribution and a fiber path is created that terminates when the local fractional anisotropy (FA) decreases below a preselected value. For each seed point, a large number of paths (typically 100 to 1,000) are created that originate from a source region. Although this model assumes only one fiber direction in each voxel, deviations from this single-fiber model (such as fiber crossing/convergence) are translated into uncertainty in the posterior distribution. This uncertainty leads then locally to an increased probability of randomly sampled fibers to diverge into multiple directions, thus allowing a certain portion of fiber paths to cross low-anisotropy areas, hence realizing also minor fiber tracks.

We have adapted the Bayesian probabilistic method to derive a measure of connectivity strength between cortical regions. To calculate the connectivity strength between a source and target region, the average probability p_i is calculated for each individual fiber path i of length N_i (equation 1 in Fig. 15.11), where p_{ij} is the randomly sampled probability of voxel j (j = 1,.N_i). Because only a subset of fibers originating from the seed region will terminate in the target region, all path probabilities p_i are subsequently normalized to the sampling space (total number of fiber paths k = 1,...,M) as p_i' (equation 2 in Fig. 15.11). Finally, the normalized probability score of connection between two regions A

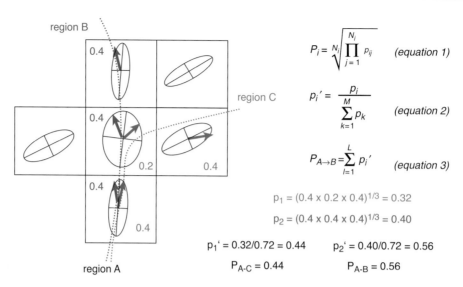

$$P_i = \sqrt[N_i]{\prod_{j=1}^{N_i} p_{ij}} \qquad \textit{(equation 1)}$$

$$p_i' = \frac{p_i}{\sum_{k=1}^{M} p_k} \qquad \textit{(equation 2)}$$

$$P_{A \to B} = \sum_{l=1}^{L} p_i' \qquad \textit{(equation 3)}$$

$p_1 = (0.4 \times 0.2 \times 0.4)^{1/3} = 0.32$

$p_2 = (0.4 \times 0.4 \times 0.4)^{1/3} = 0.40$

$p_1' = 0.32/0.72 = 0.44 \qquad p_2' = 0.40/0.72 = 0.56$

$P_{A\text{-}C} = 0.44 \qquad\qquad P_{A\text{-}B} = 0.56$

Figure 15.11 Assessment of the connectivity strength between cortical regions using probabilistic fiber tracking. Starting from a seed region (region A), random samples are drawn from the calculated probability distribution function in each image voxel, yielding ~10,000 paths originating from the source region. The average probability p_i for each path is calculated (equation 1) and subsequently normalized so that the total probability to reach any brain region equals to 1 (p_i', equation 2). The connectivity strength between two cortical regions (A-B or A-C) is then calculated as the sum of all path probabilities terminating in the particular target region ($P_{A\text{-}B}$ or $P_{A\text{-}C}$). In the example above, the total probability for the two fibers is 0.72 (= 0.32 + 0.40) and the connectivity strength to reach region B is higher than to reach region C (0.56 > 0.44).

and B is obtained as $P_{A\text{-}B}$ (equation 3 in Fig. 15.11) with the index 1 (L < M) representing all fiber paths connecting the two regions.

In preliminary studies, we have applied this approach to the study of structural connectivity between cortical areas representing seizure onset and cortical areas showing remote functional abnormalities on FDG PET. Initially, finite cortical elements were defined representing primary and remote functional abnormalities (Fig. 15.12A–C). As fiber tracts originate and terminate from the border between gray and white matter, a white matter mask was initially created from a high-resolution T1-weighted MR volume and a white matter border zone of 5-mm thickness was created (Fig. 15.12D). Finite surface elements were subsequently extended 30 mm into the brain and their overlap with the white matter border zone constituted white matter seed/target regions. The connectivity strength between the primary seizure focus and the remote functional abnormalities was then calculated using Eq. (3) in the ipsilateral hemisphere as well as for corresponding finite elements in the contralateral hemisphere. Fiber paths were color-coded according to their probability from red (low-probability fiber) to white (high-probability fiber) (Fig. 15.12E,F). Results of this study showed that connectivity strength between the primary seizure focus and remote cortical abnormalities is decreased ipsilaterally, as compared to corresponding areas in the contralateral hemisphere (Fig. 15.12E,F). Although further work is required to validate this finding, the observed decrease in structural connectivity ipsilaterally is possibly due to

protective mechanisms, causing a functional disconnect of the focus from connected cortical areas.

MULTIMODALITY DATABASES

The creation of databases that allow storage, integration, and sharing of both imaging and non-imaging data between investigators with different scientific backgrounds in easily accessible archives is one of the main goals of the newly emerging field of neuroinformatics. Neuroinformatics is becoming increasingly important in the brain imaging field, as an unprecedented amount of data is acquired using complementing modalities that need to be analyzed based on an overarching strategy (Barinaga et al. 2003; Van Horn et al. 2001, 2004). Following the model of other scientific fields that were revolutionized through the implementation of powerful database structures and associated mining techniques—such as the GenBank (www.ncbi.nlm.nih.gov) for the field of genomics or the Protein Data Bank (www.rcsb.org/pdb) for the field of proteomics—several neuroimaging databases have been generated in the past decade to fully mine the information present in the acquired data sets. Prominent examples are the ICBM database (www.loni.ucla.edu) that includes PET, MRI, fMRI, EEG, and MEG modalities (Toga et al. 2002) and the BrainMapDBJ (www.brainmapDBJ.org) and the ECHBD (www.dhbr.neuro.ki.se/ECHBD) databases, which both integrate PET and fMRI image data (Fox and Lancaster 2002).

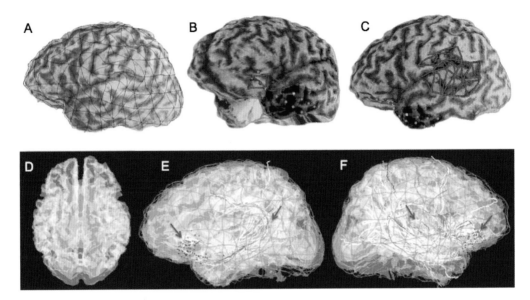

Figure 15.12 Integration of PET, EEG, and DTI data to study cortico-cortical connectivity between the primary seizure focus and electrophysiologically normal functional abnormalities. (A) Surface-rendered FDG PET tracer concentration in finite cortical elements of a representative patient. (B) Abnormally decreased FDG uptake highlighted in blue together with an intracranial 8 × 2 EEG grid showing onset (red), early spread (yellow), and electrophysiologically normal (green) electrodes. (C) Cortical elements representing remote functional abnormality that were shown to be electrophysiologically normal. (D) White matter mantle of 5-mm thickness underlying the cortex. Finite elements defined on the cortical surface are extended into the brain and their cross-section with the white matter mantle identifies the seed/target regions. (E) Fiber paths originating from seeds in white matter beneath the seizure onset zone (red arrow) and terminating in white matter beneath the remote functional abnormality (blue arrow). The connectivity score was calculated as 0.045. (F) Corresponding fiber paths in the contralateral hemisphere. The connectivity score was calculated as 0.107, which is more than twice as large as in the ipsilateral hemisphere.

These databases were designed with the goal of combining the expertise of computer programmers, statisticians, and basic researchers in an attempt to develop neuroinformatics tools for interdisciplinary collaborations in brain research.

In addition to these large multi-institutional archives that aim at standardization of a large amount of collected data sets, there is a need for smaller, locally managed multimodality database structures that are specific to a particular project using the various imaging modalities summarized in this volume. As an example, local database structures are beginning to be routinely used in the context of patient preparation for epilepsy surgery that incorporate a whole array of available image data volumes (PET, SPECT, MR, DTI, fMRI), electrophysiologic data sets (electrode positions, location of seizure onset and frequent spiking electrodes), and clinical information (e.g., seizure semiology, epilepsy duration, age of seizure onset). An important feature of these newly emerging databases is the fast and highly integrative display of processed 3D-rendered image volumes that visualizes a combination of diverse datasets in native space. Moreover, within this framework the user also has access to a whole suite of computational tools for the quantitative analysis of spatial/temporal relationships among the

diverse multimodal parameter sets. Advanced statistical methods are then applied to quantitatively relate the different datasets both within the patient as well as across other patient or normative groups. Consequently, such 3D image database structures have the potential to generate quantitative information that characterize the abnormal state of the brain in much finer detail than would be possible using each individual modality, and are likely to contribute to the discovery of new causal relationships between the various abnormalities associated with epilepsy.

To demonstrate the basic concepts of small-scale multimodality databases, we describe here the design of a clinically managed database structure developed at our institution that was developed to study relationships between functional and electrophysiologic parameters in epilepsy patients who are being evaluated for resective surgery (Muzik et al. 2007). An important design focus was the easy-to-navigate access to the data via a 3D display module, so that users could grasp the results of their queries in an intuitive way (Fig. 15.13). Conceptually, the database is structured into three hierarchical levels, consisting of a patient, cluster, and cortical element level. At the highest level (patient level), clinical variables are stored such as age of patient, age at first seizure, seizure type, seizure

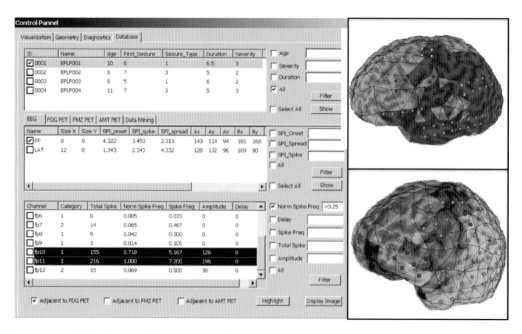

Figure 15.13 Integration of PET, MR, and EEG data into an XML-based database. A focus of the database was an easy-to-navigate visual representation of relationships between PET and EEG data in 3D space. The database is conceptually structured into a patient level carrying clinical data, an intermediate cluster level representing large-scale anatomical information, and the lowest, finite cortical element level. On the right, two representative brains are shown where the relationship between onset electrodes (red) and functional PET abnormalities (blue) can be assessed in 3D space. Electrodes representing early spread are rendered in yellow and electrophysiologically normal electrodes in green. Using such integrative 3D display, one can appreciate that onset electrodes are preferably located at the border zone of PET abnormalities.

severity or seizure duration. As the cortical distribution of each PET tracer for detection of epileptic foci (e.g., FDG, FMZ, AMT) is distinct, the database includes separate entries for the different PET tracers. The lowest level is given by the cortical element level, which provides information with regard to the location of functional data in finite cortical elements at different resolution levels. Moreover, the surface coordinates of each EEG grid electrode are also stored at this lowest level. Electrophysiologic parameters representing seizure category (onset, spread, spiking), interictal spike frequency, or normalized interictal spike frequency can be then mapped onto a particular grid electrode. Given the location of each electrode, this environment automatically determines the corresponding cortical element at various resolution levels and reports the corresponding SPI values for seizure onset, seizure spread, and interictal spiking. Lastly, the intermediate cluster level allows the grouping of cortical volume elements either into anatomical territories (e.g., lobes) or into functional clusters according to PET or EEG data. To accommodate the flexibility of an evolving database schema, an XML-based approach was employed. In this way, the database not only allows a graceful inclusion of additional modalities at each of the three levels, but also ensures easy scalability of the system.

FUTURE DIRECTIONS IN MULTIMODALITY DATA INTEGRATION

Present trends in multimodality neuroimaging point in two directions that are likely to have an impact on the efficiency and increased information content of both data acquisition and analysis of neuroimaging data. The first is the development of newly emerging hybrid PET/MR scanners that are able to acquire both PET and MR data simultaneously. The second important development is the emergence of advanced database structures that include interactive 3D visualization and powerful data-mining tools. These advanced databases will provide an overarching data-integration structure for all information, thereby allowing quantitative assessment of relationships among qualitatively diverse parameter sets (image-based, electrophysiology-based, and clinical) both within a patient as well as across well-defined patient groups.

Simultaneous PET/MR Acquisition

In the past decade PET/CT showed the added value of multimodality image acquisition for cancer research, and this form of imaging became within a few years the state of the art in diagnostic oncology. In fact, since 2000, the world market share of PET/CT scanners increased from less than 5% to more than 95%, thereby completely replacing dedicated PET scanners. The added value provided by combined PET and CT imaging has improved both the localization and staging of tumors in addition to significantly increasing patient throughput. Although current PET/CT scanners acquire the image data sequentially (initial helical CT scan is followed by multiple-bed-position PET imaging), this is usually of little consequence for tumor assessment, as only the overall PET tracer distribution, established following an extended uptake period, is of clinical interest. In contrast, there are fundamental advantages to the *simultaneous* acquisition of PET and MR data for neuroimaging that reach far beyond simple co-registration of PET and MR image volumes (which can be relatively easily performed for rigid objects such as the brain within a skull). The true advantage of simultaneous PET/MR acquisition is that limitations of one modality (e.g., limited resolution in PET or the limited functional information inherent in MR) can be offset by data derived from the complementing modality. This exchange of complementary information can be taken into account already at a very basic hardware level, so that many issues, at present only poorly accounted for during image post-processing, become irrelevant. There has also been a paucity of research focused on direct comparisons of imaging capabilities in PET and MR when it comes to brain function. The opportunity, for example, to compare perfusion measures, cerebral vascular hemodynamics, and brain metabolism directly under the same circumstances will likely lead to new concepts and a deeper understanding of the various physiologic mechanisms that accompany the origin of epileptic seizures.

Specifically in the context of pediatric epilepsy patient management, the relevance of simultaneous PET and MR acquisition is extraordinary. At present, all epilepsy patients undergo MR and PET imaging on two separate occasions, doubling the time/frequency of sedation (important in pediatric patients) and on-scanner time. The simultaneous acquisition of PET and MR will allow a more efficient use of both patient time and staff resources and would significantly improve the logistics of patient scheduling as well as enrollment into research studies. More importantly, the combination of various PET tracers with DTI (fiber tract connectivity), MR volumetry (morphology), and BOLD MR (blood flow) acquired simultaneously is likely to bring new insights into the study of seizure generation and propagation. As an example, PET/MR imaging could provide the unique opportunity to measure simultaneously both presynaptic (short echo proton MR spectroscopy) and postsynaptic (^{11}C-flumazenil PET) aspects of GABA neurotransmission during interictal (and possibly ictal) periods. Moreover, the

combination of PET with high-resolution MR spectroscopy (MRS) could provide a significant advantage, as a preliminary PET image (reconstructed using data from the initial part of the PET study) could be used to guide the definition of several large MRS regions. This approach would be more efficient than whole brain coverage of MRS, especially in the case of substances such as GABA or glutamate that require a prohibitively long MRS scan time to yield clinically acceptable sensitivity.

In addition, simultaneous acquisition of anatomical and functional data opens the door to significant methodological improvements, which will become common even in clinical routine. Among these improvements is the automated correction of patient motion, correction of partial volume effects, and the noninvasive determination of the blood input function as a prerequisite for absolute PET quantification. With regard to motion correction, the simultaneous acquisition of dynamic PET data together with short MR navigator sequences is able to account almost completely for motion in pediatric image scans. For example, a whole brain anatomical EPI MR scan can be easily acquired in about 5 seconds; this can be timed so that these scans coincide with the dynamic frames of a PET study. As the EPI scans show anatomical (T2-weighted) images that are identical in time (unlike PET images, in which the image pattern changes according to tracer kinetics), automated algorithms can be implemented that automatically account for motion of each frame at a very basic sinogram level. As a result, dynamic PET images can be reconstructed that are largely free of motion artifacts. Moreover, due to the limited spatial resolution of PET scanners, it is currently difficult to account for partial volume effects in reconstructed PET images. Using a high-resolution structural MR image and applying reasonable assumptions (e.g., that the concentration of tracer is homogeneously distributed in white matter), the spillover of white matter into gray matter structures can be calculated and the true concentration in gray matter structures obtained (Baete et al. 2000, 2004; Lipinski et al. 1997). Again, such a correction can be implemented directly in the reconstruction algorithm, so that the resulting images are largely free of white matter partial volume effects. Finally, structural information from an inversion recovery MR sequence, optimized for blood flow, can be used to exactly determine geometric factors for large brain vessels (e.g., carotid artery or venous sinus), which in turn can be used to model partial volume distortions of the vessels. Correction of partial volume of the vessels then allows the noninvasive determination of a correct arterial input function in every pediatric patient for subsequent full absolute quantification of kinetic PET data using compartmental modeling.

Instrumentation Challenges

At present, the main technical challenge in the construction of a commercial PET/MR scanner is the problem of converting scintillation events into electrical signals with subsequent amplification in the presence of a high magnetic field. Typically this functionality is performed by photomultiplier tubes (PMTs) that feature high gain (~10^6) and low excess noise and are insensitive to temperature fluctuations. Unfortunately, PMTs cannot operate in a magnetic field, and a new generation of photo amplifiers needs to be developed that are insensitive to high magnetic fields. The most promising of the newly, MR compatible, photo amplifiers are avalanche photo diodes (APDs) and silicon photo multipliers (SiPM). APDs are cheap and can be produced in large size and numbers but have only a small gain (<10^3) and are extremely sensitive to temperature and voltage fluctuation. Although SiPM have a gain similar to PMTs, they are small (detection area ~1 mm^2), expensive, and sensitive to both bias voltage and temperature fluctuations and require corrections for crosstalk between the microcells. The first prototype PET/MR scanner was built by Siemens in 2008 using a 3T TIM Trio MR device with a PET brain insert (BrainPET, 36-cm aperture, Fig. 15.14) using lutetium oxy-orthosilicate (LSO) scintillation crystals and APD technology. A newer design (projected to be commercially available in 2012) will feature an integrated PET/MR system, where the LSO PET detector ring is placed within the gradient coils. This system will have a 60-cm aperture

and will allow both brain and whole body PET/MR imaging. Although uncertain at present, it can be expected that the impact of simultaneous PET/MR acquisition for neuroimaging will be comparable to that of PET/CT for oncology and will lead to new paradigms in brain research.

Integrative Databases

Newly emerging database structures will allow integration of quantitative results obtained from a wide range of modalities into one consistent framework for advanced data mining and 3D visualization. The goal of these advanced databases is to include virtually all data associated with a patient in a consistent and searchable computational framework. Modalities included are patient history records, seizure semiology, multiple processed 3D image volumes, histology data, genetic information as well as constantly updated outcome data. An important characteristic of these emerging database structures is that they are highly dynamic so they adjust gracefully to new requirements as they arise, instead of being based on a fixed design common to traditional database systems. The leading candidate for generating such flexible database structures is the XML (eXtensible Markup Language) model (Chebotko et al. 2004; Lu et al. 2003; Muzik et al. 2007) due to its flexibility, extensibility, and scalability. The flexibility of XML database structures will subsequently allow the combination of patients with similar disease within a common reference frame,

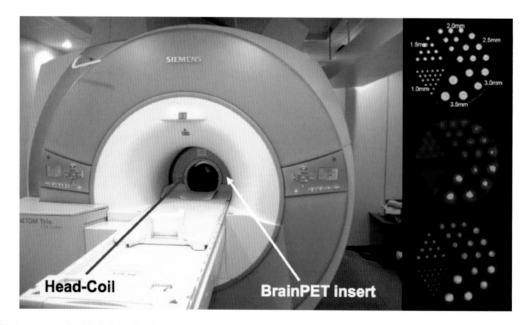

Figure 15.14 Prototype of a PET/MR device from Siemens featuring a 3T TIM Trio scanner with a brain PET insert. The insert (BrainPET) uses lutetium oxy-orthosilicate (LSO) scintillation crystals and avalanche photo diode (APD) technology to allow simultaneous acquisition of MR and PET data. The insert on the right shows simultaneously acquired MR and FDG PET images of a Derenzo phantom.

allowing meta-analysis of data patterns distributed over many modalities.

SUMMARY AND CONCLUSIONS

Advances in imaging technologies such as molecular imaging using multiple-tracer PET studies, SPECT, structural and functional MR imaging, and quantitative electrophysiologic cortical mapping provide today an abundance of qualitatively diverse brain datasets. In the past, qualitatively different datasets have been analyzed largely independently, and results of such studies have been integrated merely qualitatively. As it becomes more and more appreciated that normal brain function is dependent on the interactions between specialized cortical regions that process information within local and global networks, current efforts focus on the improved quantitative integration of the acquired multimodality data sets to obtain a more detailed understanding about process interaction in a complex biological system.

Current software developments in the medical field concentrate on the design of cohesive computational frameworks that are directed towards an understanding of qualitatively different measurements in a larger context. Important features of these newly emerging integrative computational frameworks are the advanced 3D visualization of processed image volumes and the quantitative description of data properties, so that relationships in anatomical and functional domains between complementing modalities can be expressed mathematically. It is believed that such an approach is not simply additive but possesses an amplifying effect, as the information entailed in one modality is used to both enhance and re-interpret information derived from complementing modalities. By taking advantage of these advanced data-integration schemes, quantitative results are subsequently combined into data structures that provide a consistent framework for the application of advanced data-mining techniques. Such multimodality database structures hold promise of providing new insights into the formation, identification, and maturation of epileptic foci. A better understanding of the relationship between structural, functional, and electrophysiologic data might lead to new approaches in epilepsy surgery and will likely improve the clinical management of patients suffering from intractable epilepsy.

REFERENCES

Alkonyi, B., C. Juhasz, O. Muzik, et al. 2009. Quantitative brain surface mapping of cortical hypometabolism in neocortical epilepsy. *Epilepsia* 87: 77–87.

Asano, E., D. C. Chugani, O. Muzik, et al. 2000. Multimodality imaging for improved detection of epileptogenic foci in tuberous sclerosis complex. *Neurology* 54(10): 1976–84.

Asano, E., O. Muzik, A. Shah, et al. 2003. Quantitative interictal subdural EEG analyses in children with neocortical epilepsy. *Epilepsia* 44(3): 425–34.

Asano, E., C. Juhász, A. Shah, et al. 2005. Origin and propagation of epileptic spasms delineated on electrocorticography. *Epilepsia* 46(7): 1086–97.

Baete, K., J. Nuyts, K. Van Laere, et al. 2000. Evaluation of anatomy based reconstruction for partial volume correction in brain FDG-PET. *Neuroimage* 23(1): 305–17.

Baete, K., J. Nuyts, W. Van Paesschen, et al. 2004. Anatomical-based FDG-PET reconstruction for the detection of hypo-metabolic regions in epilepsy. *IEEE Transactions Medical Imaging* 23(4): 510–9.

Barinaga, M. 2003. Still debated, brain image archives are catching on. *Science* 300 (5616): 43–5.

Basser, P. J., and C. Pierpaoli. 1998. A simplified method to measure the diffusion tensor from seven MR images. *Magnetic Resonance in Medicine* 39: 928–34.

Behrens, T. E., M. W. Woolrich, M. Jenkinson, et al. 2003. Characterization and propagation of uncertainty in diffusion-weighted MR imaging. *Magnetic Resonance in Medicine* 50(5): 1077–88.

Bruggemann, J. M., S. S. Som, J. A. Lawson, et al. 2004. Application of statistical parametric mapping to SPET in the assessment of intractable childhood epilepsy. *European Journal of Nuclear Medicine Molecular Imaging* 31(3): 369–77.

Caselles, V., R. Kimmel, and G. Sapiro. 1997. Geodesic active contours. *International Journal of Computer Vision* 22: 61–79.

Chebotko, A., D. Liu, M. Atay, et al. 2005. *Reconstructing XML sub-trees from relational storage of XML documents.* In: Proceedings of the 2nd International Workshop on XML Schema and Data Management (XSDM), 78–87.

Conturo, T. E., N. F. Lori, T. S. Cull TS, et al. 1999. Tracking neuronal fiber pathways in the living human brain. *Proceedings of the National Academy of Sciences U S A* 96(18): 10422–7.

Cootes, T. F., and C. I. Taylor. 2001. *Statistical models of appearance for computer vision.* Technical report, University of Manchester, 2001. http://www.isbe.man.ac.uk/bim/refs.html

Dale, A. M., B. Fischl, and M. I. Sereno. 1999. Cortical surface-based analysis. I. Segmentation and surface reconstruction. *Neuroimage* 9(2): 179–94.

Drury, Heather A., et al. 1999. In Arthur W. Toga (Ed.), *Brain warping.* Academic Press, 337–63.

Edelsbrunner, H., and E. P. Mucke. 1994. Three-dimensional alpha shapes. *ACM Transactions on Graphics* 13(1): 43–72.

Engel, J, Jr., T. R. Henry, M. W. Risinger, et al. 1990. Presurgical evaluation for partial epilepsy: relative contributions of chronic depth-electrode recordings versus FDG-PET and scalp-sphenoidal ictal EEG. *Neurology* 40: 1670–77.

Fischl, B., M. I. Sereno, and A. M. Dale. 1999. Cortical surface-based analysis. II: Inflation, flattening, and a surface-based coordinate system. *Neuroimage* 9(2): 195–207.

Fischl, B., D. H. Salat, E. Busa, et al. 2002. Whole brain segmentation: automated labeling of neuroanatomical structures in the human brain. *Neuron* 33(3): 341–55.

Fischl, B., A. van der Kouwe, C. Destrieux, et al. 2004. Automatically parcellating the human cerebral cortex. *Cerebral Cortex* 14(1): 11–22.

Fox, P., and J. Lancaster. 2002. Mapping context and content: the BrainMap model. *Nature Reviews Neuroscience* 3: 319–21.

Friman, O., G. Farnebäck, and C. F. Westin. 2006. A Bayesian approach for stochastic white matter tractography. *IEEE Transactions Medical Imaging* 25(8): 965–78.

Friston, K. J., C. D. Frith, P. F. Liddle, et al. 1991. Comparing functional (PET) images: the assessment of significant change. *Journal of Cerebral Blood Flow Metabolism* 11(4): 690–9.

Gu, X. Y., T. F. Wang, P. M. Chan, et al. 2004. Genus zero surface conformal mapping and its application to brain surface mapping. *IEEE Transactions Medical Imaging* 23(8): 949–58.

Hurdal, M., and K. Stephenson. 2004. Cortical cartography using the discrete conformal approach of circle packings. *Neuroimage* 23: S119–S28.

Juhász, C., D. C. Chugani, O. Muzik, et al. 2000. Electroclinical correlates of flumazenil and fluorodeoxyglucose PET abnormalities in lesional epilepsy. *Neurology* 55(6): 825–34.

Juhász, C., D. C. Chugani, O. Muzik, et al. 2000b. Is epileptogenic cortex truly hypometabolic on interictal positron emission tomography? *Annals of Neurology* 48, 1: 88–96.

Juhász, C., M. E. Behen, O. Muzik, et al. 2001. Bilateral prefrontal and temporal neocortical hypometabolism in children with epilepsy and aggression. *Epilepsia* 42: 991–1001.

Juhász, C., E. Asano, A. Shah, et al. 2009. Focal decreases of cortical GABAA receptor binding remote from the primary seizure focus: what do they indicate? *Epilepsia* 50(2): 240–50.

Kagawa, K., D. C. Chugani, E. Asano, et al. 2005. Epilepsy surgery outcome in children with tuberous sclerosis complex evaluated with alpha-[11C]methyl-L-tryptophan positron emission tomography (PET). *Journal of Child Neurology* 20(5): 429–38.

Kim, Y. K., D. S. Lee, S. K. Lee, et al. 2002. (18)F-FDG PET in localization of frontal lobe epilepsy: comparison of visual and SPM analysis. *Journal of Nuclear Medicine* 43: 1167–74.

Koch, M. A., D. G. Norris, and M. Hund-Georgiadis. 2002. An investigation of functional and anatomical connectivity using magnetic resonance imaging. *Neuroimage* 16: 241–50.

Lee, J. J., W. J. Kang, D. S. Lee, et al. 2005. Diagnostic performance of 18F-FDG PET and ictal 99mTc-HMPAO SPET in pediatric temporal lobe epilepsy: quantitative analysis by statistical parametric mapping, statistical probabilistic anatomical map, and subtraction ictal SPET. *Seizure* 14: 213–20.

Liang, F., and E. G. Jones. 1997. Zif268 and Fos-like immunoreactivity in tetanus toxin-induced epilepsy: reciprocal changes in the epileptic focus and the surround. *Brain Research* 778, 281–92.

Liang, F., L. D. Le, and E. G. Jones. 1998. Reciprocal up- and down-regulation of BDNF mRNA in tetanus toxin-induced epileptic focus and inhibitory surround in cerebral cortex. *Cerebral Cortex* 8, 481–91.

Lipinski, B., H. Herzog, E. Rota Kops, et al. 1997. Expectation maximization reconstruction of positron emission tomography images using anatomical magnetic resonance information. *IEEE Transactions Medical Imaging* 16(2): 129–36.

Lohmann, G. 1998. Extracting line representations of sulcal gyral patterns in MR images of the human brain. *IEEE Transactions Medical Imaging* 17:1040–8.

Lu, S., M. Atay, D. Liu, et al. 2003. A new inlining algorithm for mapping XML DTDs to relational schemas. In: *Proceedings of the 1st International Workshop on XML Schema and Data Management*, 167–84.

Luat, A. F., E. Asano, C. Juhász, et al. 2005. Relationship between brain glucose metabolism positron emission tomography (PET) and electroencephalography (EEG) in children with continuous spike-and-wave activity during slow-wave sleep. *Journal of Child Neurology* 20: 682–90.

Malladi, R., J. A. Sethian, and B. C. Vemuri, 1995. Shape modeling with front propogation: A level set approach. *IEEE Transactions on Pattern Analysis and Machine Intelligence* 17(2), 158–75.

Miller M., A. Banerjee, G. Christensen, et al. 1997. Statistical methods in computational anatomy. *Statistical Methods in Medical Research* 6: 267–99.

Minoshima, S., K. A. Frey, R. A. Koeppe, et al. 1995. A diagnostic approach in Alzheimer's disease using three-dimensional stereotactic surface projections of fluorine–18-FDG PET. *Journal of Nuclear Medicine* 36: 1238–48.

Mori, S., B. J. Crain, V. P. Chacko, et al. 1999. Three dimensional tracking of axonal projection in the brain by magnetic resonance imaging. *Annals of Neurology* 45: 265–9.

Mori, S., W. E. Kaufmann, C. Davatzikos, et al. 2002. Imaging cortical association tracts in the human brain using diffusion-tensor-based axonal tracking. *Magnetic Resonance in Medicine* 47: 215–23.

Morris, K., F. Bardenhagen, T. J. O'Brien, et al. 2000. An anatomical correlation between language mapping by functional MRI with that by electrical cortical stimulation mapping. *Neurology* 54 (Suppl 3): A108.

Murphy, M. A., T. J. O'Brien, K. Morris, et al. 2004. Multimodality image-guided surgery for the treatment of medically refractory epilepsy. *Journal of Neurosurgery* 100: 452–62.

Muzik, O., D. C. Chugani, C. Shen, et al. 1998. An objective method for localization of cortical asymmetries using positron emission tomography to aid in surgical resection of epileptic foci. *Computer Aided Surgery* 3: 74–82.

Muzik, O., D. C. Chugani, C. Juhász, et al. 2000. Statistical parametric mapping: assessment of application in children. *Neuroimage* 12(5): 538–49.

Muzik, O., E. A. da Silva, C. Juhász, et al. 2000b. Intracranial EEG versus flumazenil and glucose PET in children with extratemporal lobe epilepsy. *Neurology* 54(1): 171–9.

Muzik, O., D. C. Chugani, G. Zou, et al. 2007. Multimodality data integration in epilepsy. *International Journal of Biomedical Imaging* 2007: 139–63.

Osher, S., and J. Sethian. 1988. Fronts propagating with curvature-dependent speed: Algorithms based on Hamilton-Jacobi formulations. *Journal of Computers in Physics* 79: 12–49.

Poliakov, A., K. Hinshaw, C. Rosse, et al. 1999. Integration and visualization of multimodality brain data for language mapping. *Proceedings of the AMIA Symposium* 349–53.

Redecker, C., M. Lutzenburg, P. Gressens, et al. 1998. Excitability changes and glucose metabolism in experimentally induced focal cortical dysplasias. *Cerebral Cortex* 8, 623–34.

Richardson, M. P., M. J. Koepp, D. J. Brooks, et al. 1998. 11C-flumazenil PET in neocortical epilepsy. *Neurology* 51: 485–92.

Rosenberger, L. R., J. Zeck, M. M. Berl, et al. 2009. Interhemispheric and intrahemispheric language reorganization in complex partial epilepsy. *Neurology* 72(21): 1830–6.

Rye, D. B. 1999. Tracking neural pathways with MRI. *Trends Neuroscience* 22(9): 373–4.

Sisodiya, S. M., J. M. Stevens, D. R. Fish, et al. 1996. The demonstration of gyral abnormalities in patients with cryptogenic partial epilepsy using three-dimensional MRI. *Archives of Neurology* 53(1): 28–34.

Sherwin, A., F. Quesney, S. Gauthier, et al. 1984. Enzyme changes in actively spiking areas of human epileptic cerebral cortex. *Neurology* 34: 927–33.

Smith, S. M., M. Jenkinson, M. W. Woolrich, et al. 2004. Advances in functional and structural MR image analysis and implementation as FSL. *Neuroimage* 23 Suppl 1: S208–19.

Shattuck, D. W., S. R. Sandor-Leahy, K. A. Schaper, et al. 2001. Magnetic resonance image tissue classification using a partial volume model. *Neuroimage* 13 (5): 856–76.

So, E. L. 2002. Role of neuroimaging in the management of seizure disorders. *Mayo Clinic Proceedings* 77(11): 1251–64.

Terzopoulos D, et al. 1987. Elastically deformable models. *Computer Graphics* 21(4): 205–14.

Thiel, A., K. Herholz, H-M. Von Stockhausen, et al. 1998. Localization of language-related cortex with 15O-labeled water PET in patients with gliomas. *Neuroimage* 7(4): 284–95.

Thompson, P. M., and A. W. Toga. 2002. A framework for computational anatomy. *Computing and Visualization in Science* 5: 13–34.

Thompson, P. M., C. Schwartz, and A. W. Toga. 1996. High-resolution random mesh algorithms for creating a probabilistic 3-D surface atlas of the human brain. *Neuroimage* 3: 19–34.

Toga, A. 2002. Neuroimage databases: The good, the bad and the ugly. *Nature Reviews Neuroscience* 3: 302–9.

Tuch, D. S., T. G. Reese, M. R. Wiegell, et al. 2002. High angular resolution diffusion imaging reveals intravoxel white matter fiber heterogeneity. *Magnetic Resonance in Medicine* 48(4): 577–82.

Valiant, M., C. Davatzikos, and B. N. Bryan. 1996. *Finding 3-D parametric representations of the deep cortical folds. IEEE Mathematical Methods in Biomedical Image Analysis workshop*, San Francisco.

Van Bogaert, P., P. David, C. A. Gillain, et al. 1998. Perisylvian dysgenesis. Clinical, EEG, MRI and glucose metabolism features in 10 patients. *Brain* 121: 2229–38.

Van Horn, J. D., J. S. Grethe, P. Kostelec, et al. 2001. The Functional Magnetic Resonance Imaging Data Center (fMRIDC): the challenges and rewards of large-scale databasing of neuroimaging studies. *Philosophical Transactions of the Royal Society of London B Biological Sciences* 356: 1323–39.

Van Horn, J. D., S. T. Grafton, D. Rockmore, et al. 2004. Sharing neuroimaging studies of human cognition. *Nature Neuroscience* 7: 473–81.

Wang, Y., L. M. Lui, T. F. Chan, et al. 2005a. Optimization of brain conformal mapping with landmarks. *Proceedings of MICCAI* 675–683.

Wang, Y., L. M. Lui, T. F. Chan, et al. 2005b. Combination of brain conformal mapping and landmarks: a variational approach. *Computer Graphics and Imaging* 70–5.

Whitaker, R. T. 1998. A level-set approach to 3D reconstruction from range data. *International Journal of Computer Vision* 29(3): 203–31.

Witte, O. W., C. Bruehl, G. Schlaug, et al. 1994. Dynamic changes of focal hypometabolism in relation to epileptic activity. *Journal of Neurological Science* 124: 188–97.

Zou, G., G. Heckenberg, Y. Xi, et al. 2006a. Integrated modeling of PET and DTI information based on conformal brain mapping. In *SPIE Medical Imaging'06 Proceedings*.

Zou, G., J. Hua, X. Gu, et al. 2006b. An approach for 3D brain function analysis based on statistical conformal geometry. In: *Proceedings of International Conference on Image Processing*.

Zou, G., J. Hua, and O. Muzik. 2007. Non-rigid surface registration using spherical thin-plate splines. *Medical Imaging and Computers* 10: 367–74.

Index

Note: Page numbers followed by "*f*" and "*t*" denote figures and tables, respectively.

A

Abnormal cortical organization, malformation due to, 38*t*
Abnormal neuronal migration, malformation due to, 38*t*, 39*t*
Abnormal white matter regions, identification of, 101
Acquired lesions
    and [¹¹C]flumazenil PET, 177
Activation patterns, heterogeneity of, 86
ADD1020 [¹¹C]FMZ PET images, 175
Adenosine triphosphate (ATP)
    for bioenergetic status, 63
    -sensitive potassium channels, 169
Adrenocortical hormone (ACTH), 159
Aicardi syndrome, 50, 50*f*
Alpha4-Ser248Phe mutation, 205
Alpha-[¹¹C]methyl-L-tryptophan (AMT) PET, 161–162, 186
    clinical applications, 188
        cortical development, malformation of, 191–192
        nonlesional epilepsy, 193–194
        reoperation, 194–195
        tuberous sclerosis complex (TSC), 188–191, 189*f*, 190*f*
        tumors, 192–193
    kynurenine pathway, 195–196
    methodology, 186–188
Alpha-methyl-serotonin, 187
Alpha-methyl-tryptophan, 123*t*
Altered membrane turnover, 63
Amygdala, 158
Amygdalo-hippocampectomy, 11, 20
Angioma, 162
Anisotropic diffusion, 93, 95
Antiepileptic drugs (AEDs), 204
    effects of, 125
Apparent diffusion coefficient (ADC), 93, 94*f*, 96–97
    reversal of, 96
Arachnoid cysts, 23
Architectural dysplasia, 38
    seizure freedom, post surgery, 42
Arterial lines, 174
Arterial spin labeling techniques, 77, 86
Arterial thromboses
    in Sturge-Weber syndrome, 4
Astrocytomas, ependymomas, 3
Asymmetry indices (AIs), 203
ATP. *See* Adenosine triphosphate (ATP)
Atypical language representation, 83, 84

Auditory cortex, identification of, 79
Auditory processing, 78, 81
Autoradiography, 187
Autosomal dominant nocturnal frontal lobe epilepsy
        (ADNFLE), 205, 206
Avalanche photo diodes (APDs), 242
Azathioprine, 206

B

Balloon-cell focal cortical dysplasia, 26
Barbiturates, 125
Bayesian probabilistic method, 237
Beck Depression Inventory (BDI) scores, 203, 204*f*
Benzodiazepine, 125
Benzodiazepine receptors, 176*f*, 180, 182
Bifrontal ECT, 217
Bifrontal hypometabolism, 151
Bilateral activation, 79, 81–82, 84
Bilateral diffuse hypometabolism, 167
Bilateral frontal cortical hypometabolism, 160
Bilateral hippocampal atrophy, 133
Bilateral hypoperfusion, 219
Bilateral language activity, 118
Bilateral occipital cortico-subcortical calcifications
    and cutaneous stigmata of Sturge-Weber syndrome, 6
Bilateral symmetric hypermetabolism, 160, 161*f*
Bilateral temporal lobe hypometabolism, 125, 160
Bitemporal ECT, 217
Blood–brain barrier, 187, 211
Blood flow-based brain mapping techniques, 77
Blood oxygen-labeled dependent (BOLD)
        technique, 77, 78
    response, 83
Brain
    calcification, 3, 4*f*
    erosion, 3, 4*f*
    structural abnormalities
        and NAA levels, 68
    tumor
        and epilepsy, 192–193
        language source localizations in patients with, 116*f*
Brain energy metabolism, 169
Brain glucose metabolism in humans, 157
Brain histamine receptors, 206
Brain ictal SPECT imaging, 211

BrainPET insert, 242, 242*f*
BrainSuite, 233
Brain surface parcellation, problem of, 227
Brodman area (BA), activation of, 81
Brownian motion, 92

C
^{11}C, 122, 123*t*
^{11}C-alpha-methyl-L-tryptophan (AMT) PET imaging, 234
Carbamazepine, 204
Carfentanil, 123*t*
^{11}C-carfentanil, 199–200, 201
^{11}C-DASB PET, 205*f*
^{14}C–2-deoxyglucose, 150
^{11}C-diprenorphine, 199, 200, 201*f*
^{11}C-doxepin, 206
Cerebral blood flow (CBF), 77, 86, 133, 200
    and cerebral glucose metabolism, 131
    dynamic [^{15}O]H$_2$O PET imaging of, 124
    and seizures, history of, 210
Cerebral cortex, 37, 191
Cerebral glucose metabolism
    and CBF, 131
    in neonates, PET studies of, 158
Cerebral glucose utilization, on PET scans, 157*f*
Cerebral metabolic rate for glucose (CMRglc), 199, 200, 206
Cerebral MRI. *See* Magnetic resonance imaging (MRI)
[^{11}C]flumazenil, 146, 207
[^{11}C]flumazenil positron emission tomography, 165, 174
    acquired lesions, 177
    benzodiazepine receptor ligands, 182
    data acquisition and analysis, 174–175
    focal epilepsies
        clinical utility in, 179–180
        extratemporal origin,, 178
    in gene mutations associated with epilepsy, 182
    in idiopathic generalized epilepsies, 181–182
    malformations of cortical development (MCD), 176–177
    outcome, 180–181
    in temporal lobe epilepsy, 175
        with normal MRI, 175–176
[^{11}C]flumazenil VD, 1784
Chlorokynurenine, 196
Choline
    in gliosis, 63
Choroid fissure cysts, 23
Classic type lissencephaly (cLIS), 46
Clinical cyclotron, 122
^{11}C-(S)-[N-methyl]ketamine, 206
^{11}C-methylnaltrindole (^{11}C-MeNTI), 200
Cobblestone brain malformations, 49–50
    Fukuyama congenital muscular dystrophy, 49–50
    muscle-eye-brain disease, 49–50
    Walker-Warburg syndrome, 49–50
Cobblestone complex (CBSC), lissencephaly, 46
Cockayne disease
    intracranial calcification, 3
Cognitive evoked fields, measuring, 117
Cognitive functional imaging techniques, 114
Color-coded fractional anisotropy, 94*f*

Commission on Classification and Terminology, 166
Complex multilayered realistic head models, 107
Computer field pattern, 107
Conformal mapping techniques, 227
Continuous spike-and-wave discharges during slow-wave sleep
        (CSWS), 164–166
Contrast resolution, of PET imaging, 123
Co-registration of high-resolution MRI, 150
Cortical development, malformation of. See Malformation of
        cortical development (MCD)
Cortical dysplasia, 159, 177*f*
    detection of, 143
Cortical glucose metabolism, 150
Cortical hypermetabolism, 142, 144, 147–148, 160, 163
Cortical malformation, 191
Cortical tubers, 161
^{11}C-PK11195 specific binding, 206
Cranial ultrasound, 157
Craniopharyngiomas, 3
Creatinine, total
    in gliosis, 63
Crossed cerebellar diaschisis, 142*f*, 147
Cryptogenic epileptic spasms, 159, 160
Current Procedural Terminology (CPT), 106
^{11}C-verapamil, 207
^{11}C-WAY binding potential, 203
Cyclofoxy, 123*t*
Cytoarchitectural dysplasia, 38
    seizure freedom, post surgery, 41
Cytotoxic edema, 96

D
2-Deoxy-2-[^{18}F]fluoro-D-glucose (FDG) PET
        123, 123*t*, 123–124, 132–133, 141, 156, 170, 230
    in extratemporal lobe epilepsy, 141–143
        cortical hypometabolism, 147–148
    ictal FDG PET scans and epileptic spasms, 160
    in lesional epilepsy, 146
    Sturge-Weber syndrome (SWS) in, 162
Deprenyl, 202
Depression, 134, 203–204
Deuterium-deprenyl, 123*t*
Diaschisis, 146–147
Differential SPECT perfusion patterns
    in temporal lobe epilepsy, 212
Diffuse cortical hypometabolism, 160
Diffusion abnormalities, in interictal period, 98
Diffusion anisotropy, 93, 95
Diffusion MRI, in epilepsy, 92–93
    Brownian motion, 92
    DWI and DTI, 93–94
    future applications, 102
    ictal and postictal diffusion changes, 95–98
    interictal diffusion changes, 98–100
    neural tissue, diffusion in, 94–95
    tractography, 100–102
Diffusion tensor imaging (DTI; DT-MRI), 40, 84, 92, 93–94,
        229, 237
Diffusion-weighted images, 94*f*
Diffusion weighted imaging (DWI), 93–94, 95

diffusion abnormalities in entire right hemisphere, 99*f*
ipsilateral hippocampal diffusion, 99*f*
ipsilateral thalamic diffusion abnormalities, 99*f*
during post-ictal period, 98*f*
Dipole localizations, 114
Dipole modeling, 107, 109
Diprenorphine, 123*t*
Direct cortical electrical stimulation mapping, 134
Discrete mapping approach, 227
Distal Wallerian degeneration of axons, 98
Distributed source modeling, 107, 113
Dopamine receptors, 204–205
Down syndrome
intracranial calcification, 3
Dravet syndrome
and PET scan, 168–169
DTI fiber-tracking, 27
"DtiStudio", 101*f*
Dual pathology
FCD, 40, 42*f*
MLTE, 19–20
intracranial EEG, 20
Dynamic [^{15}O]H$_2$O PET imaging, of cerebral
blood flow, 124
Dystonia, 222

E

Early infantile epileptic encephalopathy. *See* Ohtahara
syndrome
ECD. *See* Equivalent current dipole (ECD) modeling
EEG. *See* Electroencephalogram (EEG)
Electrical status epilepticus of slow-wave sleep
(ESES), 164–165
Electroconvulsive therapy (ECT), 217
Electrocortical stimulation (ECS) studies, 82–83
Electroencephalogram (EEG)
frontal epileptic focus on, 187, 188*f*
versus MEG, 109
in MRI scanner, 86
in PET research protocols, 124–125, 132–133
prolonged imaging with, 86
with video (VEEG), 112, 113
Eloquent cortex localization, applications for, 78
language, 79–84
memory, 84–85
motor and sensory, 78–79
End-stage Rasmussen encephalitis
cortical gliosis and atrophy, 22
MR interpretation of, 25
Ependymoma
with hydrocephalus, 5*f*
Epilepsia partialis continua, 124
Epileptic focus, 141–142, 147, 148, 150, 151
Epileptogenesis in TSC, 189
Epileptogenic abnormalities, MRI of, 15–23
developmental abnormalities, 21
gliosis and miscellaneous abnormalities, 22–23
hippocampal sclerosis, 15–20
medial temporal lobe anatomy, overview of, 15–16
neoplasms and vascular malformations, 20–21

normal and sclerotic hippocampus, MRI of, 16–20
postoperative findings, 23
Epileptogenic cortex, 9, 177
AMT uptake in, 191*f*
Epileptogenic hippocampus
using MRS and tissue segmentation, 64
Epileptogenic networks
and NAA, 66
Epileptogenic tubers, 161, 188
Epileptogenic tumor, 189
Epileptogenic zone
mapping, 85–86
and secondarily generalized tonic-clonic seizures, 217–218
Equivalent current dipole (ECD) modeling, 110–111, 114
Excitatory amino acids, nicotinic and histamine receptors, 206
Expressive language cortex, activation of, 117
Extratemporal hypometabolism, neurocognitive and
behavioral correlates of, 151
Extratemporal lobe epilepsies (ETLE), 132
glucose metabolism in, 141
abnormal FDG PET for, 148–149
cortical hypometabolism, 147–148
FDG PET, localizing value of, 141–143, 146
hyper metabolism, significance of, 143–146
hypometabolism, neurocognitive and behavioral
correlates of, 151
necortical hypometabolism in epilepsy, potential
mechanisms of, 149–151
subcortical and cerebellar metabolic abnormalities,
localizing value of, 146–147
SPECT in, 212
subtraction ictal SPECT in, 215
Extratemporal lobe hyper metabolism, significance of, 143–146

F

^{18}F, 122, 123*t*
Fahr's disease, 3
Fallypride, 123*t*
False lateralization, 116
False-positive FMZ PET, 178*f*
False-positive localization, 113–114
FCWAY (trans-4-fluoro-N-2-[4-(2-methoxyphenyl)
piperazin-1-yl]ethyl]-N-(2-pyridyl)
cyclohexanecarboxamide), 123*t*, 202
^{18}F-cyclofoxy, 200
FDG PET, 113, 191, 193, 199
co-registration of, 149, 150
Febrile seizures, hippocampal sclerosis, 15
^{18}F-F-A-85380, 206
^{18}F-fallypride (^{18}F-FP), 205
^{18}F-FCWAY PET, 202–203, 203*f*,
^{18}F-FDG PET, 175, 177*f*, 202–203
5-(2'-[^{18}F]Fluoroethyl)flumazenil ([^{18}F]FEF), 182
^{18}F-fluoro-L-DOPA uptake, 204, 205
Fiber-tracking method, 100
Fibronectin gene expression, 162
Fick's first law, 92
Field strength
for performing spectroscopic imaging at 7T,
challenges for, 74

Finite surface elements on spherical surface, 228–229

FLAIR images. *See* Fluid attenuated inversion recovery (FLAIR) images

^{18}F ligands, 202

Fluoroethylflumazenil, 123t

Fluency tasks, 81

Fluid attenuated inversion recovery (FLAIR) images, 12, 38, 161
    of low-grade glioma, 192f
    superficial gliosis, detection of, 22

Flumazenil, 123t, 182

Fluoro-l-DOPA, 123t

^{18}F-MPPF PET scans, 202, 204

Focal cortical dysplasia (FCD), 27, 38–42
    balloon-cell, 26, 38
    brain pathologies, association with, 40, 42f
    clinical presentation in, 41
    cytopathologic features, 38
    histopathologic patterns of, 38
    with lesionectomy, 42
    MRI of, 28
    seizure freedom, 41

Focal cortical hypometabolism, 143, 145f, 151

Focal epilepsies
    clinical utility of FMZ PET in, 179–180
    extratemporal origin, 178

Focal evoked fields, MEG mapping of, 110

Focal glucose hypermetabolism, 166, 167

Focal hypometabolism, 142, 147, 148, 150

Focal lesions, diagnosed using CT, 6

Focally increased [^{11}C]FMZ binding, 178

Focal mesial temporal hypermetabolism, 130

Focal siderosis, detection of, 14f

Focus 220 microPET scanner, 157, 158f

Forward problem, 107

Fractional anisotropy (FA), 93, 94f, 98, 99, 237

Freesurfer software environment, 229

Frontal epileptic focus on EEG, 187, 188f

Frontal lobe epilepsy
    and FMZ PET, 177f, 178, 178f, 179f
    and NAA level, 65
    and white matter changes, 179f

Fukuyama congenital muscular dystrophy, 49–50

Functional imaging, in correlation of peri-ictal semiologic changes, 222

Functional MRI (fMRI), 3, 77, 108
    eloquent cortex localization, applications for, 78
        language, 79–84
        memory, 84–85
        motor and sensory, 78–79
    epileptogenic zone, 85–86
    individual activation maps, 78
    motor mapping studies, 79f
    principles, 77–78
    region-of-interest (ROI) approach, 78, 81

Functional neuroimaging with FDG PET, 162–163

G

GABA, 148
    dose-escalation study, 72
    neurotransmitters, 63
        intracellular alterations in, 70–72

GABA$_A$ receptor, 150, 175, 177, 180

GABA$_A$ receptor binding, PET scanning of, 146

Gabapentin, 72

Gadolinium enhancement on MRI, 193

Gamma amino-butyric acid (GABA), 174
    synthesis, 169

Ganglioglioma, 21f

Gaussian displacement distribution model of diffusion, 92

Gene mutations associated with epilepsy, 182

Generalized epilepsy with febrile seizure plus (GEFS+), 169, 170f

Glial fibrillary acidic protein (GFAP)
    in neuronal injury, 67

Glial proliferation, malformation due to, 38t, 39t

Gliomas, 10–11, 192
    grade II to IV, 193

Glioneuronal tumors, 193

Gliosis, 22–23, 63
    intractable drug-resistant epilepsy, 22
    post-traumatic seizures, risk factors of, 22

Glucose hypermetabolism, 162, 165

Glucose hypometabolism, 160, 161, 162f, 163, 165, 169f

Glucose metabolism, in TLE
    basal and lateral (neocortical) TLE, 131–132
    mesial TLE, 125–131
    using positron emission tomography (PET), 66

Glucose metabolism PET scanning, 156, 161, 165
    in children on ketogenic diet, 169–170
    in children with Rasmussen's encephalitis, 167
    in neonates and infants, 157

Glucose transporter 1 (GLUT1), 149

Glutamate, 149
    and neurotransmitter metabolism, 63
    neurotransmitters, intracellular alterations in, 70–72
    in TLE patients, 70–71

Glyceraldehyde–3-phosphate dehydrogenase (GADPH), 150

Gray matter
    diffusion abnormalities in, 98
    diffusion properties of, 94

Gray matter heterotopia, 50–52
    assigned to known genes or loci, 39t
    periventricular heterotopia, 51–52
        epilepsy, 52
    subcortical nodular heterotopia, 52

Greater-than-90-second group, 219

Grid implantation, postoperative MRI, 12

H

Healing, of cellular process
    and NAA levels, 68

Hemimegalencephaly, 6, 42–43
    and associated disorders, 42–43
    children with, 43f
    continuous focal seizures, children, 43
    histopathologic characteristics of, 42
    and PET scan, 168

Hemispheric asymmetry, 233

Hemispheric atrophy, 22
    hippocampal sclerosis

diffuse, 17
symmetric bilateral, 18
Hemispheric dominance, determining, 116
Hemodynamic response function, 77, 78, 86
High field MRI, 13–15, 72–74
disadvantages of, 73
enhanced lesion detection, 14
MRS and diffusion and perfusion imaging, 14
RF energy deposition, 14
signal-to-noise ratio, 13
High-resolution cerebrospinal fluid enhanced CT scans
and surgical findings, in medial temporal sclerosis, 4–5
High-resolution EEG recording, 106
High-resolution MRI, co-registration of, 150
Hippocampal pathology, 12, 84, 85
Hippocampal sclerosis (HS), 15–20
and [^{11}C]FMZ PET, 179
ectopic neurons and perivascular oligodendrocytic
infiltrates, 15
gliosis and neuronal loss, 15
medial temporal lobe anatomy, overview of, 15–16
MRI findings in, 18
normal and sclerotic hippocampus, MRI of, 16–20
amygdala and hippocampus, 16
FDG-PET findings, 18
hippocampal atrophy, 17
inversion recovery (IR) sequences, 17
quantitative hippocampal volumetry, 18
Hippocampal sulcus remnant, 23
Hippocampal volumetry and T2 relaxometry, 18
Histamine receptors, 206
Histiocytosis, 3, 4f
^{1}H MRS imaging
and spectroscopic imaging, 64
and TLE, 64–65
5HT$_{1A}$ receptors, 202, 203–204
5HT transport, 204
5-Hydroxyindole acetic acid (5-HIAA), 186
3-Hydroxykynurenine, 188
Hypermetabolism, 163
Hyperperfusion, 95, 216–217, 222
-dominant SISCOM images, 216
Hypoperfusion, 216–217, 222
postictal, 213
Hypoperfusion-dominant SISCOM images, 216
Hypothalamic hamartomas, types of, 21
Hypoxia, 162
hippocampal sclerosis, 15
Hypsarrhythmia, 160

I
^{123}I-based radiopharmaceuticals, 211
Ictal/peri-ictal FDG scans, 130–131
Ictal and interictal scalp VEEG, 112, 113
Ictal dystonia, 222
Ictal FDG PET, 144
and epileptic spasms, 160
Ictal hyperperfusion, 214
Ictal–interictal subtraction SPECT studies, 214, 220
Ictal period, diffusion abnormalities, 98
Ictal scalp EEG recordings, 113

Ictal scalp-sphenoidal EEG recordings, 133
Ictal SPECT, 113, 133, 134. See also SPECT
Ictal subtraction SPECT, 218
Idiopathic epileptic spasms, 159
Idiopathic generalized epilepsies, FMZ PET in, 181–182
Imaging, seizure disorders, 8–9. See also specific imaging
indications for, 9t
inflammation due to, 206
intractable epilepsy, 9, 10
medial temporal lobe structures, optimal
imaging of, 12f
misinterpretations, 24–25
symptomatic causes, new-onset seizure patients with, 8
Implanted dipoles, locations of, 111
Indoleamine 2,3-dioxygenase (IDO), 188
Infantile hemiplegia, cortical gliosis and atrophy, 22
Infantile spasms. See epileptic spasms
Inferior frontal gyrus (IFG), activation of, 81
Injection systems, automated, 216
Inorganic phosphate, for bioenergetic status, 63
Interictal cortical hypermetabolism, 145
Interictal deep temporal hypermetabolism, 130
Interictal diffusion changes, 98–100
Interictal FDG PET
of basal and lateral (neocortical) TLE, 131, 132f, 133
in epilepsy research, 123
of limbic TLE, 124f
of mesial TLE, 126f–128f, 129
Interictal glucose metabolism PET, 158, 168
Interictal hypermetabolism, 163
Interictal PET scan, 166
Interictal regional hypometabolism, 134
Interictal source localization, 86
Interictal SPECT localization, 211
International League Against Epilepsy (ILAE), 156, 165
Intracarotid amobarbital test (IAT), 79, 80, 83, 115
comparison with fMRI, 80
Intracellular pH, for bioenergetic status, 63
Intracortical lesion, sagittal reformatted volumetric
SPGR of, 20
Intracranial EEG (icEEG), 107, 108, 111, 112f, 113, 141
integration of, 230–236
Intracranial electrode placements, 133
Intracranial infection, hippocampal sclerosis, 15
Intracranial vascular malformations, seizures, 20
Intractable drug-resistant epilepsy, 22
Intractable epilepsy, 158, 162f, 169, 190, 192f
Intractable epilepsy, chronic, 10
Intractable seizures, 21, 192
Intrahypothalamic hamartoma, 21
Inverse problem, 107
examination, 106
Ipsilateral basal ganglia hyperperfusion, 220
Ipsilateral lentiform nucleus, AMT uptake in, 194
[^{123}I]Ro 43-0463, 202
Irreversible injury, 97
Ischemia, chronic, 162

J
John Hughlings-Jackson, 222
Juvenile myoclonic epilepsy (JME), 181, 181f

K

K-complex factor, 187
Ketogenic diet, 169–170
Kynurenine pathway, 187–188, 195–196

L

Lamotrigine, 72, 204
Landau-Kleffner syndrome (LKS) and PET,
        164–166, 165*f*, 167*f*
Language cortex, 79–84
Language mapping with MEG, 107–108, 114–118
Late-onset epilepsy, 10, 22
Left mesial temporal sclerosis (left MTS), 119
Lennox-Gastaut syndrome (LGS), 6, 10, 69, 130
    and PET scan, 166–167
Lesional epilepsy. *See* Epilepsy, lesional
Levetiracetam (LEV), 72, 201, 204
Linear regression analyses
    tissue heterogeneity, 66
Lissencephalies, 45–49
    assigned to known genes or loci, 39*t*, 46
    callosum agenesis and abnormal (or ambiguous)
            genitalia (XLAG), X-linked, 49
    with cerebellar hypoplasia due to mutations of the
            RELN Gene, 49
    and subcortical band heterotopia, 45–49
Listening to tones, 81
Lobar atrophy, 22
Localization, of epileptic source, 102
Localization-related epilepsy, 85
    planning surgery of, 132–134
Longitudinal DTI studies, 100
Low-grade tumor cells, 192
Lutetium oxy-orthosilicate (LSO) scintillation crystals, 242

M

Magnetic resonance imaging (MRI), 156
    bilateral parietooccipital polymicrogyria on, 54*f*
    bilateral perisylvian polymicrogyria on, 53*f*
    cerebral MRI, 133
    of common epileptogenic abnormalities, 15–23
        developmental abnormalities, 21
        gliosis and miscellaneous abnormalities, 22–23
        hippocampal sclerosis, 15–20
        neoplasms and vascular malformations, 20–21
        postoperative findings, 23
    and computed tomography (CT), seizure, 8
    cortical development, malformations of, 37
    and diffusion MR, 27
    enhanced detection of epileptogenic pathology,
            MRI post-processing techniques for, 27–28
    and epilepsy surgery, 9–12
        postoperative MRI, 11–13
        and surgical navigation, 11
    on FCD patient, features of, 39, 40
    of hemimegalencephaly, 42
    hippocampal sclerosis, and FMZ PET, 179
    lissencephaly on, 47*f*
    magnetic resonance spectroscopy (MRS), 26–27
    negativity, 178, 179

Ohtahara syndrome, 158
    periventricular nodular heterotopia on, 51*f*
    strategies and technical issues, 13–15
        high-field MRI in epilepsy, 13–15
    subcortical band heterotopia (SBH) on, 48*f*, 49*f*
    successful interpretation of, 23–26
    tuberous sclerosis complex (TSC) on, 44*f*, 45
Magnetic resonance spectroscopy (MRS), 26–27, 241
    as clinical tool, 63–64
    DTI fiber-tracking, 27
    nonlesional epilepsy and, 26
    proton MRS, 27
    single-voxel spectroscopy, 26
    and standard magnetic resonance imaging (MRI), 63
Magnetic source imaging (MSI), 106, 148
    clinical utility, in epilepsy surgery, 113
    language mapping, 107–108, 114–118
Magnetoencephalography (MEG), 3, 106
    accuracy, 109–111
    versus EEG, 109
    five-point rating scale, 112
    memory mapping, 119
    presurgical brain mapping, 107
    sensitivity, 109
    spike source localization, 108, 111
    validation, 111–113
Magnetoencephalography-magnetic source imaging
        (MEG-MSI), 10
Malformations of cortical development (MCD), 143, 176–177,
        191–192
    Aicardi syndrome, 50
    assigned to known genes or loci, 39*t*
    cobblestone brain malformations, 49–50
    focal cortical dysplasia, 38–42
    gray matter heterotopia, 50–52
        periventricular heterotopia, 51–52
        subcortical nodular heterotopia, 52
    hemimegalencephaly, 42–43
    lissencephalies, 45–49
    and NAA level, 65
    polymicrogyria, 52–55
    schizencephaly, 55–56
    tuberous sclerosis complex (TSC), 43–45
Marginal glioneuronal heterotopia, 38*t*
Mean diffusivity (MD), 93
Medial temporal sclerosis, 15
    in temporal lobe epilepsy, 4
MEG-based source localization, see Magnetic source
        imaging (MSI)
Memory systems, 84–85
Mental navigation tasks, 85
Mesial cortex, 233
Mesial structures, lesions in, 83
Mesial temporal lobe epilepsy (MTLE), 10
    and dual pathology, 19
    endfolium sclerosis and, 19
    due to hippocampal sclerosis, 15
    imaging techniques, 10–11
        structural MRI, 16
    localization of, 16

due to medial temporal sclerosis, 15
  paradoxical TLE, 18–19
Mesial temporal sclerosis, 83, 86
Mesial TLE, 125–131
Mesio-basal limbic pattern, 221
Metabolic imaging, 64
(S)-[N-Methyl-^{11}C]ketamine, 123*t*
Metrizamide-enhanced CT
  for medial temporal structure abnormalities, 5
Meyer's loop, tractography of, 102
mGluR5 ligands, 206
Microdysgenesis, 38*t*, 176
MicroPET scanner, 157–158, 201, 207
  Focus 220 scanner, 157, 158*f*
Miller-Dieker syndrome, 48
Mitochondrial poison studies, 68
m-nitrobenzoylalanine, 195
Möbius transformation, 228
Monoamine oxidase type B inhibitor (MAO-B), 202
Monte Carlo simulations, 237
Montgomery-Asberg mood rating scale, 203
Motor cortex, 78–79
Motor mapping studies using fMRI, 79*f*
MPPF (2'-methoxyphenyl-(N-2'-pyridinyl)-p-18F-fluoro-
    benzamidoethylpiperazine), 123*t*, 202
MR-FOCUSS, 117
MRI. *See* Magnetic resonance imaging (MRI)
MRIcro, 233
MR techniques. *See specific MR techniques*
^{99m}Tc-bicisate (Tc-ECD), 211
^{99m}Tc-hexamethylpropylene amine oxime
    (Tc-HMPAO), 211
^{99m}Tc-pertechnetate brain scans, 4
Multidetector array systems, 106
Multimodality neuroimaging, 161, 226
  brain surface parcellation, problem of, 227
  future directions, 240
    instrumentation challenges242
    integrative databases, 242–243
    simultaneous PET/MR acquisition, 240–241
  integration of multimodality data sets, 229–230
  multimodality data, 238–240
    integration in native space, 227–229
  PET and intracranial EEG, integration of, 230–236
  structural connectivity, 236–238
  template versus space analysis, 227
Multiple tissue microstructural changes, 96
Multiple tissue structural components, 99
Mu-opiate receptors, 199
Muscle-eye-brain disease, 49–50
Myelination, advanced, 168

N
^{13}N, 122
N-acetyl aspartate (NAA), 129
  for acetate transfer, 68
  in contralateral hemisphere, 65
  decreased level, interpretation of, 66–68
  and epileptogenic networks, 66
  NAA/Cr abnormality

  in ipsilateral hippocampus, 65
  in MRI-negative patients, 65
  and neocortical epilepsy, 65–66
  in neuronal mitochondria, 63
Naloxone, 200
Native-space approach, 227
  multimodality data integration in, 227–229
Necortical hypometabolism in epilepsy, potential
    mechanisms of, 149–151
Neocortical and nonlesional epilepsy patients,
    heterogeneity of, 113
Neocortical epilepsies, 82, 213
  MEG in, 108, 109
  and NAA, 65–66
Neocortical TLE, 131–132
Neonatal intensive care units (NICUs), 157
Neonatal seizures, 43*f*
  and PET, 157–158
Neoplasms
  diagnosed using CT, 4
  and vascular malformations, 20–21
    ganglioglioma, 21*f*
    hemangiomas, 21
    tumors in eloquent cortex, fMRI and DTI
        techniques for, 21
Network inhibition hypothesis, in TLE, 222
Neural tissue, diffusion in, 94–95
Neuroimaging, 157
Neuronal injury
  and glial fibrillary acidic protein (GFAP), 67
  and NAA level, 66
Neuronal proliferation, malformation due to, 38*t*, 39*t*
Neurotransmitters
  intracellular alterations in
    GABA, 70–72
    glutamate, 70–72
  positron-emitter-labeled ligands and
      precursors of, 123*f*, 125
New-onset seizure patients, CT and, 8
  symptomatic causes, 8
Nicotinic acetylcholine receptors (nAChRs), 206
N-methyl-D-aspartate (NMDA), 188, 206
N-methyl piperidyl benzilate, 123*t*
Non-epileptogenic epileptogenic tumor, 189
Non-invasive language mapping, utility of, 117
Nonlesional epilepsy. *See* Epilepsy, nonlesional
Nonlocalization SISCOM and false localization, 216
Nonlocalized results, 113
Normalization, of cellular process
  and NAA levels, 68
Noun–verb task, 81
Nuclear medicine techniques, conventional, 4

O
^{15}O, 122, 123*t*
Object naming, 80, 82
Occipital biopsy, 206
Ohtahara syndrome, PET scans for, 158–159, 159*f*
Oligodendrogliomas, 3, 193
o-methoxybenzoylalanine, 195

Opiate receptors, 199–201
Oro-alimentary behavior, 221
[15]O-water positron emission tomography, 77, 82, 86
Oxcarbazepine, 204

P

Paced fluency, 81
Paradoxical TLE, 18–19
Parahypothalamic hamartoma, 21
Parenchymal depth electrodes, 11
Partial epilepsy, 221
Partial epilepsy, ictal SPECT in, 214
Partial epilepsy. *See* Epilepsy, Partial
Partial seizures, 210
Patlak analysis, 170, 187
PCr. *See* Phosphocreatine (PCr)
Pediatric epilepsy
    findings in, 84
    surgery centers, 159
Pediatric new-onset seizures, 8
Perfusion, "postictal switch" of, 213
Perifocal hypometabolism, 150
Peri-ictal [^{18}F]FDG PET studies, 130
Peri-ictal semiologic changes, 222
Perilesional epileptic cortex, 146
Perilesional epileptogenic cortex, 177
Perilesional hypometabolism, 146
Peripheral benzodiazepine receptor, 206, 207
Periventricular calcifications, 6f
Periventricular nodular heterotopia, 192
PET/MR acquisition, 240–241
PET and intracranial EEG, integration of, 230–236
PET-CT, 123
PET ligands used in epilepsy, 199
    depression, epilepsy, and 5HT 1A receptor
        binding, 203–204
    dopamine receptors, 204–205
    excitatory amino acids, nicotinic and histamine
        receptors, 206
    imaging inflammation, 206
    monoamine oxidase type B inhibitor (MAO-B), 202
    opiate receptors, 199–201
    p-glycoprotein, 206–207
    receptor PET in epilepsy, 207
    serotonin receptors, 202–203
PET–MRI co-registration, 125
p-glycoprotein, 206–207
Phenytoin, 123t, 204
Phonological tasks, 81
Phosphocreatine (PCr)
    for bioenergetic status, 63
    PCr/ATP
        Lennox-Gastaut syndrome, 69
        [31]P metabolism, 70
Photomultiplier tubes (PMTs), 242
Picture encoding tasks, 85
Pineal tumor, calcified, 5f
PK-11195, 123t
[31]P metabolism
    in epilepsy, alterations in, 70

Polymicrogyria, 52–55
    assigned to known genes/loci, 39–40t
    bilateral, 38t
    bilateral parasagittal parieto-occipital, 54
    bilateral perisylvian, 53
        speech production impairment, 53
    clinical sequelae of, 53
Porencephalies, diagnosed using CT, 4
Positron emission tomography (PET), 3, 40, 122, 141, 156
    abnormal FDG PET for extratemporal epilepsy surgery
        outcome, significance of, 148–149
    continuous spike-and-wave discharges during
        slow-wave sleep (CSWS), 164–166
    contrast resolution, 123
    cortical hypometabolism, 147–148
    Dravet syndrome, 168–169
    epileptic spasms, 159–161
    extratemporal hypometabolism, neurocognitive and
        behavioral correlates of, 151
    extratemporal lobe hyper metabolism, significance of,
        143–146
    FDG PET
        in extratemporal lobe epilepsy, localizing value of,
            141–143
        in lesional epilepsy, localization value of, 146
    fusion with X-ray computed tomographs, 122–123
    glucose metabolism, in TLE, 66
    hemimegalencephaly, 168
    ketogenic diet, 169–170
    Landau-Kleffner syndrome (LKS), 164
    Lennox-Gastaut syndrome (LGS), 166–167
    methodology, 122–125
    necortical hypometabolism in epilepsy, potential
        mechanisms of, 149–151
    neonatal seizures, 157–158
    Ohtahara syndrome, 158–159
    process resolution, 123
    radiopharmaceuticals, in epilepsy studies, 123t
    Rasmussen's encephalitis, 167–168
    requirements, 122
    spatial resolution, 123
    Sturge-Weber syndrome (SWS), 162–163
    subcortical and cerebellar metabolic abnormalities,
        localizing value of, 146–147
    temporal lobe epilepsy (TLE) studies with glucose
        metabolic imaging
        basal and lateral (neocortical) TLE, 131–132
        mesial (limbic) TLE, 125–131
        presurgical evaluation, 132–134
    temporal resolution, 123
    tuberous sclerosis complex (TSC), 161–162
Positron-emitting isotopes, 122
Posterior lateral temporal sources, 109
Postoperative seizure recurrence, 10
Posttraumatic amnesia, 22
Prednisone, 206
Primary sensory cortex, mapping of, 114
Process resolution, of PET imaging, 123
Progressive degenerative changes, during interictal period,
    98–99

Proof-of-principal clinical validation, 111
PROPELLER (Periodically Rotated Overlapping
　　ParallEL Lines with Enhanced Reconstruction)
　　technique, 12, 13
Proteus syndrome, 43
Proton MRS, 27
^{31}P spectroscopy
　in human epilepsy, 68–69
　interpretation, and factors affecting, 69–70

Q
Quinolinic acid, 188

R
Radiofrequency signals, 63
Radiopharmaceuticals,216
　　in PET, 123*t*
　　in SPECT, 210–211
Radiotracer injection, 215–216
Raphe nuclei, 160
Rasmussen's encephalitis, 206
　and PET scan, 167–168, 168*f*
Reading tasks, 81, 82*f*
Receiver operating characteristics (ROC) analysis, 232
Receptive language cortex, activation of, 117
Receptor PET in epilepsy, 207
Recordings with implanted dipoles, 111
Refractory epilepsy, role of MRI in surgical
　　management of, 11*t*
Region-of-interest (ROI) approach, 78, 81, 175
"Release" phenomenon, 222
Reoperation, 194–195, 218
Resective surgery, 22–23
Resolution elements (RESELS), 229
Resting FDG PET abnormalities, 134
Reversed language "dominance" activation patterns, 84
Reverse speech, 78, 81
RF shimming, 73
Right-dominant subjects, studying, 117

S
Scalp electroencephalogram (EEG), 109, 141
Scatchard analysis, 199
Schizencephaly, 55–56
　clinical findings in, 55–56
　left-sided open-lip, 56*f*
　unilateral, 56
Secondarily generalized tonic-clonic seizures and
　　epileptogenic zone, 217–218
Seizure activity, 96
Seizure focus localization, 86
Seizure freedom, 10
Seizures, 210
　recommended MRI protocol for, 12*t*
Seizure semiology, 141
Selective serotonin reuptake inhibitors (SSRIs), 204
Sensitivity for spikes, 109
Sensory cortex, 78–79
Serotonin (5HT) receptors, 202–203
Serotonin synthesis capacity, 186

Severe myoclonic epilepsy of infancy.
　　See Dravet syndrome
Severity index, 234
Side-to-side asymmetry indices (AIs), 203
Signal-to-noise ratios, 123
　for performing spectroscopic imaging at 7T,
　　challenges for, 74
Silicon photo multipliers (SiPM), 242
Single photon emission computed tomography
　　(SPECT), 3, 148, 165, 202, 210
　cerebral blood flow and seizures, history of, 210
　and consciousness, 222–223
　epileptogenic zone and secondarily generalized
　　tonic-clonic seizures, 217–218
　in extratemporal lobe epilepsy (ETLE), 212
　false localization and nonlocalization SISCOM, 216
　lateralization, 211*t*
　parametric mapping of, 218–221
　and pathophysiology of epileptic seizures, 221–222
　radiopharmaceuticals, 210–211
　radiotracer, early injection of, 215–216
　repeat epilepsy surgery, evaluating the need for, 218
　SISCOM in postictal state, 216
　subtraction ictal SPECT, 214–215
　　in ETLE, 215
　in temporal lobe epilepsy (TLE), 211–212
　　differential SPECT perfusion patterns, 212
Single-voxel spectroscopy, 26
Skull X-ray, 3–4
Source analysis, 106
Source localization, 106
　accuracy, 109–111
　dipole modeling, 107
　distributed source modeling, 107, 110*f*, 117
　validation, 111–113
Source of spike, 107
Spatial proximity index (SPI), 232–233
Spatial resolution, of PET imaging, 123
Spatial-temporal dipole model, 113
SPECT. *See* Single photon emission computed tomography
　　(SPECT)
Spectral resolution
　for performing spectroscopic imaging at 7T, 74
Spectroscopic imaging
　and ^{1}H MRS imaging, 64
SPECT-to-SPECT coregistration, 214
Spike-and-wave activity, 166
Spike-related fMRI, 86
Spike source localization, 108
Spin-echo phase, 93*f*
Split pulse diffusion weighting gradient, 93*f*
Statistical parametric mapping (SPM), 101, 125, 148, 175, 176*f*,
　　202, 227
Structural MRI
　electroclinical features of MTLE, patients with, 16
Structural neuroimaging, 156, 169
　and Sturge-Weber syndrome (SWS), 162
Sturge-Weber syndrome (SWS), 130
　and angiomatosis distribution, 5
　cortical gliosis and atrophy, 22

Sturge-Weber syndrome (SWS) (*cont'd*)
  diagnosis
    using CT scan, 5–6
    using skull X-ray, 3
  hemispheric atrophy and calcification, changes of, 6*f*
  and PET, 162–163, 163*f*
  recurrent seizures and, 23
  tramtrack-like calcifications, 5*f*
Subcortical/periventricular heterotopias, 143
Subcortical and cerebellar metabolic abnormalities, localizing
      value of, 146–147
Subcortical band heterotopia, 48*f*, 49*f*
  mental retardation and epilepsy, association with, 49
Subcortical Virchow-Robin spaces, 24
Subdural depth electrodes, 11
Subependymal heterotopia, 38*t*
Subtraction ictal SPECT, 214–215
  in extratemporal lobe epilepsy (ETLE), 215
Subtraction ictal SPECT co-registered to MRI (SISCOM), 215,
      218, 219–220
  in extratemporal lobe epilepsy (ETLE) patients, 215
  nonlocalization SISCOM and false localization, 216
  in postictal state, 216
Succinic semialdehyde dehydrogenase (SSADH)
      deficiency, 182
Surgery, 9, 10, 11
  planning, 132–134
  resective surgery, 22–23
Surround inhibition, 150
Susceptibility weighted imaging (SWI), 162
Symptomatic epileptic spasms, 159

T
T1 or T2 images, 95
T1-weighted gadolinium-enhanced axial
      MRI images, 164, 169*f*
Task-dependent dominance, 81
Taylor-type cortical dysplasia, 38
  seizure freedom, post surgery, 41
TBSS, 101
Template versus space analysis, multimodality
      neuroimaging, 227
Temporal lobe astrocytoma, 6
Temporal lobe epilepsy (TLE), 63, 147, 175, 199, 202, 211,
      218, 219–220
  [^{11}C]FMZ PET in, 175
  differential SPECT perfusion patterns in, 212
  glucose metabolism studies in, 122
    basal and lateral (neocortical) TLE, 131–132
    mesial (limbic) TLE, 125–131
    positron emission imaging methods, 122–125
    presurgical evaluation, 132–134
    radiopharmaceutical tracers, 123*t*
  and NAA level, 65
  normal MRI, 175–176
  SPECT in, 211–212
Temporal lobe hypometabolism, 127, 129, 134
Temporal lobe resection, 133, 134
Temporal lobe seizures, 212, 212*f*, 213
Temporal resolution, of PET imaging, 123, 124
Temporal versus extratemporal lobe epilepsy, 112–113

Temporo-polar region, 221
Tensor-derived parameters, 93–94
Tensor ellipsoids, graphic representation of, 95*f*
Test–retest [^{11}C]FMZ PET study, 180
Thalamic atrophy, 147
Thalamus, glucose metabolism in, 147
Three-dimensional brain location, 106
Thrombosis, 162
Tissue heterogeneity
  linear regression analyses for, 66
Tonic hyperpolarization, 150
Topiramate, 72, 83
TORCH infection, 6*f*
Tractographic methods, 94, 100
  diffusion properties, studying, 100–101
  future studies, 102
  morphological studies, 101
  neuronavigational uses, 102
  unreliability, 102
Tramtrack-like calcifications
  Sturge-Weber syndrome, 5*f*
Trauma, hippocampal sclerosis, 15
Traumatic brain injury, symptomatic epilepsy, 22
Tryptophan, 186, 193
Tryptophan-hydroxylase immunocytochemistry, 187
TSC 1 and 2 genes, 161, 162*f*
Tuberous sclerosis, 6
Tuberous sclerosis and epilepsy, MRI of, 44*f*
Tuberous sclerosis complex (TSC), 188–191, 189*f*, 190*f*
  characteristic intracranial lesions of, 44
  clinical triad, 43–44
  nonconventional MRI techniques and, 45
  and PET, 161–162
  seizures, children, 44
  subependymal hamartomas, location of, 44–45
  TSC1 or TSC2 mutations, 43
Tumors, 20–21, 192–193
  in eloquent cortex, fMRI and DTI techniques for, 21
  ganglioglioma, 21*f*
  hemangiomas, 21
Two-dimensional scalp-recorded waveforms, 106
Type 1 cannabinoid receptor (CB1R), 201
Type I errors, 179
Typical language development, 83

U
Uncertain epileptogenic tumor, 189
Unilateral temporal hypometabolism, 125
Unilateral temporal lobe epilepsy, 125
Unilateral temporal lobe hypometabolism, 132, 133

V
Valproate (VPA), 123*t*, 201, 204
Vasogenic edema, 96
Venous angioma, 23
Venous stasis, 162
Vent-related designs, 84, 86
Verbal encoding, 85
Verbal fluency, 80, 82*f*, 83
Verbal recognition language task, 118*f*
Verbal recognition stimulation paradigm, 114

Vigabatrin, 72, 159, 182
Visual presentation of fMRI, 81
Volume of distribution (VD)
    images, 174, 175
    parameter, 187
Voxel-based analysis, 100*f*, 101, 175, 227
Voxel-based morphometry (VBM), 28, 40
Voxel-by-voxel analysis of SPM, 175
Voxel-by-voxel basis, 78

W
Wada language lateralization, 117
Wada test, 115, 116, 119, 134
Walker-Warburg syndrome, 49–50
Water diffusion, 94
WAY100635, 123*t*, 203

Wernicke's area activity, 117
West syndrome, 159
White matter
    abnormal regions identification, 101
    diffusion abnormalities in, 99
    diffusion properties of, 94
    FMZ-VD in, 176
    isolation of tracts, 100, 101*f*
    progressive loss of integrity, 101
Whole-head detector arrays, 106

X
Xenon 133, 211
XML (eXtensible Markup Language) model, 242
X-ray image, 230